Stories and the Brain

Stories and the Brain

The Neuroscience of Narrative

PAUL B. ARMSTRONG

Johns Hopkins University Press

Baltimore

© 2020 Johns Hopkins University Press
All rights reserved. Published 2020
Printed in the United States of America on acid-free paper
9 8 7 6 5 4 3 2 1

Johns Hopkins University Press
2715 North Charles Street
Baltimore, Maryland 21218-4363
www.press.jhu.edu

Library of Congress Cataloging-in-Publication Data

Names: Armstrong, Paul B., 1949– author.
Title: Stories and the brain : the neuroscience of narrative / Paul B. Armstrong.
Description: Baltimore : Johns Hopkins University Press, 2020. |
    Includes bibliographical references and index.
Identifiers: LCCN 2019031189 | ISBN 9781421437743 (hardcover) |
    ISBN 9781421437750 (paperback) | ISBN 9781421437767 (ebook)
Subjects: LCSH: Narration (Rhetoric)—Psychological aspects. |
    Neurosciences and the arts.
Classification: LCC P301.5.P75 A76 2020 | DDC 809.9/23—dc23
LC record available at https://lccn.loc.gov/2019031189

A catalog record for this book is available from the British Library.

Special discounts are available for bulk purchases of this book. For more information,
please contact Special Sales at specialsales@press.jhu.edu.

Johns Hopkins University Press uses environmentally friendly book materials,
including recycled text paper that is composed of at least 30 percent post-
consumer waste, whenever possible.

For Tim, Maggie, and Jack

CONTENTS

ACKNOWLEDGMENTS

I am glad to thank the many colleagues, students, and friends who generously helped me with this book. Its errors and shortcomings are of course my own. Terence Cave, Jakob Lothe, and Jim Phelan responded to my earliest ideas with welcome encouragement and important criticisms and suggestions that had a formative influence on the shape this project eventually took. Nancy Easterlin asked hard questions about my argument at an early stage that forced me to think more rigorously and precisely about a number of key issues, and I am deeply in her debt. As the project neared completion, Steve Mailloux and Don Wehrs took time from their overcommitted lives to read the entire manuscript, and their responses at this late stage were invaluable. Among the many other friends and colleagues with whom I have discussed the ideas in this book, I am especially grateful to Marty Hoffman, Ann Kaplan, Sowon Park, Ben Morgan, Kay Young, Ellen Esrock, Karin Kukkonen, Elaine Auyoung, John Lutterbie, Richard Gerrig, Rita Charon, and George Smith. I also benefited greatly from the careful readings the manuscript received from the two anonymous referees as well as from the faculty editorial board at Johns Hopkins University Press. Their suggestions as well as good advice from my editor, Catherine Goldstead, provided important guidance to my final round of revision and rewriting.

My research and teaching have always informed each other, and that was especially the case with this project. Working with neuroscience concentrators in my undergraduate seminar on neuroaesthetics and reading at Brown has been one of the ways in which I have stayed in touch with the scientific community. These young scientists are smart and very well trained, and I have learned much from their knowledge of the field as well as from their sharp eye for the weaknesses of a scientific argument or the limitations of a particular experiment. I have also been gratified by their enthusiasm for conducting interdisciplinary conversations about big issues concerning art, culture, and our cognitive lives that go beyond the focus of their laboratory work. Directing Carolyn Rachofsky's honors thesis on the neuroscience of metaphor for her biology concentration started me thinking about the contradictions in this research that I analyze in this book. I have also learned much from the graduate students whose research on cognitive topics I've had the privilege to advise, especially Dorin Smith, Sarah Brown, and Fadwa Ahmed. The students in my courses on narrative theory, phenomenology, and the novel may also recognize in this book many ideas that I have tested on them over the years.

I also learned much from the thoughtful questions I received from various audiences who heard presentations from my work in progress. I am especially grateful to the Cognitive Futures in the Humanities community, whose meetings in Durham, Oxford, and Stony Brook provided forums for trying out my ideas and opportunities for discovering exciting research I might not otherwise have encountered. I also benefited from questions and conversations after talks I gave at the International Association of Literary Semantics meeting in Krakow, the English Language and Literature Association of Korea conference in Seoul, the meeting of the Crisis and Beyond research group in Uppsala, and the "Future of Literary Studies" conference at the Norwegian Academy of Science and Letters in Oslo. I am grateful as well for the chance to present my work to the Literature and the Mind group at the University of California, Santa Barbara, and at the Robert J. and Nancy D. Carney Institute for Brain Science at Brown.

It is harder to express what I owe to my children, Tim, Maggie, and Jack, to whom I have dedicated this book. I have been surprised to discover over the years that being a parent is a more important part of who I am than I ever thought it would be. I owe most, however, to Beverly, for many things besides what she contributed to this project. The play of her mind has taught me what a joy conversation can be.

Stories and the Brain

Prologue

How STORIES CONFIGURE experience and organize events in time is an especially intriguing and important example of how literature plays with the brain. As I argued in my previous book on neuroscience and art (2013), reading a literary work typically sets in motion to-and-fro interactions between experiences of harmony and dissonance. A novel, poem, or play may reinforce and refine our sense of the world's patterns through the symmetry, balance, and unity of its forms, or it may disrupt and overturn our customary syntheses by transgressing established conventions and refusing to satisfy our expectations about how parts fit together into wholes. These kinds of interaction between harmony and dissonance in aesthetic experiences help to negotiate a basic contradiction that is fundamental to our cognitive lives—the contradiction between our need for pattern and constancy and our equally crucial need for flexibility and openness to change. The ability of the brain to play with these competing imperatives is also evident in our capacity to tell and follow stories. For example, plots convert the one thing after another of passing moments into meaningful patterns that draw on, support, and shape our cognitive habits for building consistency and making connections. But the twists and turns in a story also hold our attention by surprising us and compelling us to remain open to the possibility that we may need to reconsider and revise our sense of the order of things. The productive imbalances between the formation and dissolution of patterns in the brain make possible this play between the building and breaking of patterns in narrative, even as the construction and disruption of patterns in the stories we tell each other contribute to the brain's balancing act between pattern and openness to change.

This book offers a neurophenomenological model of narrative that charts the correlations between our lived, embodied experiences as tellers and followers of stories and the neurobiological processes that underlie and constrain these interactions. Building on the work of phenomenological theorists of reading and narrative (especially Wolfgang Iser and Paul Ricoeur), I construct an account of narrative as an experience-based interaction between the production and reception of figurative patterns. As I explain in the first chapter, experience is already prefigured because understanding is always a process of seeing-as—a recursive, configurative operation of pattern building that characterizes vision, reading, and all other cognitive processes. Narratives take up prefigured aspects of experience (including culturally shared conventions, assumptions, and practices) and reconfigure them into as-if patterns of various kinds ("Once upon a time . . ." and "they lived happily ever after"—or not!). The experience of reading or listening to a story may in turn prompt the recipient to refigure his or her understanding of the world, and the cycle can then begin again through which storytellers and audiences shape, exchange, and reshape their experiences.

This phenomenological account of the production and reception of narrative has a long and varied history on which I draw in the following pages as I explore different, much-discussed topics in narrative theory having to do with the relation between stories and experience: for example, how narrative organizes and plays with the disjunctions of our experience of time (the focus of chapter 2), how plots construct patterns of action (chapter 3), and how the exchange of stories brings different worlds into relation with one another (chapter 4). My contribution to this tradition is the addition of the perspective of neuroscience. What neurobiological processes, functions, and structures underlie these interactions? How is our capacity to tell and follow stories constrained and enabled by our embodied brains? In short, what kind of brains do we have that we are able to tell each other stories, and how do stories affect our brains?

The aim of such an exercise in neurophenomenology is to clarify the correlations between cognitive experience and its biological underpinnings. Correlations are not causation, however. As one introduction to neurophenomenology (Thompson, Lutz, and Cosmelli 2005, 40) observes: "Although neuroscientists have supplied neural models of various aspects of consciousness, and have uncovered evidence about the neural correlates of consciousness (or NCCs), there nonetheless remains an 'explanatory gap' in our understanding of how to relate neurobiological and phenomenological features of consciousness." This gap is evident in the much-discussed hard problem of how to account for first-person experiences in the third-person language of science (whether an analysis of neuronal activity can explain what it is like to see the color red, for example, a question I take up in chapter 4). It is also central to the problem of emergence, the mystery of how electro-chemical processes in the brain give rise to consciousness (see Deacon 2012 and Nagel 2012).

On the one hand, biologically based processes obviously constrain consciousness and cognition. Members of our species can convert only a limited portion of the electromagnetic spectrum into perceivable experiences of light and color, for example, and our auditory cortex similarly is limited in the acoustical wavelengths it can recognize as sounds. As is well known, the auditory capacities of dogs and bats enable them to hear much higher frequencies than we respond to, and elephants and whales are sensitive to low-frequency sounds that we don't notice (hence the speculation that some animals may be able to predict an earthquake by picking up low-frequency seismic vibrations [see Bear, Connors, and Paradiso 2007, 346]). On the other hand, describing these constraints and correlating what we can see and hear to our visual and auditory equipment is not the same as explaining causally how experiences emerge. Nor do these constraints and correlations explain what it is like to have visual and auditory experiences. The aim of neurophenomenology is "not to close the explanatory gap (in the sense of conceptual or ontological reduction), but rather to bridge the gap by establishing dynamic reciprocal constraints between subjective experience and neurobiology" (Thompson, Lutz, and Cosmelli 2005, 89). This gap should caution us from jumping from correlation to causation, but it is nevertheless a productive difference rather than a disabling divide, and that is because it allows for comparisons that can be mutually illuminating. As I have argued previously (see Armstrong 2013, 1–12, 175–82) and try again to show in this book, the inability of literary theorists and neuroscientists to overcome the differences between their perspectives is not a bad thing because it gives them the opportunity to exchange insights about matters of mutual concern from distinctive disciplinary vantage points.

We could not tell each other stories if our brains and bodies did not have some of the characteristics I explore in this book, but neuronal activity alone is not sufficient to produce and sustain narrative activity. A brain in a vat could not tell or understand stories. I am referring, of course, to the classic thought experiment in which a brain is imagined to exist in a tub of fluid with sensors attached to it, and the question is asked: 'Could you (or your) brain tell the difference?' Evan Thompson (2007, 242) explains: "As conscious subjects we are not brains in cranial vats; we are neurally enlivened beings in the world." Without a body situating us in a social world, the cognitive equipment provided by our brains could not generate the experiences we exchange in the stories we tell each other. But the features and capabilities of that equipment also constrain and enable the construction of stories.

The brain's paradoxical temporal processes that I explore in chapter 2 are a particularly good example of this. The timing of various neuronal and cortical processes is curiously disjunctive and nonsimultaneous, with different parts of the cortex reacting at different rates and neuronal assemblies forming and dissolving at different speeds (connections between different parts of the cortex take longer to form than linkages within a specific region of the brain). As Benjamin Libet's well-known mind-time experiments demonstrate (Libet 2004), one consequence of these disjunctions is that consciousness always lags by as much as a half second behind events to which our perceptual equipment has already responded before we are aware that we've done so (as when we slam on the brakes to avoid a child chasing a ball across the street before we are fully cognizant of the danger we've already avoided). The experiential correlatives of these neural disjunctions are the kinds of paradoxes that famously make Augustine find time bewildering. As Ricoeur points out, Aristotle's theory of plots transforms such aporias into stories. If cortical processes were not temporally various and nonsimultaneous, we could not tell stories. Such simultaneity occurs in what neuroscientists call "hypersynchrony," which characterizes states like sleep and epilepsy (see Baars and Gage 2010, 245–47), and hypersynchrony obviously paralyzes the construction and exchange of stories (among other things).

Elucidating the correlations between the nonsimultaneity of cortical temporality, the paradoxes of experienced time, and the much-discussed contradictions of narrative activity, as I do in chapter 2, can tell us much about the brain-body-world interactions that generate stories. But charting these correlations does not mean that neuronal processes in the brain are by themselves sufficient to produce stories. They aren't. The experiences we have as embodied social beings are constrained by the kinds of brains we have, and it's those experiences we exchange when we tell and follow stories. We couldn't do that, however, if we didn't have brains, and how we do it depends on various brain-based cognitive capacities that narrative sets in motion.

My analysis of the relations between brain, body, and world in narrative interactions is meant to correct the one-sidedness of some versions of so-called 4e cognition that view consciousness as (count the *es*) embodied, enactive, embedded, and extended. This movement has made important contributions to the project of integrating bodily processes, social constructs, and technological equipment into accounts of cognition. I regard this as a worthy attempt to do justice to the bodily, cultural, and historical dimensions of experience that the later Husserl, the early Heidegger, Merleau-Ponty, and various existential and hermeneutic phenomenologists also emphasize, as do such pragmatists as William James, Charles Sanders Peirce, and John Dewey—all figures in whose tradition I work in this book. But as I argue in chapter 1, the embeddedness and extendedness of cognition matter because of the ways in which our brains are connected to the world, and those connections go both ways—from the world to the brain and from the brain to the world. In the words of one of the anonymous referees who reviewed this book for Johns Hopkins University press, it is important "not to throw the brain out with the bathwater, so to speak" (a point this reviewer acknowledged while confessing to hold to a more radical view of enactivism than I propose). In their zeal to reject a Cartesian splitting of mind and body, some proponents of 4e cognition go too far in the other direction and neglect brain-based processes that are necessary for socially situated, embodied cognition to do its work. A corrective to such one-sidedness, my neurophenomenological account of narrative offers a model of embodied neuroscience that incorporates brain-based concepts.

Although I am opposed to neural reductionism, I believe that there is much to learn from comparing lived experience and the neural correlates of consciousness, and the aim of this book is to show what such correlations reveal about narrative. The following chapters chart a variety of correlations between our experiences as tellers and followers of stories and the neuronal processes that enable and constrain these interactions, correlations that have various consequences for narrative theory. Not all problems in narratology can be solved by turning to the science, by any means, but some narrative theories are inconsistent with the science, and those discrepancies should give narratologists pause. As the science of cognition and language has changed, so too must narrative theory.

For example, as I explain in chapter 1, the recursive, nonlinear dynamics of the cortical processes and brain-body-world interactions responsible for language call for jettisoning the structuralist assumptions that still haunt some versions of cognitive narratology. Contemporary neuroscience has discarded the formalist, modular explanation of linguistic development and brain functioning on which the project of identifying orderly, universal structures of mind and language was based. The formalist model of innate, orderly, rule-governed structures for language is inconsistent with what we now know about the unstable equilibrium of the temporally decentered brain and the probabilistic processes through which neuronal assemblies synchronize, desynchronize, and resynchronize. The taxonomic ambitions of some kinds of cognitive narratology that aim to identify and classify the frames, scripts, and preference rules that purportedly underlie our ability to tell and understand stories should be treated skeptically because this program oversimplifies and reifies the interactive neurobiological processes at work in language and cognition.

Narratologists love to build classificatory schemes, taxonomies that sometimes leave even the most devoted students of narrative theory lost in a terminological fog. Rather than reject classification altogether, we should ask whether a given scheme has heuristic value for pointing out aspects of narrative experience that might otherwise be invisible. But a taxonomic model and its accompanying terminology should not be reified or ontologized. Cognitive formalism is not consistent with the best science and should be abandoned in favor of the kind of pragmatic, interactionist approach that I describe in the first chapter. As I explain there, a number of promising versions of such an approach are gaining prominence on the narratological scene, and one of the reasons for favoring them over the models proposed by formalist cognitive narratology is that they line up better with the science.

Chapter 2 explores the neuronal and cortical underpinnings of the ways in which narrative organizes our experience of time. The asynchronies of neuronal and cortical timing processes are curiously correlated to many of the much-discussed paradoxes of narrative temporality—the interactions of the time of the telling and the time of the told, for example, and the different chronological permutations that Gérard Genette (1980) has famously analyzed. Our experiences of narrative temporality are correlated to the temporality of brain processes on multiple levels, from short-term millisecond interactions among neuronal assemblies up to long-term interactions of memory and imagination. These correlations suggest how the work of narrative in organizing our experience of time goes up and down and across multiple dimensions of embodied temporality that are dynamically, recursively, mutually formative. Narratives play with our experience of time in how they emplot events (the level of story) as well as in how they are told (the orderings of the discourse), and these interactions can be powerfully formative because of the many kinds and levels of cognitive timing processes they coordinate and relate to one another.

Chapter 3 examines the relation between the role of action in cognition and the organization of action in narration and emplotment. Ample, well-known experimental evidence demonstrates that the brain is responsive to linguistic representations of action (the same sections of the motor cortex firing, for example, when we read about kicking or throwing a ball as when we perform those actions [see Pulvermüller and Fadiga 2010]). Motor equivalence and action understanding are by themselves not sufficient to account for language, however, inasmuch as people who suffer from different kinds of physical incapacities can still make sense of actions they cannot perform. But narrative imitations of action can profoundly influence cognitive processes in many areas remote from motor control because our capacity to act in the world is intimately and inextricably involved in our ability to understand the world. As this chapter explains, the pervasive role of action in perception and cognition undergirds the power of represented patterns of action to reinforce or reconfigure patterns of cognitive activity. The ways in which action coordinates different modalities of perception in our everyday experience of the world help to explain the interaction of different kinds of action in narrative—the interaction between emplotted actions (the story), the act of narrating (the discourse), and the activity of reception (reading, listening to, and making sense of narrative).

Some influential 4e models describe cognition as simulation because it is grounded in embodied experiences that are reactivated when analogous situations recur. Chapter 3 shows that this process of reenactment is more paradoxical than is often understood because a simulation is an as-relation, both like and not like what it recreates. Mechanical and causally deterministic models of simulation do not do justice to the variability of these as-relations—how, for example, a prior experience can be reconfigured to meet a novel cognitive challenge, its traces recombined in not entirely predetermined or predictable ways. As this chapter also demonstrates, a causal model is similarly unable to explain the heterogeneity of the different metaphors for embodied experiences like pain and anger that make us biocultural hybrids. Some of these figures are grounded in widely shared, bodily based experiences, but others are unique to the conventions of the cultural and historical world we happen to inhabit and may be at odds with the configurations that prevail in another culture or period even though we have the same bodies and brains.

As chapter 4 explains, similar problems call into question the frequently heard claim that simulating social experience by reading or listening to a story predictably and automatically increases empathy or improves our ability to understand other minds. Narrative reconfigurations of experience may produce many different effects, some pro- and some antisocial, which they would not do if the process of fictional simulation were a linear, one-way causal mechanism. Narratives entail doubling processes whereby my world is brought into relation with a world it is not, and this is not a cause-effect relationship. The contradiction of such doubling, whereby I use my cognitive powers to animate a world that is both like and not like my own, enacts what phenomenology calls the paradox of the alter ego. Social relations of all kinds, including the telling and following of stories, are fundamentally paradoxical because they are inextricably both intersubjective and solipsistic. As phenomenologists from Husserl to Merleau-Ponty have explained, we are always intersubjectively involved with others in a world we share because we assume, for example, that the view of another perceiver will fill out what we cannot see in a manner consistent with our perspective, even as the inescapably solipsistic my ownness of experience prevents us from ever knowing another person's self-for-themselves (what Heidegger calls the *Jemeinigkeit* of an unshareable experience like death [his example] or childbirth [my wife's]).

Because reading or listening to stories entails a doubling of worlds, it can take many different, unpredictable forms. A mechanistic model of cognitive simulation fails to recognize the variety and unpredictability of these doublings. The circuit of figuration through which we exchange experiences as we tell each other stories may indeed shape and reshape our lives, but it does not necessarily have uniformly beneficial effects, as some psychologists and philosophers wishfully proclaim. The experimental findings about the moral and cognitive effects of reading are consequently interestingly contradictory, as the fourth chapter explains. A phenomenological account of the paradoxes of self-other relations in narrative interactions explains how stories can promote either conflict or care, aggression or compassion, imitative violence or an expansion of our capacity for sympathy. The doubling of as-if relations in narrative simulations of experience can also shed light on some of the contradictions in collaborative interactions that a growing number of neurobiologists have begun to explore as recognition spreads in the scientific community that studying a single brain in the isolated confines of an fMRI machine oversimplifies the real-life interactions of embodied brains in a social world.

As much as students of narrative have to learn from neuroscience, so neuroscience stands to learn from narrative theory. Some of the most advanced work in neuroaesthetics has been accomplished in the field of the neuroscience of music because these two-way exchanges across the explanatory gap have been so successful there. Many neuroscientists who have studied music are themselves musicians, and they consequently understand and respect the need to let their research be instructed by concepts drawn from music theory (for example, see Patel 2008 on language, music, and the brain and Koelsch 2012 on music and perception). By contrast, the neuroaesthetics of the visual arts is often marred by basic mistakes that are a consequence of the presumption and naivete of vision scientists who go into a museum and think that their knowledge about the neurobiology of vision is sufficient to explain what they see (for critiques of some prominent instances, see Conway and Rehding 2013 and Hyman 2010). Neuroaesthetics requires good aesthetics as well as good science.

The neuroaesthetics of literature has lagged behind other areas of neuroscientific study of the arts in part because literature is such a complicated and heterogeneous state of affairs but also because an adequate theoretical framework has been lacking (for attempts to remedy this deficiency see Starr 2013, Zeman et al. 2013, and Jacobs 2015). As I show, structuralist cognitive narratology cannot provide such a framework because its assumptions about language and the brain are inconsistent with the best science. A neurophenomenological model of how reading and narrative play with the brain may begin to address this need, however. The rich and diverse resources of phenomenological theories of reading, interpretation, and narrative on which this book draws may provide the sort of aesthetic framework to guide such investigations that music theory offers the neuroscience of music.

This book attempts to speak to multiple audiences, from readers with a general interest in the cognitive humanities to narratologists and neuroscientists. Students and scholars interested in cognitive criticism and literary theory will find, I hope, that this book sheds light on the age-old question of what our ability to tell stories reveals about language and the mind. That is an issue that has fascinated generations of specialist and nonspecialist readers alike. For cognitive critics, as I have explained, the book corrects the mistake of neglecting brain-based concepts in analyzing embodied cognitive processes, and it provides instead a neuroscientifically informed model of embodied, enactive cognition. For narratologists and narrative theorists, the book offers many large and small suggestions for how to refine our understanding of narrative interactions in light of the findings of neuroscience. For neuroscientists, last but not least, the book aims to provide a theoretically informed framework for studying the cognitive processes involved in narrative that is necessary to guide the formulation of research questions that are based not only on good science but also on good aesthetics.

Such a framework may be helpful to cognitive scientists who recognize the importance of stories as evidence for studying brain-to-brain coupling and the nonlinear dynamics of what Stanislas Dehaene (2009) calls our "bushy" brains. The to-and-fro play with pattern that characterizes reading and narrative is potentially fertile territory for exploring the dynamics of the brain web and the connectome that are increasingly at the center of neuroscientific investigation (for example, see Varela et al. 2001 and Raichle 2011). Narrative is a much-underutilized model for studying such processes, and neuroscience is impoverished by neglecting it. A scientist who happens upon the arcane, often bewildering world of narratology and narrative theory might not immediately see how the technical terms and concepts that circulate there could be of use to neuroscientific research, but perhaps this book can point the way.

CHAPTER ONE

Neuroscience and Narrative Theory

THE ABILITY TO tell and follow a story requires cognitive capacities that are basic to the neurobiology of mental functioning. Neuroscience cannot of course reveal everything we might want to know about stories, but it is also true that our species would probably not produce narratives so prolifically if they weren't somehow good for our brains and our embodied interactions with the world. What kind of brains do we have that enable us to tell each other stories? And how do stories configure our brains? Neuroscience and narrative theory have much to say to each other about our species' facility and fascination with stories. How plots order events in time, how stories imitate actions, and how narratives relate us to other lives, whether in pity or in fear—these central concerns of narratologists from Aristotle to Paul Ricoeur are perhaps surprisingly aligned with hot topics in contemporary neuroscience that I explore: temporal synchrony and the binding problem, the action-perception circuit in cognition, and the mirroring processes of embodied intersubjectivity. The ways in which stories coordinate time, represent embodied action, and promote social collaboration are fundamental to the brain-body interactions through which our species has evolved and has constructed the cultures we inhabit. Crucial questions about how the brain works—how it assembles neuronal syntheses without a central controller—have to do with issues concerning time, action, and self-other relations that are central to narrative. The purpose of this book is to explore and explain these convergences.

Stories help the brain negotiate the never-ending conflict between its need for pattern, synthesis, and constancy and its need for flexibility, adaptability, and openness to change. The brain's remarkable, paradoxical ability to play in a to-and-fro manner between these competing imperatives is a consequence of its decentered organization as a network of reciprocal top-down, bottom-up connections among its interacting parts. Narrative theorist Seymour Chatman (1978, 47, 45) attributes plot-formation to "the disposition of our minds to hook things together"; as he notes, "our minds inveterately seek structure." This is, indeed, a basic axiom of contemporary neuroscience. Against the cognitive need for consistency, however, the psychologist William James (1950 [1890], 1:139) describes the brain as "an organ whose natural state is one of unstable equilibrium," constantly fluctuating in ways that enable its "possessor to adapt his conduct to the minutest alterations in the environing circumstances." The brain knows the world by forming and dissolving assemblies of neurons, establishing the patterns that through repeated firing become our habitual ways of interacting with the environment, even as ongoing fluctuations in these syntheses combat their tendency to rigidify and promote the possibility of new cortical connections. The brain's ceaseless balancing act between the formation and dissolution of patterns makes possible the exploratory play between past equilibria and the indeterminacies of the future that is essential for successful mental functioning and the survival of our species.

Stories contribute to this balancing act by playing with consonance and dissonance. Borrowing Frank Kermode's (1967) well-known terms, Paul Ricoeur (1984a, 65–66) describes emplotment as "concordant discordance"—"a synthesis of the heterogeneous" that configures parts into a whole by transforming the "diversity of events or incidents" into a coherent story. According to Ricoeur, the act of "composing plots" converts "the existential burden of discordance" (33, 31) into narrative syntheses that give meaning to life's disjunctions by constructing patterns of action. Even in the simplest narratives that approach what Gérard Genette (1980, 35–36) calls the hypothetical "zero degree" of difference between the order of events in the telling and their order in the told, the conjunctions that join together the elements of the plot are invariably disrupted by twists and turns on the way to resolution. What Genette calls temporal "anachronies" (flash-forwards and flashbacks, for example, that disrupt the correspondence between the telling and the told) further play with the competing impulses toward consonance and dissonance that are basic to narrative. The imbalances between pattern formation and dissolution in the brain make possible this narrative play between concord and discord, even as the construction and disruption of patterns in the stories we tell each other play with the tensions in the brain between the competing imperatives of order and flexibility. The neuroscience of these interactions is part of the explanation of how stories give shape to our lives even as our lives give rise to stories.

Stories can draw on experience, transform it into plots, and then reshape the lives of listeners and readers because different processes of figuration traverse the circuit of interactions and exchanges that constitute narrative activity. As I explain in chapter 2, the neural underpinnings of narration start with the peculiarly decentered temporality of cognitive processes across the brain and the body—disjunctions in the timing of intracortical and brain-body interactions that not only make possible but also actually require the kind of retrospective and prospective pattern formation entailed in the narrative ordering of beginnings, middles, and ends. Next, as chapter 3 shows, the strangely pervasive involvement of processes of motor cognition not only in the understanding of action and gesture but also in other modalities of perception suggests why the work of creating plots that simulate structures of action can have such a profound effect on our patterns of configuring the world. Finally, as chapter 4 explains, if stories can promote empathy and otherwise facilitate the cointentionality required for the collaborative activity unique to our species, the power and limits of their capacity to transform social life ultimately depend on embodied processes of doubling self and other through mirroring, simulation, and identification, processes whose limitations are reflected in the strengths and weaknesses of narratives as ethical and political instruments.

Each of the following chapters explores one of these convergences in detail. In all of these areas, narratives configure lived experience by invoking brain-based processes of pattern formation that are fundamental to the neurobiology of mental functioning. To set the stage for these analyses, however, we first need to consider some preliminary questions about the relation between neuroscience and narrative theory. Why should students of narrative pay attention to neuroscientific discoveries about cognition and language, and how should the research program of narratology take account of the science?

Language, the Brain, and Cognitive Narratology

Triangulating our phenomenological experience as tellers and followers of stories with neuroscientific findings about embodied cognition and with narrative theories about plots, fiction, and reading is an attempt to understand the relation between language, cognition, and narrative—a goal that many thoughtful investigators across a variety of disciplines have pursued. One of the reasons why philosophers, literary theorists, and everyday readers have wondered about why and how we tell stories is that narrative seems to hold the key to how language and the mind work. Narratology is now at a turning point in its understanding of the relation between language, cognition, and narrative, poised between (on the one hand) the formalist models of schemes, scripts, and preference rules inherited from structuralism and (on the other hand) pragmatically oriented theories of narrative as embodied, intersubjective interaction. Whether these models can be reconciled and if so how are important, unsettled questions. Understanding the neurobiological bases of narrative may help answer them by showing how the ability to tell and follow stories aligns with how the brain processes language. Not all of the conflicts among students of narrative can be settled by the discoveries of science, but some claims turn out to be stronger than others, and others are just plain wrong. The aims and methods of narratology need to be adjusted in light of what we know about the neuroscience of language and the brain.

The goal of classical narratology was to construct the ideal taxonomy— the classificatory scheme that would identify the fundamental elements of narrative and their rules of combination, based on the model of how grammar and syntax determine meaning by establishing the structural relations between the constituent parts of a logical, ordered system.[1] Whether inspired by Saussure's prioritization of *langue* over *parole* (the presumably stable, orderly structures of language as opposed to the contingencies of speech) or Chomsky's claims about universal grammar (the inborn cognitive structures that constitute what Pinker [1994] memorably calls the "language instinct"), the assumption was that the structures of mind, language, and narrative are homologous, innate, and universal. Classical narratologist Ann Banfield (1982, 234) expressed a view shared by many narrative theorists, for example, when she asserted that "the ingredients for represented speech and thought" in a story "are . . . given in universal grammar" and that the ease with which we create and understand stories is explained by fundamental homologies between the structures of narrative and "the speaker's internalized grammar."

Some versions of cognitive narratology still operate within the structuralist paradigm, either tacitly or explicitly. For example, the editors of the recent anthology *Stories and Minds: Cognitive Approaches to Literary Narrative* assert that "rather than turning away from structuralist narratology, cognitive narratologists . . . build on the insights of structuralism and combine them with cognitive studies" (Bernaerts et al. 2013a, 13). As James Phelan (2006, 286) explains, "cognitive narratology . . . shares with [structural narratology] the same goal of developing a comprehensive formal account of the nature of narrative" and "conceives of its formal system as the components of the mental models that narratives depend on in their production and consumption." These "mental models" are the frames, scripts, and preference rules that Manfred Jahn defines and explains in his authoritative account of cognitive narratology in the *Routledge Encyclopedia of Narrative Theory* (2005, 67–71). Articulating the aims of "post-classical narratology," Jan Alber and Monika Fludernik (2010b, 11) endorse this project: "Cognitive narratologists . . . show that the recipient uses his or her world knowledge to project fictional worlds, and this knowledge is stored in cognitive schemata called frames and scripts."

Whether these mental constructs can do justice to the cognitive processes they purport to describe is highly questionable, however. The formalist goal of identifying orderly, universal structures of mind, language, and narrative does not match up well with the unstable equilibrium of the temporally de-centered brain or the probabilistic processes through which cognitive connections develop and dissolve. There is a growing scientific consensus that the formalist model of language as an innate, orderly, rule-governed structure should be cast aside because it does not fit with what we know about how the brain works. As the science of cognition and language has shifted, so too must narratology revise its methods and aims.

New versions of cognitive narratology have arisen to challenge the structuralist paradigm. Advocates of the 4e (embodied, enactive, embedded, and extended) view of cognition argue that rather than "conceiv[ing] of the mind" as a structure of "abstract, propositional representations" like frames and scripts, narrative theory should understand "the human mind as shaped by our evolutionary history, bodily make-up, and sensorimotor possibilities, and as arising out of close dialogue with other minds, in intersubjective interactions and cultural practices" (Kukkonen and Caracciolo 2014, 261–62). Whereas first-generation cognitive science was "firmly grounded in a computational view of the mind," with "frames, scripts, and schemata" functioning as "mental representations that enable us to make sense of the world by serving as models of specific situations or activities," second-generation cognitive science shares with phenomenology and the pragmatism of Dewey and James an emphasis on the interactions between embodied consciousness and the world in "feedback loops" through which "experience shapes cultural practices" even as "cultural practices help the mind make sense of bodily experience" (Caracciolo 2014, 45; Kukkonen and Caracciolo 2014, 267). Rather than prioritizing the construction of taxonomies, schemata, and systems of rules to explain how the mind works and to account for narrative by disclosing its underlying cognitive structures, second-generation narratology "insist[s] on the situated, embodied quality of readers' engagement with stories and on how meaning emerges from the experiential interaction between texts and readers" (Caracciolo 2014, 4). A quest for structures and rules has been displaced by an emphasis on the interactions between embodied minds, stories, and the world.

Instead of viewing this change as a paradigm shift, some prominent narrative theorists with roots in the first generation have sought ways of reconciling embodied, enactivist narratology with schema theory and formalist, grammatically based models. For example, rejecting the idea that second-generation cognitive science has replaced earlier theories, Fludernik (2014, 406) proposes that they should be seen as informing one another: "A history of cognitive studies might perhaps better start out from an inherent duality in cognitive work—research that is static and abstract flanking research that looks at the body and human experience." Reminiscent of how structural linguistics juxtaposed synchronic and diachronic approaches to language, this proposal views frames and scripts as "static, abstract" structures that are actuated in experience, much as the structuralists thought the rules of *langue* are manifested in the speech acts of *parole*. David Herman seems to have cast aside his earlier project of constructing a "story logic" that reflects transcendental, universal "mental models" (2002, 1–24) in favor of what he calls "discursive psychology" (2010, 156). On this view, meaning is not a product of "mental processes 'behind' what people say and do"; "the mind does not preexist discourse, but is ongoingly accomplished in and through its production and interpretation" (156). Still, hoping like Fludernik to rescue formalism and schema theory, he nevertheless asks "how we might work toward a rapprochement between (1) discourse-oriented approaches to the mind as a situated interactional achievement and (2) the work in cognitive grammar and cognitive semantics that likewise promises to throw light on the mind relevance of narrative structures but that focuses on discourse productions by individual speakers" (175). Again echoing structuralism's opposition between *langue* and *parole*, Herman proposes that we think of language as having social and individual sides that could be separately but compatibly studied—but with the switch that pragmatic, interactive theories rather than formal structures would explain the social side, while grammatically based schema theory would provide models for individual mental structures.[2]

The problem with both of these proposals, however, is that the epistemological assumptions of first- and second-generation cognitive science are irreconcilably opposed: the first views meaning as a manifestation of underlying frames, scripts, and rules, while the second regards it as a product of mutually formative, historically evolving interactions between brain, body, and world. The narratological programs based on these opposing epistemologies are also fundamentally at odds. The second focuses on the figurative, interactive processes through which stories are constructed and experienced, while the first prioritizes the schemes, structures, and rules presumably underlying them.[3] The problem is not whether to emphasize what happens in interactions between the body and the world or, alternatively, what goes on in the head. What is at issue is how to correlate neuronally based, embodied cognitive processes with our experience of the social world and with our capacities to tell and follow stories. Two questions are at stake here. How are we to understand the pattern-forming capacities of our cognitive equipment that first-generation cognitive narratologies would formalize into frames, scripts, and preference rules? And how should we understand the regularities of language that formalists would systematize into orderly classificatory schemes and rule-governed structures? Cognitive narratology needs a neuroscientifically sound understanding of language that explains how neuronal and cortical processes interact with our lived experience of the social world.

Not everything, to be sure, in first-generation cognitive narratology need be abandoned. Jahn (2005, 67) describes "'seeing X as Y' as a foundational axiom" of cognitive narratology, and this idea is indeed scientifically sound. Configurative processes of categorization and pattern formation—what existential phenomenologist Martin Heidegger (1962 [1927]) similarly calls the "as-structure" ("Als-Struktur") of understanding—are crucial to embodied cognition and narrative, but they need to be understood in nonschematized, interactive form. One reason why gestalt theory has been a resource from which neuroscientists like Semir Zeki (2004), cognitive psychologists like James J. Gibson (1979), and phenomenologists like Maurice Merleau-Ponty (2012 [1945]) have all repeatedly drawn is its appreciation of the role that figuration or seeing-as plays in cognition. This is, for example, the epistemological moral of the famously ambiguous rabbit-duck gestalt (with the beak of the duck shifting if we see the shape as a rabbit, a new part-whole configuration transforming it into a pair of ears). This gestalt is a model of cognition because the circular, recursive work of configurative pattern building (seeing-as) animates not only vision but cognitive processes of all kinds. Making a case for what he calls "carnal hermeneutics," Richard Kearney (2015, 20) similarly observes that the "'as-structure' is already operative in our most basic sensations." This is because, as Merleau-Ponty (2012 [1945], 162) points out, "the slightest sensory given cannot be presented except as integrated into a configuration and as already 'articulated.'" It is consequently a basic principle of contemporary neuroscience that "categorization (or conceptualization) is a fundamental process in the human brain. . . . There are ongoing debates about how categorization works, but the fact that it works is not in question" (Lindquist et al. 2012, 124).

The as-structure of categorization—how seeing always entails seeing-as—is also evident in the circularity of literary interpretation (see Armstrong 2013, 54–90). Literary theorists have long recognized that interpretation is inherently circular because understanding a text or any state of affairs requires grasping in advance the configurative relation between part and whole. Any act of interpretation sets in motion a reciprocal interaction between part and whole because a detail makes sense only if it can be seen as somehow relating to the entire text, even as the whole can only be understood by working through its parts. This epistemological theory about the need for pattern—the idea that part and whole are reciprocally constructed and together construed as a configurative relation of some kind—is common ground between the humanities and the cognitive sciences.

It is a mistake, however, to reify these configurative processes into mental modules that bear no relation to the anatomy of the embodied brain or to posit linear logical models of cognitive decision making that do not correspond to the reciprocal, to-and-fro movements of figuration in experience, in the cortex, or in the interactions between brain, body, and world. These are some of the problems with the terminology of frames, scripts, and preference rules employed by cognitive narratology. As Jahn (2005, 69; see 1997) acknowledges, these notions were developed by artificial intelligence theorists "to replace the concept of context by more explicit and detailed constructs" that "aim at reproducing a human cogniser's knowledge and expectations about standard events and situations"—with frames referring to "situations such as seeing a room or making a promise" and scripts encompassing "standard action sequences such as . . . going to a birthday party, or eating in a restaurant." The brain is not a computer, however. As Hubert Dreyfus (1992) points out, computers lack context, background, and prior experience that we as embodied conscious beings typically employ in testing hypotheses about how to configure a situation we encounter, whether in a text or the world, and replacing this deficiency by positing preset mental constructs that do the work only displaces the problem that needs to be solved. Rather than explaining the processes whereby the embodied brain configures experiential contexts, these constructs instead call attention to what computers can't do.

Seeing-as sets in motion interactions between brain, body, and world that are fluid, reciprocal, and open ended, and preset schemata like frames and scripts are too rigid and linear to do justice to these sorts of dynamic, recursive processes. This is why psychologist Richard Gerrig (2010, 22), whose work on reading is widely (and rightly) respected among cognitive narratologists, has recently parted company from what Jahn describes as the mainstream view, in the process rejecting the term "schema" as too rigid and for-mulaic. Gerrig prefers instead to speak of "memory-based processing," a concept that recognizes that "readers' use of general knowledge" is "more fluid and more idiosyncratic" than the terminology of frames and scripts can capture.

The linear, overly tidy notion that cognition is governed by preference rules also needs to be abandoned. According to Jahn, "A preference rule is usually cast in the form *Prefer to see A as B given a set of conditions C*" (69). In its favor, the notion of preference is not absolute and leaves a little wiggle room for probabilistic variation, but the problem with structuring preferences into "rules" is that they posit a linear chain of decision making, following the form of a logical proposition: if C, then A implies B. This linear, mechanical, logical structure is not an adequate representation of how cognitive decision making happens either in neurobiology or experience. Neurobiologically, it bears little relation to the interactive, top-down, bottom-up processes of the dynamical systems of synchronization and desynchronization in the brain. Neuronal assemblies form and dissolve according to patterns of habituation that re-sult from the reciprocal reinforcement of connections that can be displaced by other syntheses, and these interactions are not like linear, mechanical al-gorithms (see Edelman 1987). Experientially, the unidirectional logic of preference rules is unable to capture the to-and-fro circularity of seeing-as in the phenomenological process of configuring part-whole relations in a text or in life. Reading is not linear logical processing, and embodied cognition cannot be adequately modeled either by ordered hierarchies of modules or mechanical, linear algorithms.

The work of seeing-as is not localizable in any particular region of the cortex but extends across the brain, the body, and the world. It is not gov-erned by rules but develops habitual patterns through repeated experiences and is consequently always open to disruption, variation, and change. The formalist goal of identifying orderly, universal structures of mind, language, and narrative doesn't match up well with the messiness of the brain or with how cognitive patterns emerge from our embodied experiences of the world. The consensus among neuroscientists is that the brain is a bushy ensemble of anatomical features whose functions are only partly fixed by genetic in-heritance and are to a considerable extent plastic and variable depending on how they connect in networks with other, often far-flung cortical areas. These connections develop and change through experience according to Hebb's law (2002 [1949]), a fundamental axiom of neuroscience: "Neurons that fire to-gether, wire together." As Stephen E. Nadeau (2012, 1) points out, "Brain order is chaotic rather than deterministic; rules are not defined but instead emerge from network behavior, constrained by network topography" and connectivity (not all parts of the cortex can do everything, and they cannot interact if they are not linked by the axons through which neurons exchange electrochemical charges). Whatever order can be found in language and cognition results, he explains, from patterns of reciprocal relationship "acquired through experience," and these patterns are attributable less to innate, genetically determined anatomical structures than to "statistical regularities of experience."[4]

The brain, in short, is not an orderly structure consisting of rule-governed relations between fixed elements like a computer with hard-wired connections between components that operate according to logical algorithms. Much messier, more fluid, and more open to unpredictable (if not unlimited) developments than the linear, mechanical model assumes, the brain is an ever-changing ensemble of reciprocally interacting parts whose functions may vary according to how they combine with other elements. Once popular when artificial intelligence concepts dominated first-generation cognitive science, modular models of the brain (see Fodor 1983) have fallen out of favor because cortical regions are not autonomous and orderly. As Shaun Gallagher (2012, 36) observes, the brain is "a dynamical system [that] cannot be explained on the basis of the behavior of its separate components or in terms of an analysis that focuses on the synchronic, or static, or purely mechanical interactions of its parts"; "the parts of a dynamical system do not interact in a linear fashion" but rather "in a non-linear way, reciprocally determining each other's behavior" (see Kelso 1995, 2000). Patterns of relationship can become established over time as particular interactions recur and reinforce existing connections or propagate and strengthen new ones, but how repeated experiences lead to the formation of habits through Hebbian "firing and wiring" is a better model for understanding these patterns than the genetically fixed, orderly structures assumed by the epistemological formalists. Preprogrammed modules and linear algorithms are not a good model for understanding the workings of the brain.

The structures of neural anatomy are limiting but not ultimately defining. Different cortical locations have particular functions that can be disabled if they are damaged, but no region works alone, and the role of each region can vary according to how it reciprocally interacts with other areas. Function and connectivity can change with experience. The visual cortex of a blind person, for example, can adapt and become responsive to touch when he or she is reading braille (see Changeux 2012, 208), and some sight-deprived people as well as animals have been shown to have superior sound localization because the unused parts of their visual cortex are recruited for auditory functions (see Rauscheker 2003). These instances of plasticity may seem exceptional, but they are examples of the general rule that, as a study by Kristen A. Lindquist and colleagues (2012, 123) explains, the "function of individual brain regions is determined, in part, by the network of brain regions it is firing with." According to Lindquist's group, this is why there is "little evidence that discrete emotion categories can be consistently and specifically localized to distinct brain regions" (121). Their review of the experimental evidence shows, for example, that the amygdala is not uniquely and exclusively associated with fear but is also active "in orienting responses to motivationally relevant stimuli" that are "novel," "uncertain," and "unusual" (130). Various studies have similarly shown, they point out, that the anterior cingulate cortex, typically connected with disgust, "is observed in a number of tasks that involve awareness of body states," including "body movement," "gastric distention," and even orgasm (133–34).

This research calls into question Patrick Colm Hogan's claim (2010, 255; see 2011a, 2011b) that "emotion is . . . the response of dedicated neurobiological systems to concrete experiences, not a function of the evaluation of changing situations relative to goals." Lindquist is a member of Lisa Feldman Barrett's laboratory that has led the challenge to the theory of basic emotions promulgated by Paul Ekman and Silvan Tomkins (also see Colombetti 2014, 26–52). As Barrett (2017, 22, 23, 33) explains, a large and growing body of neuroscientific and psychological research has challenged the view that emotions are universal classes with objective biological markers:

> Overall, we found that no brain region contained the fingerprint for any single emotion. . . . Emotions arise from firing neurons, but no neurons are exclusively dedicated to emotion. . . . [A]n emotion word, like "anger," does not refer to a specific response with a unique physical fingerprint but to a group of highly variable instances that are tied to specific situations. . . . [T]he emotions you experience and perceive are not an inevitable consequence of your genes. . . . Your familiar emotion concepts are built-in only because you grew up in a particular social context where those emotion concepts are meaningful and useful, and your brain applies them outside your awareness to construct your experiences.

Emotions are mixed products of biology and culture that are better thought of as variable, internally heterogenous populations than logical categories or universal classes with fixed neurobiological foundations.

Anatomical location and cortical structure alone cannot explain embodied cognition. Brain-body-world interactions can affect not only internal connectivity but also the functions of particular cortical regions. To understand a complex cognitive phenomenon like vision, emotion, or language, it is not enough to identify structure and modularity (as the formalist models assume); it is necessary, rather, to trace the configurative, nonlinear, to-and-fro processes through which various components of our dynamic cognitive systems interact and reciprocally constitute each other.

A good example of the brain's combination of anatomical specialization and openness to change through experience is the manner in which the visual cortex adapts inherited functionalities in order to support the unnatural, culturally acquired capacity to read written texts (see Armstrong 2013, 26–53). As Stanislas Dehaene (2009, 4) points out, we learn to read Shakespeare by adapting cortical capacities that our species acquired on the African savannah. This is an instance of what M. L. Anderson (2010) calls "neural reuse"—the capacity of cortical regions to acquire functions for which they did not first evolve. New, unpredictable experiences with the world may set in motion variable interactions between different areas of the brain and the body as well as with other members of our species that can produce fundamental changes in cortical structure and functionality. As the visual and auditory cortices interact during the often arduous processes through which beginning readers learn to associate word shapes with phonetic sounds (also activating parts of the motor cortex associated with the mouth and the lips that fire not only in the articulation but also during the recognition of speech), connections get established and reinforced between different regions of the brain that have the effect of converting a specific area of the visual cortex to a culturally specific use (the recognition of visual word forms) for which it was not innately, genetically predetermined. The acquisition of the ability to read may be an extraordinary cultural and neurobiological accomplishment, but as an example of neural reuse, it is simply an illustration of what Anderson calls "a fundamental organizational principle of the brain" (245).

Our species' development of the capacity to read illustrates the dual historicity of cognitive functions (see Armstrong 2015). Some of our epistemological equipment is based on long-term, evolutionarily stable capacities like the responsiveness of the visual system to edges, orientation, lines, and shapes, but these capacities are open to change depending on learning and experience—they can be recruited, in this case, to identify alphabetic signs—because the function of a cortical region depends on how it interacts with other components of the dynamical system in which it is engaged. The brain can be molded by cultural institutions (like literacy) that adapt particular areas and capacities for their purposes, but as with reading, these capabilities need to be relearned with each generation until or unless the neural reuse through which they are repurposed becomes evolutionarily adapted into the biological makeup of the species. The structures and functions of the brain are historical, not universal, because they are the products of evolution, but some capacities are more enduring than others and are shared by members of our species across time and around the globe, even as they get reshaped and repurposed through particular, historical, culturally situated experiences of learning.

Language is what neuroscientists call "a biocultural hybrid" (Evans and Levinson 2009, 446) that develops through the interaction of inherited functions and anatomical structures in the brain with culturally variable experiences of communication and education. Although some parts of the brain are known to be linked to language (lesions in Broca's and Wernicke's areas, for example, can disrupt syntactical or semantic processes), Nadeau points out that "linguistic function taps the entire cerebrum" (83), and recent fMRI-based research has confirmed that language entails far-flung syntheses of cortical areas and connections between the brain and the body (see Huth et al. 2016). There is no single module that governs language and no discrete, anatomically identifiable set of regions that would constitute the grammar unit predicted by structural linguistics. As Nadeau explains, "The grammar anyone of us uses is not intrinsically universal. . . . Instead it is based on the statistical regularities of our own linguistic experience (instantiated in neural connectivity), which have been determined by the modest community of people we have conversed with or read" (164–65). Cases of aphasia in different languages reveal not an anatomically based, universal grammar system that gets knocked out with the loss of language function but rather what Nadeau calls "graceful degradation" (17). Everything doesn't simply collapse and disappear, but some functions are more or less strongly preserved in different patterns of vulnerability that depend on cross-cerebral connections and redundancies and that vary between linguistic communities. This evidence is better accounted for by the stochastic, probabilistic regularities established through Hebbian connections and developed through experience than by a logically ordered, innate grammar.

Such a probabilistic model also helps to explain the duality of language as a set of regularities open to innovation, variation, and change. As Jean-Pierre Changeux argues, the Hebbian explanation of stochastic regularities offers a better account of the creative capacities of language than prefixed formal systems can provide (see 2012, 206–7, 316–17). On the one hand, language is a set of shared codes, evident in its recurring patterns, that support intersubjective communication and well-formed sentences. On the other hand, the irregularities of language are also vitally important because they make possible unpredictable if constrained linguistic innovation through rule-governed or rule-breaking creativity. In accord with a probabilistic model, structures do not completely decide in advance all the ways they can be used (innovation within the rules is possible), and sometimes new configurations can emerge as previous connections are replaced by new ones (transgressing existing rules is not always wrong, as with a novel metaphor that at first may seem like a mistake but then becomes accepted and gets adopted into the lexicon [see Ricoeur 1977]).

If language and narrative are biocultural hybrids, any transcultural, transhistorical regularities in their functions and forms are a product of variable but constrained interactions between brain, body, and world and not universals that are homologous to logical structures of the mind. The sources of these regularities are typically both biology and culture; it's not simply that nature is fixed and culture variable. Similarly, any recurring patterns in the stories we typically tell each other are the mixed products of interactions between our species' neurobiological equipment and repeated experiences we are likely to undergo. If stories across the world have recurrent forms, this is not a result of narrative structures that reflect universal cognitive schemata. Rather, as biocultural hybrids, the patterns identified by various narrative theories have probably developed because evolved cognitive proclivities shared by members of our species have interacted with recurrent, typical experiences to produce configurative relations between brain, body, and world that demonstrate statistical regularities. These patterns are not logical structures but habitual configurations that are variable but constrained within limits that are attributable to the regularities of both biology and experience.

Consider, for example, Hogan's claim (2003, 230–38) that certain narrative universals characterize the mind and its stories—story structures that he identifies as the romantic, the heroic, and the sacrificial. How to understand cross-cultural "universals" is a notoriously difficult matter. For example, arguing that the claims of relativism overstate the differences between cultures, Donald E. Brown (1991, 9–38) carefully distinguishes between different kinds and degrees of universality—universals of "essence," attributable to the biological characteristics of our species, as opposed to universals of "accident," produced by widely shared experiences, some of which may be "near universals," probably all encompassing but at least broadly evident, and "statistical universals" that may not be omnipresent but are more common than would be predicted by chance. Hogan (2010, 48–49) admits different kinds and degrees of universality, but he thinks and talks like a structuralist: "Hierarchies of universals are defined not only by the schematization of techniques and by a receding series of explanatory abstractions but by a series of conditional relations. . . . Much as unconditional universals may be subsumed into hierarchies of abstraction, implicational universals may be organized into typologies." This kind of logical formalism is not a good way of thinking about the messy, probabilistic development of regularities that characterize biocultural hybrids like language and narrative.

If narrative patterns like those identified by Hogan recur across cultures, that is not because they reflect universal cognitive structures. They are better understood as biocultural hybrids—recurrent configurations that develop because certain repeated characteristics of our species' shared experiences of birth and death, collaboration and competition, propagation and violence interact with biologically based cognitive proclivities to produce statistically discoverable regularities in cultural institutions, including the stories we circulate in our communities. Given the commonalities in the basic experiences members of our species typically undergo in their journeys from birth to death, it would be surprising if the cognitive configurations established through Hebbian connectivity between our brains, bodies, and worlds did not demonstrate various regularities that would show up in our narratives. Members of our species fall in love and have sexual relations, engage in conflicts that produce winners and losers, and form communities that join some members and exclude others, and the configurative powers of pattern formation based on the connective capacities of our embodied brains build narratives about these experiences that may evince various regularities (Hogan's stories of romance, heroism, and sacrifice).

It is misleading to call these "narrative universals" or to attribute them to a structural logic of "the mind and its stories," because these terms are too static, orderly, and ahistorical to do justice to the messy, dynamic processes through which biocultural hybrids get produced in the interactions of brain, body, and world. These interactions may produce patterns that demonstrate regularities because habitual connections are established through Hebbian processing and neural reuse that are then passed on by cultural sharing of the kind through which, for example, literacy is developed and handed down. But formalist terminology and structuralist models are not good tools for describing these processes because such concepts misrepresent the way habitual patterns of connection and configuration get made and transformed in experience and in the brain. Formal taxonomies are not sufficient to explain these interactions.

Figuration in Narrative and Cognition

Figuration, or seeing-as, is the key concept joining cognitive science and narrative theory, and it is central to the neurophenomenological model of narrative that I construct in the following chapters. The configurative powers of embodied cognition are a primary concern of phenomenological theories of how we tell and follow stories, from Roman Ingarden's early analysis of the polyphonic concretization of the multiple strata of a literary work to the theory of reading as a process of consistency building and gap filling developed by Konstanz School theorists Wolfgang Iser and Hans Robert Jauss.[5] Paul Ricoeur's monumental work on time and narrative similarly foregrounds the role of configurative processes in cognition and aesthetic experience.[6] Explaining the figurative processes at work in a phenomenological model of narrative is one of the aims of this section.

A second, related aim is to show what a focus on cognitive figuration can contribute to narrative theory. Sometimes narrative theory can seem like an exercise in the generation of classificatory schemes for their own sake, without regard for their practical purpose, unfortunately resulting in what James Phelan (2006, 283) describes as "the large Terminological Beastie looming over the field." Even if we need to reject the structural, formalist epistemology implicit in the taxonomical project, that does not mean we have to discard all narrative terms as useless. Challenging this epistemology should, rather, foreground the question of what their uses are, and triangulating narrative theory, our experience with stories, and the neuroscience of embodied cognition is a way of posing that question. Many of the ambiguities in the lexicon of narrative theory are a result of the ways in which figurative activity crosses back and forth between aspects of narrative that narratological distinctions attempt to discriminate but can't always keep tidily in place. Attending to the passage of figurative activity across different aspects of narrative with the help of a phenomenological model can clarify some of these ambiguities.

Ricoeur describes emplotment as a response to the enigmas of time that famously troubled Augustine (1961 [397–400], 264): "What, then, is time? I know well enough what it is, provided that nobody asks me; but if I am asked what it is and try to explain, I am baffled." Time is a scandal for speculative thought because various aporias and paradoxes immediately arise as soon as we try to provide a rigorous theoretical account of the lived experience of time passing. "How can time exist," Ricoeur asks, "if the past is no longer, if the future is not yet, and if the present is not always?" (1984a, 7). What William James calls "the specious present" (1950 [1890], 1:609)—our everyday sense of the moment as "a duration, with a bow and a stern, as it were—a rearward- and a forward-looking end"—is more bewildering than we ordinarily realize. As Merleau-Ponty (2012 [1945], 441) points out, "My present transcends itself toward an imminent future and a recent past, and touches them there where they are, in the past and in the future themselves." Hence Husserl's (1964 [1928], 48–63) description of the passing moment as bounded by "retentional and protential horizons," a metaphor meant to suggest the paradoxical connectedness of the present to past and future experiences that we sense across its borders even if we cannot reach them. But the horizon metaphor describes what still needs to be explained: how can the present "actually" touch the past and the future? Or, as Shaun Gallagher and Dan Zahavi (2008, 75) ask, "How can we be conscious of that which is no longer or not yet?" We respond to these enigmas, according to Ricoeur, by telling and following stories. Finding in Aristotle an answer to Augustine's question, Ricoeur argues that "speculation on time is an inconclusive rumination to which narrative activity alone can respond," not by resolving these aporias theoretically but by making them productive—"put[ing them] to work—poetically—by producing" plots that transform the paradoxical disjunctions and connections of lived time into coherent figures of "discordance and concordance" (6, 22).

According to Ricoeur, this work of transforming temporal aporias into structures of discordant concordance is evident in each of the three parts of Aristotle's well-known definition of a plot as 1) an imitation of an action that 2) combines a beginning, middle, and an end into a unified whole, which then, in the case of tragedy, 3) induces pity and fear in the audience. "It is only in the plot that action has a contour" and "a magnitude," Ricoeur argues, as the immediacy of lived experience is shaped into dramatic form (39). Plots configure action by negotiating the competing claims of change and pattern in the tensions (for example) between the accidental and the necessary in decisions about what is probable (and not merely possible) or in the opposition between the expected and the unexpected in the resolution of a story's conflicts. Similarly, Ricoeur claims, "it is only in virtue of poetic composition that something counts as a beginning, middle, or end" (38). This structuration of succession into a logic of connection governed not by chance but by "conformity to the requirements of necessity or probability" (39) transforms the one thing after another of lived time into a differentiated order that endows some events with the status of beginnings that meaningfully project us forward toward other moments that relate backward to them as ends. Finally, whatever the much-disputed term "catharsis" may entail, the emotions of pity and fear it arouses also provoke opposed movements of relatedness and disconnection as we empathize with the travails of the characters only to undergo the repulsions of terror, in both cases experiencing the paradoxical doubleness of an identification of ourselves with who we are not. In each of these dimensions of emplotment, the disjunctions and connections between the horizonal moments of time passing make possible the formation of narrative configurations that synthesize the heterogeneous.

Narrative is a productive response to the aporias of time because stories reorganize what Ricoeur (1984b, 338) calls "the ordinary experience of time, borne by daily acting and suffering." Stories give intelligible form to the lived immediacy of our interactions with the world, embodied experiences that are already meaningful but that we may not fully comprehend. The work of narrative, according to Ricoeur (1980a, 151), is "the unceasing passage . . . from a prefigured world to a transfigured world through the mediation of a configured world"—a circuit of reciprocal, mutually transformative interactions that he calls "mimesis$_1$," "mimesis$_2$," and "mimesis$_3$" (see 1984a, 52–87). "Mimesis" is, Ricoeur acknowledges, a potentially misleading term for what he has in mind. "If we continue to translate mimesis by 'imitation,'" he explains, "we have to understand something completely contrary to a copy of some preexisting reality" or "some redoubling of presence" through representation because "artisans who work with words produce not things but quasi-things; they invent the as-if" (1984a, 45), "a kind of simulacre, . . . in the sense precisely that fiction is *fingere*, to feign and figure, or better configure" (1980a, 139; also see Iser 1993). The language of figuration, configuration, and refiguration is preferable to the terminology of imitation, representation, and copying not only because the latter terms are heavily freighted with referential associations but also because the term "figure" suggests the activity of constructing gestalts or patterns that is basic to embodied cognition at all levels—from neuronal assemblies to the interactions of brain, body, and world—and that is also integral to the process of telling and following stories.

Different processes of figuration cross and interact as stories transform experience into narrative patterns. Mimesis$_2$ is the configurative work of creating stories by fashioning incidents and events from life into plots, but it in turn draws on prefigurative patterns of experience (mimesis$_1$), the intentional activity of our nonreflective being-in-the world that includes the "implicit categorization of the practical field" by the "cultural stock" of inherited norms and prior narratives that the poet utilizes (1984a, 47). Because action itself is characterized by preinscribed "temporal structures that evoke narration," Ricoeur describes "life as an activity and a desire in search of a narrative" (1987, 434). But life is always also culturally and symbolically mediated, he notes, and "without myths that have been passed on, there would be nothing to transform poetically" (1984a, 47). This configuration of life into plots and stories is, however, not an end in itself but only a stage along the way: "Structuration is an oriented activity that is only completed in the spectator or the reader" (48) through the potentially transfigurative experience of comprehending the narrative (mimesis$_3$). The reception of the narrative can in turn bring about a reshaping of the audience's emotional, embodied, and culturally mediated sense of its world.

And so the circuit is completed, only to stand ready to begin again, as culturally shared and shaped patterns of being-in-the-world (mimesis$_1$) are taken up and refashioned by poets, writers, and storytellers of all kinds (mimesis$_2$) who offer refigured narratives to ever-new audiences that may play with and transform the configurations through which they experience the world (mimesis$_3$). It may be, as Ricoeur observes, that "stories are told and not lived" whereas "life is lived and not told" (1987, 425), but there is a circuit between living and telling that is mutually formative and potentially transformative, and that is because the work of figuration crosses and joins the three modalities of mimesis. Stories have the power to pattern and repattern our brains because the configurative activity of narration across the circuit of the three types of mimesis sets in motion and can shape and reshape fundamental processes of embodied cognition.

An analysis of the configurative powers of narrative and the embodied brain can clarify a number of conundrums in narrative theory. Focusing on the ability of stories to forge patterns of concordant discordance out of our heterogeneous temporal experience can dissipate at least some of the terminological fog by showing what matters experientially and cognitively in some notorious disputes. Consider, for example, E. M. Forster's (1927) well-known but highly problematic distinction between a story and a plot. These simple terms can seem hopelessly confusing until one understands their relation to the production of concordant discordance.[7] According to Forster's oft-quoted definition, "The king died and then the queen died" is a story because it recounts events in time, whereas "the king died and then the queen died of grief" is a plot because it supplies motivation and causality. Whether the report of the king's and queen's successive deaths is by itself a story is unclear, however. Anyone hearing of these events would want to know "why?" Is there a connection? Or are these deaths merely accidents, contingencies, random happenings? What is missing from the initial, question-begging account is the as-structure of figuration. The one thing after the other of temporal succession only becomes a story when the sequence of events is made meaningful and understandable by answering these questions, thereby configuring them into a pattern that makes the discordant concordant.

As Ricoeur (1980b, 171; original emphasis) compactly if somewhat cryptically explains: "A story is *made out of* events to the extent that plot *makes events into* a story." In other words, a story needs a plot in order to become a story because emplotment synthesizes the heterogeneous—building figurative consistency between elements that otherwise sit inertly side by side, awaiting connection and explanation. When plot transforms a mere sequence of events into a story, a narrative pattern makes concordant the juxtaposition of events (like these two deaths) that might otherwise seem random, accidental, and discordant—and this configurative connection is what the addition "of grief" supplies. Other explanations would produce different stories by arranging the events into different patterns—for example: "as the assassin turned his gun from the monarch to his bride" or "as the poison they had taken gradually did its lethal work." Each of these potential plots configures events into a different story by projecting a different mode of seeing-as.

Another related ambiguity that often troubles narrative theorists is whether the plot is an element of the telling or the told. The arrangement of events in the telling is typically regarded as belonging to the discourse, borrowing Seymour Chatman's well-known terminology, whereas the story consists of the events that are told. Similarly, narratologists sometimes employ the terms "fabula" and "sjužet," first introduced by the Russian formalists, to differentiate between "the order of events referred to by the narrative" and "the order of events presented in the narrative discourse" (Brooks 1984, 12). The problem with these distinctions, of course, is that we only know the story through the discourse, and the telling shapes the told. Is the explanation of the queen's grief part of the telling or the told, the *sjužet* or the *fabula*? Is it an interpretation added by the discourse or a key element of the story? A narrator's insertion of a psychological inference as he or she recounts what happened or a crucial connecting element between otherwise inexplicable events in what is told? As Peter Brooks observes, "the apparent priority of *fabula* to *sjužet* is . . . a mimetic illusion, in that the *fabula*—'what really happened'—is in fact a mental construction that the reader derives from the *sjužet*, which is all that he ever directly knows" (13).

It is easy to get lost in the terminological fog here. Once again, however, the key issue to keep in mind is how narratives perform the work of figuration. Because the arrangement of events in the discourse is itself a way of creating syntheses of the heterogeneous, the boundary between story and discourse is inherently blurry and unstable. Both entail configurative processes (modes of seeing-as) that can mix, mingle, and play off of each other. Discordant concordance is a characteristic not only of emplotment (how events in the story are configured into meaningful patterns) but also of the act of narration (how they are organized in the recounting, with different patterns of presentation distinguishing how various storytellers see the same events). The role of seeing-as in narration also explains why Gérard Genette's much-discussed distinction between mood ("who sees") and voice ("who speaks") is notoriously slippery. The narrator's voice is itself necessarily a way of seeing—a perspective on the events he or she narrates by shaping them into one configuration or another that *sees* them *as* a particular gestalt, a reciprocal arrangement of parts in a whole.[8]

The interplay of configurative processes between the telling and the told—between the shaping, perspectival activity of narration and the patterns of action organized by the plot—is open to infinite permutations that defy the taxonomist's best efforts to sort them into separate categories. The interactions between these patterns of configuration refuse to stay neatly in one narratological box or the other. Hardly unfortunate, however, this merging and mingling is productive because the interplay of configurative processes between telling and told makes possible unlimited narrative innovation. From Homer's *Odyssey* to Joyce's *Ulysses*, for example, the same configuration of events can be repatterned in ever-changing acts of narration. The boundary crossing that confuses narratological classification is evidence of how semantic creativity occurs by reshaping configurative patterns.

The configurative work of building cognitive patterns characterizes not only the telling and the told but also the relations between them, and that is another reason why the distinction between story and discourse is so hard to pin down. To follow a story, readers not only need to understand the events and appreciate the storyteller's artful ways of presenting them; they must also align the sometimes congruent but sometimes disjunctive, even occasionally bewildering relations between the story and the discourse. Think, for example, of the difference between the *Odyssey* and *Ulysses*, where Joyce's experiments with style provide an ironic commentary on the journeys of his heroes, experiments that sometimes, in their antic playfulness, seem to take on a life of their own—hence one Joyce critic's well-known description of the novel as an "odyssey of style" (Lawrence 1981). The fun or the frustration (depending on your point of view) of reading *Ulysses* is that these levels do not line up as straightforwardly as T. S. Eliot claims in his assertion that Joyce's "mythic method" holds in parallel Homer's story and the events of Bloomsday in Dublin. The challenge of making sense of these ironic, playful allusions that typically refuse to settle down belongs neither to the story

nor to the discourse but to how they interact and align (or don't quite fit together). If reading is an activity of consistency building, as Wolfgang Iser
(1978) argues, the work of constructing configurative patterns in our experience of stories occurs not only within but also between these interconnected
domains that narrative theory only artificially separates.

Configurations of discordant concordance characterize story, discourse,
and their interactions in our experiences of narratives. Complex patterns of
figuration may occur even in Genette's so-called zero-degree narratives
(1980, 35–36)—stories where the telling seems to be a transparent reflection
of the told and the events related are interesting primarily because of the connections between them and not because of the artfulness of the telling. Meir
Sternberg's (1987) description of narrative as a construct based on curiosity, suspense, and surprise holds even for such simple tales because these responses can be evoked by the story itself—the conjunctions and disjunctions
in the patterning of the told. Hence Aristotle's (1990 [355 BCE], 12–13)
well-known concern with reversals and recognition in the construction of
plots—changes of fortune like the fall of the tragic hero, for example, or
the revelation of unexpected facts or relationships—and his claim that "the
finest recognition is the one which occurs at the same time as the reversal,
like the one in *Oedipus [Rex]*" where the hero's demise is precipitated by his
discovery of his parentage. Moments of reversal and recognition are crucially
important in the construction of plots because of their role in disrupting and
re-establishing configurative patterns. Zero-degree narratives are still narratives to the extent that they are structures of concordant discordance and
play with the competing cognitive imperatives of pattern and change that
stories set in motion and manipulate.

Another reason why the boundary between story and discourse is blurry
is that the arrangement of events in the story is itself artful, even in the case
of the simplest tales. Even in stories where the telling seeks to disappear and
the discourse does not call attention to itself, Sternberg's curiosity, suspense,
and surprise may be enhanced or spoiled by different modes of emplotment.
This is why, after all, Aristotle thinks he can give useful advice about what
makes for a better or worse plot, more or less artfully patterned. There is an
art to making good plots, and there is an art to telling good stories, and it
is sometimes difficult to tell the difference between emplotment and narration because both entail acts of configuration.

Despite these ambiguities and complications, the distinction between
story and discourse is still useful. The line separating story and discourse can
be hard to draw because the configurative work of constructing patterns of
discordant concordance crosses back and forth across it, but it is sometimes

useful to ask what side of the line we're on. Sometimes our interest in a narrative has mostly to do with one side or the other—that is, with the relations between narrated events themselves or with how they are assembled in the process of narration. The elements in what is told may seem intrinsically interesting because their connections and disjunctions seem curious, anomalous, or surprising, or the artfulness of the telling may transform an otherwise unremarkable set of events into a narration that holds us in suspense or keeps our curiosity alive by the way information is offered, implied, or withheld. The same story can be recounted more or less well by different tellers who are trying not to embellish or digress.

The opposition between story and discourse can help to disclose different modes of configuration that can interact in a variety of ways. Even if the terms themselves refuse to settle down, the distinction they suggest can make visible various typical, recurring patterns of interaction. Once again, what matters is not the construction of a logically impregnable classificatory scheme but understanding how narratives undertake the cognitive work of figuration. The interactions between these aspects of narrative matter more than precisely delimiting and controlling their boundaries.

Consider, for example, what can happen when the discourse provides patterns of explanation that complement, assist, and support the configurative work of the story—as when Balzac's omniscient narrator in *Père Goriot* declares that "all is true!" and asks us to trust him as he explains "the laws of Paris" that Rastignac must master in order to achieve the social success he strives for; or as when George Eliot's sympathetic if nevertheless critical narrative voice in *Middlemarch* guides the reader's judgments about Dorothea Brooke's noble if lamentably misplaced commitments. When the configurative patterns in the telling and the told complement each other in these ways, the result can be (as with Balzac) to encourage the reader's immersion in a lifelike world by building coherent, consistent illusions or (as with Eliot) to reinforce the pedagogical lessons of the narrative as the teller's judgments draw out the moral implications of the told. Consonant configurative patterns between the telling and the told can enhance the illusion of being transported to another world or encourage us to learn certain practices of seeing-as.

The dissonances between the various modes of figuration set in motion by a narrative can also be productive even if (or sometimes especially when) it is difficult to determine whether to attribute them to the story or the discourse. For example, the interaction between different story lines in a multiple-plot novel like *Anna Karenina* can be artfully constructed so that its effects go beyond what can be traced back to either of the stories alone or to the discursive pronouncements of the narrator. The famous opening line of this novel ("All happy families are alike") is an authoritative declaration by what Isaiah Berlin memorably calls the voice of the "hedgehog" in Tolstoy, who knows simple, singular truths, but the interplay of the Anna plot and the Levin plot resists these reductions and produces a counterpoint of sympathies pointing in different, not always mutually compatible, directions that Tolstoy the "fox" seems to recognize cannot be easily reconciled. This novel would be much less interesting if the two plots were disentangled and published separately—the decline and fall of the adulteress in one volume and the moral triumph of the happily married man in the other. As the two plots interact and play off each other, the flaws and virtues of these two characters, the pressures on their lives, and the opportunities open to them can be differently configured by readers in ways that the novel's narrative structure sets in motion but cannot predict or completely control. Each story offers a perspective through which to view the other, and the interaction of seeing-as in this interplay of perspectives is not attributable to either story alone. Nor is it simply a product of the narrator's discourse. The interaction between the plots occurs in the figurative space of reading, where story and discourse meet and the reader attempts to align the patterns they offer.

The consonances or disjunctions between discourse and story can have a variety of effects by playing with the figurative workings of cognition. If congruent processes of figuration in the telling and the told can facilitate immersion or instruction, disjunctions between discourse and story can defamiliarize and foreground cognitive processes that may ordinarily go unnoticed in reading or in life because we are absorbed by our habitual ways of knowing. In *Lord Jim*, for example, Joseph Conrad juxtaposes Marlow's telling and the titular hero's tale in ways that call attention to the role of configurative patterns in cognition by blocking the narrator's (and the reader's) attempts to formulate them. The inconsistencies between the different perspectives Marlow receives on the enigmatic title character resist synthesis into a coherent point of view and consequently leave him frustrated and bewildered: "The views he let me have of himself were like those glimpses through the shifting rents in a thick fog—bits of vivid and vanishing detail, giving no connected idea of the general aspect of the country" (1996 [1900], 49).

Conrad's narrator presents Jim to the reader through fragmentary and disconnected perspectives—conflicting interpretations offered by multiple informants that refuse to coalesce, pieces of evidence with opposing implications that cannot be reconciled—and these disjunctions in the discourse prevent a single, coherent story from emerging. Is Jim a romantic hero or an egotistical coward? Is Marlow's sympathy for him a noble example of fellow feeling or an unconsciously motivated wish for the wrongdoer to escape punishment?[9] The refusal of these perspectives to synthesize foregrounds the drive to build consistency among elements in a pattern that is necessary for lucid comprehension. The incongruities between Marlow's fragmentary, disjointed discourse and Jim's elusive story produce an ambiguous text that resembles the classic rabbit-duck figure, oscillating between possible configurations, interrupting the building of an illusion in order to call attention to the processes of pattern formation it sets in motion but prevents from settling down. Once again, the value of the distinction between story and discourse has less to do with its ability to support a classificatory scheme than with its usefulness as a tool for analyzing the configurative workings of narrative.

The examples I have been discussing illustrate how this distinction relates to narrative configurations of action, but it is also relevant to temporality and intersubjectivity, the two other dimensions of narrative that are the topics of the following chapters. For example, the relation between discourse and story is often complicated by the anachronies (to use Genette's terminology) that disrupt the temporal correspondence between the telling and the told. If simple, zero-degree tales unfold seamlessly from beginning to end, artful telling can manipulate chronology to provoke curiosity, suspense, or surprise through temporal disjunctions that play further with the tension between concord and discord. Conrad's sometime collaborator Ford Madox Ford (1924, 136) complained that "what was the matter with the Novel, and with the British novel in particular, was that it went straight forward, whereas in your gradual making acquaintanceship with your fellows you never do go straight forward." By keeping a rough parallel between the chronology of presentation and the sequential order of events, however, the novels Ford criticizes assist the reader's efforts to discover and build patterns and thereby actually encourage the immersion in an illusion on which realism depends. Ford's point, however, is that this continuity disguises the processes it manipulates. In getting to know any state of affairs, we "never do go straight forward" inasmuch as we are always going back and forth between expectations about what lies beyond our horizons and corrections of previous guesses in light of evidence that has since come into view.

Temporal anachronies can serve many purposes, one of which is to foreground the temporal processes of consistency building that otherwise go unnoticed in the configurative work of storytelling or everyday cognition. In Ford's novel *The Good Soldier*, for example, the narrator John Dowell crisscrosses back and forth over his past as he tries to make sense of events and relationships that, as he is surprised to find, he had completely misconstrued, and the result is a bewildering narration that constantly jumps around in time, challenging the reader to piece together in an orderly way the shifting, disconnected, incomplete perspectives it offers: "I have, I am aware, told this story in a very rambling way so that it may be difficult for anyone to find their path through what may be a sort of maze. I cannot help it. . . . I console myself with thinking that this is a real story and that, after all, real stories are probably told best in the way a person telling a story would tell them. They will then seem most real" (1990 [1915], 213). As with many other things, Dowell is probably not right about this. The notorious time-shifts in *The Good Soldier* may actually thwart the consistency building necessary to create illusions that can "seem real" because their coherence encourages our suspension of disbelief—but the gain from these disruptions is the opportunity they afford to reflect about temporal processes of cognition that are invisible when they function smoothly. By making the bewildered reader work harder and more reflectively than with continuous narration to build coherent story patterns out of the scattered bits and pieces in Dowell's discourse, Ford transforms anticipation and retrospection from implicit cognitive processes into explicit issues in the experience of reading. Where consonance between the temporalities of story and discourse can facilitate mimetic immersion, disruptions to the temporal work of pattern formation can expose how configuration works.

Different degrees of consonance and dissonance between discourse and story can similarly be deployed to play games with the intersubjectivity of stories. According to Henry James (1970b [1883], 237–38), reading a narrative "makes it appear to us for the time that we have lived another life— that we have had a miraculous enlargement of experience." Narratives whose consonances encourage immersion in an illusion can promote such identifications of self and other. The experience of following a story does not collapse the differences between selves, however, but entails a doubling of my consciousness with the intentionality held ready by the narrative, thereby enacting the paradoxical combination of community and solipsism that characterizes intersubjectivity. Such an identification is a paradoxical experience in which I configure another world as if it were my own—which, of course, it is not, so that a sense of the foreignness of the cognitive patterns I am temporarily inhabiting invariably shadows my immersion in them, even when I feel them in my own body in the fears and tears and other impassioned responses the story may set in motion. The pity or fear I may feel for the tragic hero is an identification with a quasi person who is not identical to me, after all, and is (strangely) not even a real human being, although I may intensely care about what happens to her (and may shed actual tears about her misfortunes).

Playing off the odd if everyday sensation that other worlds are both complementary and inaccessible to our own, various kinds of congruences and dissonances in the ways narratives stage these configurations may seek either to disguise or to foreground the doubleness of my world with another that occurs when I identify with lives that are not mine. James's own famous experiments with point of view are marked by a peculiar doubleness that exploits this ability of narratives to transport us outside of ourselves even as he calls for reflection about the epistemological limits it oversteps. By projecting the reader into the world of the character whose perspective he re-creates (Strether's bewildered fascination with the Parisian Babylon, for example, as he begins his ambassadorial mission), James gives us a rare view of another life from the inside, experienced by another for him- or herself. But in projecting ourselves into this other life, we experience as well the gap between its perspective and other points of view that remain obscure and mysterious to varying degrees (we never know but can imagine what Mrs. Newsome thinks back in Woollett, Massachusetts, about the no doubt alarming letters Strether sends home). This double movement of transcending and reencountering the gap between selves dramatizes in the reader's own experience the combination of relatedness and opacity that makes the alter ego paradoxical.

Narratives double self and other by configuring and reconfiguring the relations between worlds in to-and-fro interactions between storytellers and their recipients. This can be done variously by first- and third-person narrations and by different kinds of focalization (the narratological term for point of view) or narrative voice (narrators with different attitudes or degrees of authority). The person of the narrator or the particular technical device that sets this doubling in motion matters little in itself. The same linguistic or narratological structure can be deployed for a variety of purposes. What counts is how the exchanges between storyteller, story, and recipient put into play various interactions between worlds, and these are dynamic, back-and-forth processes of configuration and refiguration that cannot be adequately accounted for by constructing a static classificatory scheme or by mapping narrative techniques onto a taxonomic grid. Naming a technique or a structure is only the first step in analyzing the configurative processes of pattern formation and disruption it sets in motion in any particular narrative and in describing the cognitive purposes these interactions serve.

Lived Worlds and Narrative Worldmaking

The term "world" is often employed in narrative theory to describe these interactions, but it is a slippery notion that deserves some analysis. For theorists in the traditions of phenomenology and pragmatism, the term refers to the configurations of meaning-making activity that characterize experience— what Merleau-Ponty calls the unreflective, "operative intentionality" that we find already at work when we reflect on our lives and discover various patterns of relationship that give shape to our typical, habitual interactions with people, places, and things (see 2012 [1945], lxxxii). As Shaun Gallagher explains, this "intentionality" (a key term in the lexicon of phenomenology) has an as-structure: "All consciousness is consciousness of something *as* something" (2012, 67; original emphasis). According to Gallagher, "Actions have intentionality because they are directed at some goal or project, and this is something that we can see in the actions of others"—hence our tendency "to attribute intentionality to geometrical figures moving in certain patterns on a computer screen . . . as well as to non-human animals and human infants whom we do not regard as following specific social norms" (77, 75).

Recognizing a world entails understanding and interpreting patterns of intentionality—as-structures that configure states of affairs in a meaningful way in our own experience or in the experiences we construe others as having, analogous to our own. As Ricoeur (1984a, 61) explains in tracing the notion of world back to Heidegger's *Being and Time,* "The structure of being-in-the-world . . . is more fundamental than any relation of a subject to an object." Against Cartesian dualism, subject and object are not separate but are always already joined in patterns of configuration that make up our lived worlds. The hyphens joining "being-in-the-world" are the patterns of intentionality set in motion as we project ourselves into futures of possibility based on the circumstances in which we find ourselves situated (hence Heidegger's description of existence as a "thrown projection," or "geworfener Entwurf" [see 1962 (1927), 185]).

Narratives bring worlds into relationship as patterns of configurative activity cross back and forth in the circuit joining lived experience, the construction of stories, and their reception by listeners and readers, Ricoeur's three-fold mimesis. As Ricoeur (1987, 430–31) explains, "The intersection of the world of [the] text and the world of the reader . . . opens up a horizon of possible experience, a world in which it would be possible to dwell." The process of telling and following stories sets in motion interactions between the patterns of configuration that characterize these different worlds.

Although the term "world" may seem slippery as it passes from one domain to another, this boundary crossing is a necessary and by no means lamentable consequence of the openness of stories to experience. As Ricoeur (1984b, 349) points out, "A text, actually, is not a self-enclosed entity. It has not only a formal structure; it points beyond itself to a possible world, a world I could inhabit, where I could actualize my own possibilities in so far as I am in the world." The recurrence of the term "world" in these different contexts is an indication of the openness of stories to the experiences they reconfigure and to the existential possibilities of their recipients. Pragmatically oriented psychologist Jerome Bruner (1986, 66) similarly invokes this term to characterize stories not as logical, formal structures but as aspects of our lived experience—projections of "possible worlds in which action, thought, and self-definition are possible (or desirable)." What matters for theorists like Ricoeur and Bruner in the phenomenological and pragmatic traditions is how the patternmaking powers of stories contribute to what Nelson Goodman (1978) memorably calls our "ways of worldmaking," a concept also adopted by phenomenological reading theorist Wolfgang Iser in his "literary anthropology" (1993, 152–70).

It is a mistake to reify worldmaking, however, by reducing it to formal, schematic models of the sort sometimes proposed by cognitive narratologists to map the structures of "story worlds" or to classify the logical markers that differentiate "actual" and "possible worlds." The interactions between worlds as we tell and follow stories cannot be reduced to grids and schemes. For example, the good thing about David Herman's (2013, x–xi) somewhat awkward, confusing description of "narrative worldmaking" as "worlding the story" and "storying the world" is its recognition that the configurative work of narrative is a dynamic process. But the taxonomic drive to construct classificatory schemes to account for these processes is problematic. Herman's much-discussed book *Storytelling and the Sciences of the Mind* (2013) is filled with one classificatory scheme, diagram, and taxonomy after the other and proliferates terms, categories, and distinctions in an almost manic attempt to reduce to an orderly system the dynamism of worldmaking. This elaborate edifice of maps, grids, and definitions misrepresents the configurative activity through which worlds are projected and interact in narratives and lived experience and fails to capture the processes it attempts to reduce to static schemes.

The fundamental problem with this approach is evident in two of Herman's central claims (2013, 56) about narrative worldmaking—namely, that "interpreters map textual patterns onto WHO, WHAT, WHERE, WHEN, HOW, and WHY dimensions of storyworlds" and that "the patterns in question emanate from reasons for (text-producing) actions" that can be systematically categorized. A static map of positions on a grid charting the answers to these questions cannot do justice to the configurative processes of meaning making through which worlds are experienced and exchanged. Herman's interrogatory map is reminiscent of the stock questions that newspaper reporters are instructed to ask as they gather material for their stories, but any journalist knows that the answers they jot down in their notebooks are *not* the story but only the bits and pieces out of which it must still be put together when they return to the newsroom. What is missing from Herman's map are the configurative processes of pattern formation that connect the dots and fill in the blanks. As I read *The Ambassadors*, for example, I can chart on a grid the answers to all of these questions about Strether's mission to retrieve Chad from Paris, but I will still miss the patterns of longing, regret, and desire that animate his impassioned plea to Little Bilham in Gloriani's garden to "live all you can! It's a mistake not to." The patterns of intentionality that animate a world resist reduction to a classificatory scheme and cannot be explained by positions on a map.

A similar problem afflicts Mark Turner's (1996) diagrams of what he calls "conceptual blending," none of which can do justice to the interaction between a word and a context through which metaphorical innovation occurs. This interaction is characterized by what Nietzsche (2015 [1873]) describes as "das Gleichsetzen des Nicht-gleichen," the "setting equal" of what is "not the same." As Ricoeur (1977, 252, 197; also see 21–22, 170–71) explains, a novel metaphor is "a calculated error," "comparable to what Gilbert Ryle (2009 [1949], lx) calls [a] 'category mistake,' which consists in 'the presentation of facts belonging to one category in the idioms appropriate to another.'" According to Ricoeur, a novel metaphor is surprising and perhaps initially confusing because it "speak[s] of one thing in terms of another" (197) that is both like and not like it, in an act of comparison that transgresses the patterns of configuration to which we are accustomed. This incongruity—"a planned category mistake" (197)—is not simply dismissed as an error, however, but instead produces new meaning because of the interpreter's adjustments through which its initial incoherences are made consistent. After they are reconfigured into new patterns of similarity and difference, these incoherences may come to seem "right" in unanticipated ways. A novel metaphor can then become dead when its incongruities are so assimilated and conventionalized that they are no longer noticed. Only then is it a "blend"— but at this point its meanings are literal, not metaphorical, because the interactions set off by the incongruities between like and not like have ended and its suggestive powers have faded and died.

Turner proposes elaborate schemes to classify these interactions and develops complex spatial diagrams to map their components (also see Fauconnier and Turner 2002). These structures necessarily miss the interaction—the category mistake and the readjustments it provokes—that constitutes the metaphorical innovation. Instead of capturing the configurative activity that creates new meaning, his taxonomies reduce the processes of disruption and reorganization to a series of charts and distinctions. The mistake here, analogous to the problem with Herman's maps, is that classifying kinds of "blends" according to their structures misses the interactions through which the surprising combination of like and not like provokes new modes of consistency building. By the same token, Turner's much-used term "blending" does not convey just how necessary incongruity and discordance are to the production of new congruence. The maps, grids, and schemes that Herman and other structurally oriented narratologists use to characterize the concordant discordance of narrative are similarly destined to miss the processes of figuration, configuration, and refiguration that they reduce to static taxonomies.[10]

Herman tellingly employs a static, structural metaphor to describe worldmaking: "The process of building storyworlds . . . *scaffolds* a variety of sense-making activities" (x; emphasis added). This is a concept sometimes invoked by 4e theorists (for example, see Clark 2011, 44–60), and it is a term to which Herman repeatedly returns. To speak of the process of building storyworlds as "scaffolding" is awkward and confusing, however. A scaffold is a structure that assists in the activity of constructing the building. It does not capture the essential work of making it, and it is then discarded when the building is finished and made available to be used and inhabited, opening the way for further unpredictable, open-ended interactions with other members of our species who pass in and through its structures and repurpose them for goals, relationships, and projects that the builders may not have had in mind. The metaphor of a scaffold misrepresents the work through which narrative worlds are built and the uses to which they can be put by reducing a dynamic process to a schematic structure. This confusing locution prioritizes structures over the events of meaning that the process of employing them makes possible.

The metaphor of a scaffold may appeal to a structurally minded imagination, but its awkwardness and blindnesses are evidence of its reification of the processes through which worlds are made, remade, and interact as we live our lives and tell and follow stories. The configurative activities involved in the construction and interaction of narrative worlds are not reducible to a map of locations, a logic of reasons, or a scaffold of structures. Metaphors like these are traces of the ghost of structuralism that haunts formalist cognitive narratology. To avoid reifying the intentional activity that constitutes lived and narrated worlds, it is necessary to keep focused on the processes of pattern formation that the metaphor of world entails, figurative processes foregrounded in the phenomenological and pragmatic traditions.[11]

This schematic approach is a legacy of the first-generation prioritization of frames and structures. By contrast, various forms of second-generation narratology focus on the actions and interactions through which stories shape the patterns of our worlds. For example, Terence Cave (2016, 4, 5) describes "thinking with literature" as a collaborative process of inquiry, improvisation, and conversation that "conscript[s] our capacity for cognitive inference" and may "alter the cognitive environment of the reader in ways that are powerful, potentially disturbing, and not at all self-evident." Cave's model of reading, based on relevance theory (see Sperber and Wilson 1995 [1986]), emphasizes the "bold and highly precise modes of underspecification" (27) of literature—what a phenomenological theorist like Iser or Ingarden calls the blanks or indeterminacies that require improvisatory responses beyond what can be captured by mapping dimensions of a storyworld onto a spatial grid. For Cave, "thinking with literature" is a cocreative response to a literary work "not as [a] neutral text but as an animated affordance" (9) that encourages and makes possible but does not fully determine our interpretations. According to Cave, "What happens when we redescribe literary conventions as affordances," borrowing Gibson's (1979) well-known term, is that "what was static and merely constraining" turns out to open up "all kinds of unexpected possibilities, ways of breaking out into new territory" (55–56).

Affordance is a better metaphor than scaffolding to describe the actions and interactions in the environments that various tools and resources may be used to build, a process Andy Clark (2011, 61–68) describes as "niche construction." Building a niche creates an environment that in turn affords a variety of uses. Similarly, the storyworld that is configured by employing various techniques, conventions, and other narrative resources (the scaffold) then affords an open-ended, unpredictable history of responses by recipients who engage in activities of meaning making that it makes possible (also see the analysis of narrative affordances in chapter 3). Mapping a world as points on a grid misses this dynamism—what Cave (77, 33) calls "the human ability to think beyond the immediate demands of [our] environment" that a text invokes through its "implicatures," the various "intended meanings that can be derived inferentially from a given utterance."

Other cognitively oriented second-generation theorists similarly focus on these kinds of interaction between modes of figuration. For example, drawing on phenomenological and pragmatic theories of text-reader interaction, Marco Caracciolo's "enactivist approach" (2014, 4) emphasizes "how meaning emerges from the experiential interaction between texts and readers"— "stories offer themselves as imaginative experiences because of the way they draw on and restructure readers' familiarity with experience itself"—a to-and-fro, temporally unfolding, dynamic relationship between the world of the reader and the world of the text in a mutually formative experiential transaction. Describing narrative as "a purposeful communicative exchange between authors and readers," Phelan (2015, 121) offers a "rhetorical theory" that similarly foregrounds processes of interaction. Phelan's "rhetorical poetics of narrative" is rightly regarded as a kind of cognitive narratology (hence his inclusion in Zunshine's 2015 anthology) because of his attention to the ways audiences take up and respond to the communicative acts of the author. Carrying on and transforming the tradition of his teachers at the University of Chicago from before the days of cognitive literary criticism, Phelan develops a theory of rhetoric as a purposeful communicative exchange that deserves "second-generation" status because it foregrounds the configurative, mutually formative processes of the text-reader interaction. His definition (2017, ix) of narrative as "somebody telling somebody else on some occasion and for some purposes that something happened" traverses Ricoeur's circuit of figuration between experience, story, and recipient.[12]

The error of reifying configurative processes also undermines the formalist project of reducing narrative actions to a logic of "reasons" from which they "emanate." According to Herman (2010, 169–70), "readers are able to understand the characters' *behaviors* as *actions* in part because of the models of emotions on which they rely to interpret the text"—what he calls an "emotionology," defined as "the collective emotional standards of a culture as opposed to the experience of emotion itself": "An emotionology specifies that when an event X inducing an emotion Y occurs, an agent is likely to engage in Z sorts of actions." Once again adopting a model based on scripts, frames, and preference rules, Herman contends that "the characters' activities can be construed as more than just a series of individual, unrelated doings because of the assumption, licensed by a model of emotions, that those behaviors constitute a coherent *class*" (170; original emphasis).

There are several things wrong with this taxonomic, rule-based approach to character, action, and emotion. To begin with, as I have explained, the best contemporary neuroscience of emotions (see Barrett 2017) suggests that anger or embarrassment should be viewed not as a coherent, homologous "class" but rather as a "population" of related, overlapping, but diverse subjective states. Further, the research on the relation between real and imagined action suggests that our responses to the action staged in a text are less like the linear, logical application of a rule from a class than the sort of bodily based resonances that Guillemette Bolens (2012) describes in her kinematic theory of narrative. The intuitive, embodied resonances that emerge and unfold over our engagement with a text cannot be adequately described by a logic of models and rules. Bodily responses to the intentionality of the text are as-relations that have the power to reconfigure our sense of the world because they are not simply applications of schemata we already know. They are, rather, dynamic and unpredictable enactments of the paradox of the alter ego, the doubling of the "real me" of my kinematic sensations that I experience while reading and the "alien me" of the world I set in motion as I empathize and identify with the actions of the text.

A scheme outlining an underlying logic of actions cannot do justice to the processes through which these configurations of embodied intentionality emerge, develop, and change across the horizons joining past, present, and future in to-and-fro, reciprocal interactions. To recall James's novel *The Ambassadors*, Strether's adventure in Europe surprises him not just because his new friends are not completely honest with him but, even more, because the values and possibilities revealed to him in this new world bring out feelings he had not anticipated and is uncertain how to act on. His past sets the stage for these reactions—his regret for his "unlived life," as it is called in the James criticism—but it does not determine how he will respond to them. Furthermore, as readers of *The Ambassadors* find their worlds interacting with Strether's, no map or chart can predict whether the consonances between them will make them identify and sympathize with this poor sensitive gentleman (as I do!) or whether instead the dissonances between his reactions and theirs will lead them to fault his hesitancies, refusals, and acts of resignation (and perhaps then also blame the author for these, as many hostile critics have done).

What matters is not only where actions come from but where they are headed—not just their sources but their goals and directions—and it is the variable, often unpredictable interaction between these that make actions dynamic. For example, as Elaine Auyoung (2013, 60) observes, narrated actions can seem lifelike because their gaps and indeterminacies draw on "our readiness to contend with partial representational cues in everyday, nonliterary experience." With the actions represented in stories as in those we encounter in everyday life, she notes, we fill out what lies beyond our limited perspective by our expectations about their future course and direction. Similarly, as Karin Kukkonen (2016) points out, the various kinds of action set in motion by a text—not only the characters' behaviors (the action of the plot) but also our responses to stylistic cues (the action of the narration)—are less like the unilinear application of preference rules than affordances that make possible but do not fully prescribe our responses, guiding our actions but leaving open room for improvisation, innovation, and surprise. Drawing on a Bayesian, predictive-processing model of embodied cognition, Kukkonen explains that the narrative environment makes some actions probable and others less so, thereby motivating not only the development of the plot but also our expectations about the course of the narration in a dynamic, interactive process of feedback loops that cascade into each other, reinforcing or disrupting the patternmaking work set in motion by different kinds of narrative figuration. The eventfulness of worldmaking and the unpredictability of the interaction of worlds in the experience of narrative that these second-generation theorists are attempting to describe are essential to how storyworlds work, and these are necessarily lost in spatial maps and classificatory schemes.

A reifying, reductionist formalism sometimes similarly afflicts narrative theories of actual versus possible worlds. For example, in Marie-Laure Ryan's analysis of fictional worlds and virtual reality there is an interesting and revealing contradiction between her attempt to do justice to the dynamic processes of "immersion and interactivity" and her resort to logical frameworks to categorize the ontological differences between worlds. On the one hand, she recognizes that the effects of immersion in the simulations of virtual reality depend on their "dynamic character"—how, for example, "it takes . . . a movable point of view to acquire a full sense of the depth of an image" (2001, 53)—and she consequently invokes Merleau-Ponty's description of how "embodied consciousness" entails "both mobility and virtuality" (71) to explain how the as-if configurations of fictional worlds can acquire the illusion of plenitude. "When my actual body cannot walk around an object or grab and lift it," she explains, "it is the knowledge that my virtual body could do so that gives me a sense of its shape, volume, and materiality. Whether actual or virtual, objects are thus present to me because my actual or virtual body can interact with them" (71). This is sound phenomenological analysis of the dynamic processes and interactions through which configurative patterns emerge.

On the other hand, however, Ryan also attempts to develop "an ontological model" that schematizes "in semantic and logical terms" (99) the differences between actual and possible worlds. This model, she explains, is based on "the set-theoretical idea that reality—the sum total of the imaginable—is a universe composed of a plurality of distinct elements, or worlds, and that it is hierarchically structured by the opposition of one well-designated element, which functions as the center of the system, to all the other members of the set" (99). Here the phenomenologist is displaced by the structuralist, and an analysis of figurative interactions gives way to a quest for a well-ordered taxonomy. And so her important book *Narrative as Virtual Reality* alternates between compelling descriptions of how immersion in virtual worlds draws on configurative patterns of embodied cognition familiar from everyday experience and overly simplistic charts and schemes that reduce these processes to formal structures based on various ontological distinctions. Rather than sharpening and clarifying fictional worldmaking, as she hopes, the formal and schematic categories of the logicians obscure the phenomenological experience of immersion and interactivity by reducing it to an abstract set of hierarchically ordered structures that necessarily miss the interactions and the configurative processes of pattern formation through which worlds are constructed.

Narratology needs to break with its structuralist legacy and embrace the paradigm shift proposed by the various pragmatically oriented, phenomenological theories of narrative that have contested the formalist program. If we want to understand stories, logical structures and taxonomies won't do the job. What we need to know, rather, as the second-generation theorists recognize, is how elements combine into patterns through their interactions in lived experience and embodied cognition. How narratives participate in the formation and dissolution of patterns in the embodied brain's interactions with the world is the right question to ask if what we have is not a logically ordered, formally structured mind but a bushy brain that is an ensemble of relationships that get fixed over time but are open to a future of variation. Those interactions are the means by which stories help the brain negotiate the tension between pattern and flexibility thanks to the play of their concordant discordances. The terms in the lexicon of narrative theory are useful insofar as they help to elucidate these interactions, but concepts and locutions that obscure or misrepresent them should be discarded. The to-and-fro processes of figuration and refiguration through which we tell and follow stories is the dynamic, ever-shifting ground on which neuroscience, narrative, and narratology meet.

Natural and Unnatural Narratives

A neuroscientifically grounded account of the relation between stories, language, and the brain can clarify what's at issue in the debate about "natural" versus "unnatural" narratives. This dispute arose when advocates of cognitive narratology called attention to the so-called natural aspects of the production and comprehension of stories. The question, of course, is what counts as natural, and the science on these matters is not irrelevant. Proposing a theory of natural narratology, Monika Fludernik (1996, 12–52) argues that narrative is based on its ability to render what she calls "experientiality" through modes of exchange that reflect the "natural schemata" of embodied cognition and the "natural parameters" of language in conversational storytelling. In her model, "the term *'natural'* is not applied to texts or textual techniques," she explains, "but exclusively to the *cognitive frames* by means of which texts are interpreted" (12; original emphasis). Frames, scripts, or schemas are natural, she argues, because they are "aspects of language which appear to be regulated or motivated by cognitive parameters based on man's experience of embodiedness in a real-world context" (17), and what she calls "narrativity" is a natural process that "emerge[s] from spontaneous conversational story-telling" and "naturalizes" unfamiliar experience "by the sheer act of imposing narrativity on it" (15, 34).

This is partly wrong and partly right. As I have explained, frames and scripts are not natural features of embodied cognition. They are, rather, artifacts of an artificial intelligence model that do not match up well with the anatomy and functions of the brain except insofar as they are metaphors for the activity of seeing-as. The problem with these terms, as I have argued, is that they reify figurative activity into substantive modules and unilinear mechanisms that misrepresent the to-and-fro processes through which patterns are formed, broken, and remade in lived experience and in the neurobiology of mental functioning. The other part of Fludernik's theory has merit, however. Her emphasis on the transactional exchanges of conversational storytelling is a useful call to structurally minded narratologists to focus on the interaction between worlds that occurs in the circuit of exchanges of experience as we tell and follow stories. Although the coinages "experientiality" and "narrativity" are somewhat awkward and opaque (the terminological beast rises again), their pragmatic value is that they foreground the circuit between the configurative processes of lived experience and their refiguration in the concordant discordances of narrative that Ricoeur describes.[13]

These processes are both natural and unnatural, however, in different ways and varying degrees. The stories we tell each other are biocultural hybrids that mix together, sometimes indistinguishably, what is natural about embodied cognition and what is artificial, cultural, and learned. For example, a recent anthropological study of residents of a geographically isolated area of Turkey who had little experience with film or television found that they were baffled by some but not all film-editing techniques. Neuroscientist Arthur P. Shimamura (2013b, 19) concludes that "these findings demonstrated that our understanding of the 'syntax' of movies is to some extent a learned phenomenon." But they also suggest the opposite conclusion, namely that narrative understanding is to some extent natural.

Stephan Schwan and Sermin Ildirar (2010, 974–75), the authors of this study, reported that subjects with little or no experience watching films were able to come up with the "standard interpretation" of a film clip exhibiting a series of typical film-editing techniques only 36–41% of the time, whereas 90% of experienced viewers were able to do so. The details behind these percentages are interesting and important: "The inexperienced viewers did describe the individual shots appropriately, but they had difficulties in relating the shots to each other," and they had particular difficulty with "clips portraying a situation or an event from the visual perspective of a certain actor. . . . Thus, the notion that so-called point-of-view shots resemble natural perception to the highest degree and therefore should be easiest to understand . . . was not confirmed by our data" (975). One of their key findings, however, was that "films containing a familiar activity led to a significantly higher percentage of standard interpretations": "The presence of a familiar line of action is essential for the interpretation processes of inexperienced viewers; a line of action helps them overcome unfamiliar perceptual discontinuities" (975). Summarizing, they conclude that "it is not the similarity to the conditions of natural perception," such as point-of-view editing techniques, "but the presence of a familiar line of action that determines the comprehensibility of films for inexperienced viewers" (970).

These findings are consistent with the well-established phenomenon that modernist recreations of a character's consciousness or point of view, as in the novels of James Joyce, William Faulkner, or Virginia Woolf, although perhaps closer to "natural perception" in their methods of representation, are typically harder for most readers to understand than conventional, plot-driven dramatizations that may lack epistemological verisimilitude but that facilitate the reader's ability to follow the line of action. *Mrs. Dalloway* and *To the Lighthouse* may be more natural than *David Copperfield* or *Jane Eyre* because Woolf's stylistic experiments seek to recreate the to-and-fro of embodied cognitive processes, but readers of Dickens and Brontë typically find that the plots of these novels promote immersion in a lifelike world (and seem "natural") because they support the construction of patterns of concordant discordance. Perhaps paradoxically, techniques not only in film but also in fiction that mirror the cognitive workings of perception can seem by contrast unnatural and bewildering.

The Turkish villagers, like many readers of Faulkner and Woolf, may find it difficult to understand a narrative depicted through the point of view of a perceiver because they have not learned this convention, and it consequently may seem unnatural even though it reenacts "natural perception." This is not surprising inasmuch as techniques in films and novels that foreground how experience is perceived may interfere with emplotment by call-ing attention to how a pattern is made rather than facilitating the work of fitting things together. As Schwan and Ildirar's study suggests, however, such viewers and readers are nevertheless able to make some sense of a confus-ing state of affairs if they can follow "a familiar activity" and track "a famil-iar line of action." This, apparently, is what is natural—the ability to follow sequences of events when they are arranged in patterns of action that are recognizable from the perceiver's past experience. Emplotment, the ability to configure actions in a narrative sequence, is a natural cognitive capability that can be put to use even when the conventions of editing and narrating are unfamiliar, which explains why the Turkish villagers were still able to make sense of bewildering films more than a third of the time. Similarly, readers unacquainted with modernist techniques can still often follow the events of Clarissa Dalloway's day as she walks through London, buys flow-ers, mends her dress, and otherwise prepares for her party.

Familiarity also matters. Even when the mode of rendering seems odd or strange, finding ways of grafting the unfamiliar onto the familiar can make it comprehensible. It is a well-established neuroscientific fact that Hebbian firing and wiring can habitualize and automatize perception. Patterns may seem natural, then, either because they can be emplotted in easily recogniz-able action sequences or because their recurrence in everyday experience has made them familiar, engraining their configurations through repetition in the cognitive habits of our brains and bodies so that they become invisible. Both of these cognitive phenomena—how action sequences facilitate emplotment and how familiarity promotes comprehension—help to explain how, in Flud-ernik's terms, narrativity has the power to naturalize a state of affairs.[14]

Conventions that promote the cognitive work of constructing patterns in these ways can seem natural, then, even when they are artificial. This con-clusion is also supported by a recent eye-tracking study that Tim Smith and colleagues (2012, 107–8) conducted on "the Hollywood style of moviemak-ing," an artificial set of techniques characterized by "focused continuity" between scenes and "consistency in cues." Comparing the movement of sac-cades (rapid, jerky jumps in the eye's point of focus) in natural perception and in viewing films, this study showed that Hollywood editors have evolved editing techniques that work—that is, promote understanding and the for-mation of illusions—because their "formal conventions . . . are compatible with the natural dynamics of attention and humans' assumptions about con-tinuity of space, time, and action" (107). Observing striking parallels be-tween saccadic eye movements in ordinary seeing and in watching Holly-wood films, Smith's group concluded that, "by piggybacking on natural vision cognition, Hollywood style presents a highly artificial sequence of viewpoints in a way that is easy to comprehend, does not require specific cognitive skills, and may even be understood by viewers who have never watched film before" (108). Hollywood movies are unnatural in the sense that they are based on a stylized, artificial set of conventions, but artifices that can be naturalized as they become familiar and habitual, and this process of naturalization is all the easier when, as here, these conventions take advantage of natural ways in which the eyes move and the visual cortex constructs a scene.

The call for a "natural narratology" almost predictably produced arguments in favor of "unnatural narratives." These sorts of stories are only comprehensible, however, to the extent that their unnatural experiments have a natural foundation in biologically based cognitive processes and familiar cultural conventions. According to the editors of a recent collection of essays on the poetics of unnatural narrative (Alber, Nielsen, and Richardson 2013, 1), "unnatural narrative theorists oppose what one might call 'mimetic reductionism,' that is, the claim that the basic aspects of narrative can be explained primarily or exclusively by models based on realist parameters" (also see Richardson 2015, 3–27). As Jan Alber (2009, 79) argues, narratives "do not only mimetically reproduce the world as we know it. Many narratives confront us with bizarre story-worlds which are governed by principles that have very little to do with the real world around us." There are cognitively based limits to how far this can go, however. Experimental modern and postmodern narratives may test the extent to which dissonance can disturb the configurative activity of emplotment without lapsing into nonsense and noise, but discord without some degree of concordance is incomprehensible. Like "natural" stories, "unnatural" narratives also set into motion and play with the brain's need for patterns to make sense of the world. Their manipulation of our natural quest for cognitive coherence is how they achieve their unnatural, antimimetic effects.

One of the most unnatural narratives ever written is James Joyce's *Finnegans Wake,* but even its bizarre experiments with language and narration are only comprehensible—or enjoyable (and they are both to some readers, but not of course to all)—to the extent that readers can configure them into patterns that relate the text's many enigmas to familiar contexts and constructs and that shape its events into recognizable structures of action. The text's repeated portmanteau words, for example, are riddles that challenge the reader to decipher the components they condense by discovering and testing various possible configurations that make sense of their Jabberwocky-like non-sense (even the seemingly innocent word "Finnegan" can then be seen as a Vicoian pun on cycles that "end," from the French "fin," only to begin again, while the middle phoneme recalls the "egg" Humpty Dumpty that fell and couldn't be put back together: Finnegan=*fin*-again + egg-again).[15] The characters (such as they are) of Humphrey Chimpden Earwicker (HCE) and his family may not be lifelike personages, but they relate to one another and to other entities in the text in various configurations of action that call on readers to invoke natural patterns of affection and conflict, rising and falling, and other cycles of transformation that play with our configurative powers. From its title onward, which alludes to a well-known song about a hod carrier who is knocked out only to revive when splattered by whiskey at his own funeral party, this strange text invokes familiar stories of all kinds, from "This is the House that Jack Built" to "The Ant and the Grasshopper," encouraging readers to search out configurative patterns. Similarly, the famous "Anna Livia Plurabelle" chapter from which Joyce recorded an extended passage is a natural narrative inasmuch as it enacts an extended gossip session between washerwomen on the model of Fludernik's conversational storytelling, even as its encyclopedic allusions to the rivers of the world are an elaborate, artificial linguistic game.

Natural and unnatural narratives depend on and play off of each other, and this is not only a recent phenomenon that characterizes modernism and postmodernism. It is not accidental, for example, that the rise of the novel in the eighteenth century saw the production of mimetically realistic works like *Moll Flanders*, *Clarissa*, and *Tom Jones* and also the irreverent *Tristram Shandy*, which pokes fun at the unnaturalness of many of the conventions of realism, such as the pretense of Samuel Richardson's epistolary style to "write to the moment" and render events as they happened (Tristram lamenting that his very attempt to describe moment to moment the misfortunes and accidents marring his birth takes so long that he has fallen behind even before his narrative gets under way).

In their classic *The Nature of Narrative*, Scholes and Kellogg (2006 [1966], 4) argue that "for writing to be narrative no more and no less than a teller and a tale are required" (4). This fundamental opposition is basic to narrative because the difference between teller and tale offers all sorts of possibilities for configuring discordance into patterns of concordance not only in the story but also in the discourse and, even more, in the back and forth between them. This opposition makes possible what Scholes and Kellogg call the "disparity among viewpoints" that is fundamental to "narrative irony" (240) in its many different forms. The discordances of irony that call on the reader to synthesize their juxtapositions into patterns of concordance can be as gentle and subtle as the decorous humor of Jane Austen in the famous opening of *Pride and Prejudice* ("It is a truth universally acknowledged that a single man in possession of a good fortune must be in want of a wife"), or they can be as kaleidoscopic as the multiple styles of *Ulysses* and or as unruly as the linguistic play of the word games of *Finnegans Wake*. Narrative irony is an unnatural, artificial state of affairs that can be played with and manipulated in any number of ways. But the natural basis of its many permutations is the ability of narrative to configure concordant discordance in syntheses of the heterogeneous that play with the brain's balancing act between order and flexibility, pattern and openness to change.

Although the correlations between neuroscience, narrative theory, and our experience of stories can illuminate many matters of interest to both scientists and humanists, it is important to keep in mind what cognitive science cannot tell us about narrative. The explanatory limits of neuroscience have to do with the so-called hard problem (see Chalmers 1995) of how electrochemical activity at the neuronal level produces consciousness and embodied experience. It is undeniable that if someone is having an experience, there must be neuronal activity of some sort correlated to it. What happens across the divide between neurons firing and lived experience is mysterious, however, and how consciousness emerges from brain-body processes at the cellular level is a question no one can as yet answer. Thomas Nagel (1974) has famously argued that empirical measures alone cannot capture "what it is like" to have an experience, and he has recently (2012) speculated that the question of how neuronal activity gives rise to consciousness probably requires a disciplinary paradigm shift (à la Thomas Kuhn) that we cannot fully imagine because we are still on this side of it (how life emerges from chemical interactions is, he claims, a similar quandary awaiting an as yet inconceivable revolution in the explanatory frameworks available to science). Experience and neuronal activity can be correlated, but neither can completely explain the other or the alchemy of their interaction.

There is consequently a disjunction between the levels of analysis at which neuroscience and the humanities approach cognitive issues. This disjunction is what neurophenomenologists call the "explanatory gap" that separates neurobiological and phenomenological accounts of consciousness—the gap between the neural correlates of consciousness that neuroscience has identified and the lived experience of the perceptual world (see Thompson, Lutz, and Cosmelli 2005). This gap may be an obstacle to what E. O. Wilson (1998) calls consilience between cognitive science and the humanities, but it also makes possible conversation between them from positions of distinctive disciplinary difference (see Armstrong 2013, 7–8). We can compare and correlate experience, neuronal processes, and narrative theories across this divide, and this work can be instructive in all kinds of ways and for all sorts of reasons, but these triangulations are exactly that—comparisons that chart convergences and divergences—and not solutions to the hard problem or explanations of the mysteries of emergence.

One obstacle to undertaking such triangulations is the bogeyman of Cartesian dualism that haunts literary studies. To inquire about the cognitive workings of the brain, it is sometimes feared, is to commit the fallacy of assuming that reality is constituted in the mind of an ego that thinks, thereby overlooking the fact that the cogito is always situated in a body and a social, historical setting and that cognition entails interactions across the boundaries joining brain, body, and social world. Advocates of so-called enactive embodied cognition sometimes similarly worry that asking about processes in the brain may wrongly neglect its situation in a body and a world of natural and socially constructed affordances (for example, see Cook 2018). Enactivism risks becoming a distorting dogma, however, if it refuses to investigate cortical and neuronal processes inside the skull on the grounds that cognition is not only a matter of what happens in the head.[16] By no means mutually exclusive, these perspectives are interdependent and inextricably linked. Usefully reminding us that "the brain is one element in a complex network involving the brain, the body, and the environment," Alva Noë (2004, 214, 222) advises that we need both "to look inward, to the neural plumbing" that gives rise to experience and "to look outward, too, to the way that plumbing is hooked up to the world." Narrative offers neuroscience perspectives that open in both directions. The configurative interactions through which we tell and follow stories deploy fundamental cognitive processes that connect our brains through our bodies with the people, places, and things in our worlds. "Look both ways" is useful advice when you're at an intersection of any kind, and that includes the conjunction between neuroscience and narrative.

CHAPTER TWO

The Temporality of Narrative and the Decentered Brain

THE CONCORDANT DISCORDANCE of emplotment is curiously and intricately correlated to the decentered, asynchronous temporality of the brain. One of the many ways in which the brain differs from a computer is that its temporal processes are not instantaneous and perfectly synchronized. Unlike electrical signals that discharge simultaneously at a fraction of the speed of light, action potentials at the neuronal level take more than a millisecond to fire, and different regions of the cortex respond at varying rates.[1] For example, as Semir Zeki (2003, 215) observes, in the visual cortex "colour is perceived before motion" by approximately 80 milliseconds, and "locations are perceived before colours, which are perceived before orientations." The integration of neuronal processes through which conscious awareness emerges may require up to half a second. As Zeki points out, however, this "binding" (as it is called) is itself not perfectly homogeneous: "The binding of colour to motion occurs after the binding of colour to colour or motion to motion" because "binding between attributes takes longer than binding within attributes" (216, 217). More time is needed to integrate inputs from vision and hearing, for example, than to synthesize visual signals alone. Although we typically don't notice these disjunctions, the nonsimultaneity of the brain's cognitive processes means that consciousness is inherently out of balance and is always catching up with itself. As Antonio Damasio (1999, 127) puts it, "We are probably late for consciousness by about 500 milliseconds."

This imbalance is not a bad thing because it allows the brain to play in the ever-changing horizontal space between past patterns and the indeterminacies of the future, the space that plots organize into beginnings, middles, and ends. Concord with no trace of discord would be disabling. In waking life, as Gerald Edelman and Giulio Tononi (2000, 72) observe, "groups of neurons dynamically assemble and reassemble into continuously changing patterns of firing." The synchronization of brain waves across the cortex makes possible the formation of neuronal assemblies and coordinates the workings of different regions of the brain (see Buzsáki 2006). As Bernard Baars and Nicole Gage (2010, 246) explain, "Normal cognition requires selective, local synchrony among brain regions," "highly patterned and differentiated" oscillatory patterns in which "synchrony, desynchrony, and aperiodic 'one-shot' waveforms constantly appear and disappear." But, as Edelman and Tononi point out, "if a large number of neurons in the brain start firing in the same way, reducing the diversity of the brain's neuronal repertoires, as is the case in deep sleep and epilepsy, consciousness disappears" (36). In those conditions, "the slow, oscillatory firing of . . . distributed populations of neurons is highly synchronized globally" (72), and global hypersynchrony paralyzes normal functioning by disrupting the to and fro of synchronization and desynchronization. In contrast to sleep and epilepsy, "consciousness requires not just neural activity," Edelman and Tononi observe, "but neural activity that changes continually and is thus spatially and temporally differentiated"—"distributed, integrated, but continuously changing patterns of neural activity . . . whose rich functioning actually *requires* variability" (73, 74–75; original emphasis).

This necessary tension at the neuronal level between pattern and change, synchrony and fluctuation, coordination and differentiation is the neural correlate of the ability of a plot to join concord and discord through temporal structures that order events while holding them open to surprise, variation, and refiguration. The ability to tell and follow stories requires much more than neural activity alone, of course, but if the temporal processes through which neuronal assemblies form, dissolve, and form again were not asynchronous in these ways, our cognitive apparatus probably could not support narrative interactions.

The capacity to play with temporal differences is a defining characteristic of narrative. As Christian Metz (1974, 18) observes, "Narrative is a . . . doubly temporal sequence. . . . There is the time of the thing told and the time of the telling (the time of the signified and the time of the signifier). This duality not only renders possible all the temporal distortions that are commonplace in narratives (three years of the hero's life summed up in two sentences of a novel . . .). More basically, it invites us to consider that one of the functions of narrative is to invent one time scheme in terms of another time scheme." The opposition between "discourse time" (sometimes referred to as "Erzählzeit") and "story time" ("Erzählte Zeit") gives rise to a series of other distinctions that narrative theorist Gérard Genette (1980) magisterially analyzes in his classic study of Proust's *In Search of Lost Time*— differences in order, duration, speed, or frequency that authors manipulate to play with our sense of time. After describing the "narrative competence of the reader" as the ability to negotiate these temporal complications, Genette notes that "this very competence is what the author relies on to fool the reader by sometimes offering him false advance mentions, or *snares*," constructing a "complex system of frustrated expectations, disappointed suspicions, surprises looked forward to and finally all the more surprising in being looked forward to and occurring nonetheless" (1980, 77, original emphasis).[2] H. Porter Abbott (2002, 3) exaggerates only a little when he argues that "narrative is the principal way in which our species organizes its understanding of time." Music and dance, to be sure, also serve this end.[3] They do so, however, by invoking and manipulating the same disjunctions in the neurobiology of time and in our lived experience of time passing that make narrative possible.

The neurobiological processes underlying our experience of time are somewhat elusive, but the scientific consensus is that there is no central clock or timing mechanism in the brain, just as there is no single language module and no "homunculus" functioning as a central processor. Instead, as Valtteri Arstila and Dan Lloyd point out (2014a, 200), "the constituent processes of vision and hearing (and all the other senses) run on different schedules. Just as there is no one place where 'it all comes together,' there is no one time where cotemporal events are simultaneously represented." Dean V. Buonomano (2014, 330) argues, indeed, that "the realization that temporal processing is not a unitary neural process" is key to understanding "the neural basis of timing." As he explains, "The brain seems to have developed fundamentally different mechanisms for timing across different timescales" (337).

These mechanisms begin at the neuronal and synaptic level. As Buonomano notes, the responsiveness of neurons is "strongly dependent on their recent history of activity," just as "the strength of the synapses between neurons" similarly "varies dramatically in a use-dependent fashion," thereby providing "an ephemeral memory of what has happened in the past few hundred milliseconds" (334). Oscillatory coupling and decoupling of neuronal assemblies across the brain and between the brain and the body provide further mechanisms for processing durations at different scales. As György Buzsáki (2006, 174) observes, "Oscillatory coalitions of neurons can expand the effective window of synchronization from hundreds of milliseconds to many seconds." This is why Francisco Varela, the foremost neurophenomenologist of time, proposes three "scales of duration" to distinguish different "windows" of integration, from "basic or elementary events" (10–100 milliseconds) beneath conscious awareness, to "large-scale integration" (250 milliseconds to a few seconds) underlying the experienced moment, to the "descriptive-narrative assessments" lasting several seconds that characterize working memory and longer-term syntheses (Varela 1999, 273; see also Thompson 2007, 330–38).

The borders between these "windows" are necessarily fuzzy, and there is some controversy about where to draw them, because the processes of synchronization and desynchronization across the brain, body, and world are always shifting. As Lloyd (2016) observes, "Brain activity, like consciousness, is a radically nonstationary process, constantly changing at every scale." Or as Varela and his colleagues explain, "In the brain there is no 'settling down' but an ongoing change marked only by transient coordination among populations" of neurons (2001, 237). Not unified or centrally organized, the neurobiological bases of time are an array of distributed, fluctuating processes from the microsecond level up to the longer integrations supporting various embodied experiences of different temporal width.

According to Varela, "The fact that an assembly of coupled oscillators attains a transient synchrony and that it takes a certain time to do so is the explicit correlate" and "origin of nowness" (1999, 283). Because any "synchronization is dynamically unstable," however, and "will constantly and successively give rise to new assemblies" (283), any "now" has what Edmund Husserl calls "horizons"—a retentional horizon carrying along traces of the immediate past and a protentional horizon pointing toward assemblies to come as synchronies organize themselves in recurring (but also changing) patterns that follow particular trajectories.[4] The duration of this "now phase" may in turn differ according to the varying scales of integration, from hundreds of milliseconds to multiple seconds, that constitute what Varela calls the "window of simultaneity that corresponds to the duration of [the] lived present" (272).

Our lived experience of time is an emergent phenomenon that is based on but is not identical with or reducible to its neurobiological underpinnings. As Varela and his coauthors explain (2001, 237), "The large-scale integration of brain activity can be considered as the basis for the unity of mind familiar to us in everyday experience." Beneath this felt unity, however, are a variety of asynchronous, disjunctive processes that support the brain's ongoing balancing act between pattern and change, order and flux, synthesis and desynchronization. These disjunctions make "instability . . . the basis of normal functioning rather than a disturbance that needs to be compensated for" (Varela 1999, 285), but they are ordinarily invisible. As Bruno Mölder (2014, 222) explains, "Consciously represented temporal properties need not match with the temporal properties of the neural processes that underpin these representations"—but sometimes the disjunctions underlying them come into view. Ordinarily time seems to pass fluently and unproblematically, but occasionally the asynchrony of brain, body, and world may emerge from its cloak of invisibility in various subjective distortions, as when time seems to speed up or slow down according to our level of arousal, attention, or engagement, for example, or in certain temporal illusions like the oft-discussed phenomenon whereby a moving dot assumes the color of a location before it gets there (more on this in the next section). Distortions like these fascinate neurobiologists of time because they provide glimpses of the discrepancies in the processing of sensation that underlie our unified experience of the world.

Temporal experience is an emergent phenomenon with a neurobiological foundation. The characteristics of experienced time are not correlated in a one-to-one manner with their neural underpinnings, but they are not magical or mysterious. They have a material basis in the asynchronous, disjunctive but patterned, conjoined interactions linking brain, body, and world. Narrative configurations and refigurations of time set in motion interactions between our lived experience of the world and our embodied brains that can in turn reshape the cognitive processes of integration that give rise to our sense of time passing. According to Ricoeur (1984a, 54), in narrative "a prefigured time . . . becomes a refigured time through the mediation of a configured time." The work of narrative in invoking and repatterning the reader's sense of time through the temporal structures of stories and their ways of telling is accomplished by its enacting and manipulating various embodied cognitive processes of synchronization and desynchronization that also characterize the neural workings of time.

Anticipation and Retrospection in Stories and the Brain

The circuit between anticipation and retrospection is a pervasive feature of narrative and embodied cognition. Just as we live forward but understand backward in our everyday experience of the world, so we comprehend a story by projecting expectations that its twists and turns then modify and revise until we arrive at an ending that may overturn and completely reconfigure what we had previously assumed.[5] This is why Heidegger says that understanding has a fore-structure (*Vor-Struktur*) that always already guides interpretation, an implicit configuration of expectations that our explications (*Auslegung*) belatedly catch up with and revise, refine, and correct (see 1962

[1927], 188–95). How cognition entails retrospective adjustment of what we have already anticipated is evident even at the neuronal level, in the ways in which our brains respond to signals before we are aware of them, a gap that we then subliminally correct and smooth over so that we typically do not notice it (otherwise we would have the weird sense that our present experience had already taken place in the past—which it indeed has, in a sense, inasmuch as consciousness lags behind detection by up to half a second).

Stories play with the anticipation-retrospection circuit at various cognitive levels—at the subliminal level, for example, as we immerse ourselves unreflectively in their revelations and reversals, and at the level of conscious awareness, as we reflect on the implications of the adjustments and revisions we must make as our expectations are surprised. At whatever level, the twists and turns in our experience of stories are only possible because the temporality of brain functioning is asynchronous, ever shifting between states of equilibrium and disequilibrium. If our brains were temporally unified and homogeneous, everything firing simultaneously and in lockstep, we could not tell each other stories because there would be no temporal gaps and no disjunctions between anticipation and retrospection for their discordant concordances to play with. The ways in which stories confirm or surprise our expectations can have deep effects on the neuronal assemblies through which we know the world because those assemblies are formed through to-and-fro recursive processes of synchronization and desynchronization.

The temporal asynchronies of brain processing can cause our conscious awareness of a signal to lag behind our reaction to it in ways that can seem paradoxical and strange. Noting that "our quick reactions to sensory signals appear to be performed without any initial awareness of the signal," Benjamin Libet (2004, 93, 33) observes that "the brain needs a relatively long period of appropriate activations, up to about half a second, to elicit awareness" of an event that we may already have responded to. Libet conducted a series of well-known experiments that documented this lag by implanting probes in the brains of patients undergoing surgery to treat a neurological disorder (procedures during which they remained conscious), and these single-cell probes enabled him to measure with exceptional accuracy the difference between neuronal reactions to various signals and a subject's reported awareness of them (see Libet et al. 1979). Libet's experiments showed that "the subjective 'present' is actually of a sensory event in the past" because "our awareness of our sensory world is substantially delayed from its actual occurrence" (2004, 88, 70).

Although this may sound odd, it is quite an ordinary and in many respects a beneficial phenomenon. As Libet notes, "All quick behavioral, motor responses to a sensory signal are performed unconsciously, . . . within 100–200 msec after the signal, well before awareness of the signal could be expected," as when a tennis player returns a serve, for example, or a baseball player hits a home run (109). Marc Jeannerod (2006, 9) similarly observes that "during the playing of a musical instrument . . . finger alternations can, in certain instances, attain the frequency of 16 strokes/s[econd], which exceeds the possibility of any sensory feedback influencing the command system." Even in an ordinary activity like speaking, Libet points out, we typically talk before we are fully conscious of what we are saying: "If you try to be aware of each word before speaking it, the flow of your speech becomes slow and hesitant" (108). Similarly, if you are driving and see a child chasing a ball into the street in front of your car, Libet explains that "you are capable of slamming on the brake in about 150 msec or less," even though you would not be consciously aware of the danger for another 350 milliseconds (91). As Jeannerod observes, "We respond first and become aware later. . . . [W]e consciously see the obstacle [only] after we have avoided it" (47; also see 41, 48–49, and 60–61 on experiments confirming Libet's results).

What is perhaps surprising is that Libet's experiments showed that drivers in this last example "subjectively antedate" the experience and "report seeing the [child] immediately," without the lag that in fact occurred between response and awareness (91). Libet makes this inference based on experiments that compared a stimulus applied to the skin and another stimulus applied intracortically. Both stimuli would require 500 milliseconds to reach awareness, but the external stimulus was reported to have happened earlier, half a second before it was consciously perceived, whereas the intracortical stimulus was reported to have occurred only after the half-second lag: "In our conscious experience of a sensory event, the event seems to occur when it actually happened, instead of 0.5 sec later (when we, in fact, became aware of the event)" (81). A primary electrical potential measurable on the skin when the stimulus is applied apparently becomes the reference point that the brain uses to establish the time of the event, even though we become conscious of the stimulus only 500 milliseconds later.

What happens, according to Libet, is a subjective referral that "corrects" the "distortions . . . imposed by the way in which the cerebral neurons represent the event," analogous to how (in a well-known experiment) subjects who wore "prism spectacles that turned the visual image upside down" began after a week or so "to be able to behave as if the image were normal" (81, 82).[6] Because of this capacity for recursive cognitive adjustment, "*subjective* timing need not be identical to *neuronal* time" (72). Our sense of the present moment—of the simultaneity of an event and our perception of it—

is thus what Libet calls an "emergent property" that is not attributable to any particular element of the system but that develops out of the interactions of its parts. It results from a to-and-fro process of subjective referral that antedates what we perceive and constructs temporal unity that smooths over the asynchronies underlying it.

Although subjective referral and temporal antedating were surprising and quite controversial when Libet first reported his findings (see Libet 1993, 2002, 2003; Gomes 1998), they are evident in phenomena widely attested and extensively studied in the neuroscientific literature on time. For example, in an experiment conducted by Patrick Haggard and his group (2002), a situation where an action was perceived to cause a tone was compared with a control case where the action and the tone were presented separately. Analyzing this experiment and its significance, Kielan Yarrow and Sukhvinder Obhi (2014, 462) note that "when an intended action caused the tone, the action was perceived to occur later, and the tone was perceived to occur earlier," almost as if they were temporally attracted to each other. As Yarrow and Obhi observe, "It seems as though actions cause their delayed sensory consequences to appear earlier in time, while the perceived time of the action is also drawn toward the sensory event," a time-shift Haggard calls "intentional binding" that may "help conscious inferences of causality" (462). In this way, according to Haggard (2002, 385), "the brain . . . binds intentional actions to their effects to construct a coherent conscious experience of our own agency."

As Thomas Fraps (2014, 273) observes, this is only one of "several studies [that] have demonstrated that causes and effects mutually attract each other in subjective time." According to Fraps, this phenomenon supports the well-known claim of eighteenth-century philosopher David Hume that "our perception of causality is a mental construct, one only inferred from the sensory experience of temporal contiguity" (265). No doubt for evolutionarily understandable reasons, our brains seem to have developed a predisposition to bind cause and effect by temporally closing the gap between them through reciprocal subjective referral. This subliminal mechanism also predisposes us to link the events emplotted in a story.

The brain's proclivity to bind temporally distinct events similarly underlies the oft-discussed color phi and cutaneous rabbit phenomena. As Mölder (2014, 220–21) explains:

The color phi phenomenon is the illusion of movement that occurs when the subject is presented with flashes of two objects of different colors at different positions (e.g., a blue spot and a red spot). It seems that the spot is moving from one location to another and changes its color midway through its movement. What is puzzling . . . is that the color seems to already change in the location that precedes the actual location where the spot with a different color is presented. . . . [T]he red color seems to be present before it is actually presented.[7]

The cutaneous rabbit experiment similarly entails temporal antedating that constructs a coherent perceptual experience by reorganizing retrospectively the stimuli that give rise to it. If five taps are made at intervals of 40–60 milliseconds first at the wrist, then at the elbow, and then again at the wrist, what the subject reports perceiving is not three discrete sets of stimuli; instead, as Mölder explains (221), "the subject feels as if something moves regularly with smooth jumps up the arm, . . . not only in the locations of the stimulation"—"as if the later taps have a backward effect" on the earlier stimuli and give rise to a feeling like a bunny hopping up the subject's arm (hence the experiment's name). In both of these cases, the brain subliminally reorganizes the temporal relations between sensory stimuli to construct a coherent pattern that uses information about what came later to restructure what came earlier. This backward-looking readjustment of previous stimuli to rearrange our sense of their order and relationship may seem counterintuitive, but this recursivity is based on processes of temporal antedating, subjective referral, and intentional binding that are constantly at work in the relation between brain, body, and world, closing the gap between late-arriving perceptual awareness and the signals to which we have already responded.

These recursive processes are often misunderstood. For example, Brian Massumi and other so-called affect theorists have used (or, better, misused) Libet's experiments to posit a bodily, autonomous realm of subpersonal affective processes prior to cognition. "Thought lags behind itself," Massumi (2002, 195) claims; "it can never catch up with its own beginnings. The half-second of thought-forming is forever lost in darkness. All awareness emerges from a nonconscious thought-o-genic lapse indistinguishable from movements of matter." This is a misinterpretation of the implications of Libet's experiment. Rather than uncovering some "dark" realm of autonomous affect beneath awareness (what Massumi notoriously calls "the mystery of the missing half-second" [28]), Libet's findings demonstrate how the temporal asynchronies of the embodied brain form configurations at different scales and interact recursively—the subliminal perception of a situation prompting a driver to slam on the breaks, for example, before conscious awareness arises of the child chasing the ball across the street, the two moments interacting to antedate the now to the moment when the intuition of danger first arose. This recursivity is not a "nonconscious thought-o-genic lapse" (whatever that odd coinage might mean) but rather as Shaun Gallagher (2005, 239) argues, a "looping" process through which immediate perception and conscious awareness interact and shape each other. In phenomenological terms, this interaction is a recursive relation between two modes of meaning making—what Merleau-Ponty (2012 [1945], 441–42) calls "non-thetic" and "thetic" intentionality to distinguish unreflective perception from deliberate, consciously active meaning-creation—not a juxtaposition between an autonomous realm of subpersonal intensities and conscious thought.

Massumi errs by transforming ordinary neurobiological and epistemological processes into obscure metaphysical mysteries.[8] These processes have a material basis, but they are also instances of emergence, whereby a phenomenon (like consciousness or life) is produced by underlying activities (neurons firing, chemicals interacting) to which it is not reducible (see Deacon 2012). Contrary to what Massumi claims, emergent processes are not "indistinguishable" from the "movements of matter" out of which they arise, nor are they evidence that we are somehow controlled by subpersonal affective processes or that a "nonconscious lapse" undermines cognition. Emergence, the creation of wholes that are more than the sum of their parts, is an ordinary and ubiquitous consequence of recursive processes that are everywhere at work in our embodied brain's interactions with its world (see Kelso 1995).

Libet's mind-time experiments and other similar instances of subjective referral and intentional binding suggest that the ability of stories to emplot disparate events into coherent temporal patterns and thereby to create concord out of discord is correlated with various timing processes in the embodied brain. Across the different tempos of relationship that join our brains and the world, we are constantly configuring story-like patterns that establish concord and "correct" (so to speak) the discord between the actual occurrence of events and our awareness of them. If we live forward but understand backward, the ability to retrospectively reconfigure past and present begins at the neuronal level as we smooth out the asynchronies in the temporality of perception just as the wearers of prism spectacles adjust the inverted shapes on their retinas.

A similar process of to-and-fro reconfiguration is at work when, as Ricoeur (1984a, 67–68) observes, we find a surprising and unforeseeable conclusion to a story to be nevertheless "acceptable" because it is "congruent with the episodes brought together by the story." At such moments, he notes, "it is as though recollection inverted the so-called 'natural' order of time. In reading the ending in the beginning and the beginning in the ending, we also learn to read time itself backwards." The trick of "reading time backwards" is not such an unnatural act after all, however, because our ability to reconfigure the shape of time is also evident in the brain-based process of subjective referral that antedates what we become aware of to the moment when it occurred or in the intentional binding that draws cause and effect to each other. These recursive temporal processes are at work in the color phi and cutaneous bunny phenomena, and they are also in play when we retrospectively reconfigure narrative beginnings to align with our later sense of the ending.

Establishing congruence retrospectively between endings and the beginnings whose meaning may shift after we discover what they led to is a to-and-fro process of reciprocal configuration that is integral to our ability to follow stories. This is the reader's response (mimesis$_3$) to the narrative act of "'grasping together' the detailed actions" in the configurative construction of a plot (mimesis$_2$) that "draws from the manifold of events the unity of one temporal whole" (Ricoeur 1984a, 66). We can readily align disparate beginnings and endings because our lived experience of time (mimesis$_1$) entails a continuous series of subjective referrals that adjust our sense of the timing of present and past. We can learn to follow stories by reconfiguring relations between surprising endings and their beginnings in events we hadn't fully understood because the configurative readjustment of anticipation and retrospection is something our basic neurobiological equipment predisposes us to do.

One of the reasons why Charles Dickens's novel *Great Expectations* is a classic of narratological theory is that it illustrates these temporal paradoxes and complications in so many interlocking ways (starting with the pun in its title, which alludes both to the narrator's many epistemological errors and to the fortune he hoped to inherit). The retrospective first-person narration of older, wiser Pip recounts the many erroneous assumptions and anticipations of his younger self, and the gap between young Pip and old Pip narrows as the time of the story converges on the time of the discourse. This temporal gap is the source of much of the irony and the comedy of the novel that survives on rereading, even when we are able to identify the various snares (or false clues) that Pip misreads about his benefactor—and one of the pleasures of rereading is spotting these mistakes (misinterpretations of which we too had perhaps been guilty the first time we read the novel). Just as a magician misdirects our attention by separating the cause of an action from its effect so that we don't see their interaction, which makes it possible for us to marvel at the trick (see Fraps 2014), so Dickens constructs a masterful plot that disguises, disjoins, and displaces cause and effect, thereby masking connections that only later emerge but whose origins we hadn't previously understood. This is a temporal art that takes advantage of the asynchronies in the way our brains process signals and construct patterns that we assume are simply "natural" and "there." We are ordinarily unaware of the recursive, to-and-fro balancing acts that create stability out of the instabilities of perceptual experience, and the patterns of temporal experience may consequently seem natural and inevitable because the constructive processes underlying them are invisible. Hence our surprise when what we had expected (about Pip's benefactor or about the coin the magician pulls out of our ear) turns out to have been an erroneous construction.

Masking the contingency of the temporal connections we routinely make is also part of the narrative game Dickens plays. As we read forward and understand backward, just as Pip lives forward only to narrate backward, the links between events in the story he had told himself about his life give way to a reconfiguration that seems to have been lurking in the background all along, waiting to spring—a gestalt shift Pip recounts in a memorable comparison of his seemingly fated retrospective enlightenment to a tale in which a "heavy slab that was to fall on the bed of state" and kill an unsuspecting usurper was slowly and elaborately prepared:

> All being made ready with much labour, and the hour come, the sultan was aroused in the dead of the night, and the sharpened axe that was to sever the rope [holding the slab] from the great iron ring was put into his hand, and he struck with it, and the rope parted and rushed away, and the ceiling fell. So, in my case, all the work, near and afar, that tended to the end, had been accomplished; and in an instant the blow was struck, and the roof of my stronghold dropped upon me. (Dickens 2008 [1861], 285)[9]

Pip's revelations seem fated and inescapable when they finally arrive, but this sense of inevitability disguises the various contingencies in his life (and in Dickens's narrative)—beginning with the accident of the convict Magwitch encountering him in the graveyard—that seem like fate only when they are ordered retrospectively into a particular pattern. The paradox of a good plot is that the connections between events must seem necessary, but the twists, turns, and reversals of the narrative are only possible because these links are variable and contingent.

This paradox is evident in the oft-discussed curiosity that Dickens was able to write two opposing conclusions to the novel (one where Pip gets his girl, the other where he doesn't). He could do this because beginnings and endings are contingent, reciprocally constituting, retrospectively variable constructs, and each ending refigures previous events in the novel into a different pattern—emphasizing either its comic, often sentimental, affirmations of Victorian values or its dark recognition of the shortcomings and hypocrisies that give the lie to those platitudes (you can see which ending I prefer!). In reading, storytelling, and life, patterns of temporal connection between events are not independent, necessary givens but are recursively established in a to-and-fro manner as anticipation and retrospection mutually constitute each other. We may feel that time simply happens naturally in our experience of the world or that the order of events in the stories we follow simply had to be, but the construction of time is an ongoing, ever-shifting process at all levels, from the recursive construction of neuronal assembles to the anticipatory and retrospective interaction of beginnings and endings. The fact that time is not a line, either in experience or on the neuronal level, but a to-and-fro product of pattern formation and dissolution, is what makes *Great Expectations* possible in all of its temporal complexity.

Questions of time, fate, and freedom often go hand in hand.[10] One implication of Libet's mind-time experiments that sparked particular controversy was that acts we may think result from the voluntary, conscious exercise of free will are in fact initiated by cerebral activity of which we are unaware: "That is, the brain starts the voluntary process unconsciously" (2004, 93). Measuring neuronal activity through probes implanted in the motor cortex of patients undergoing brain surgery, Libet found that "the brain exhibited an initiating process, beginning 550 msec before the freely voluntary act; but awareness of the conscious will to perform the act appeared only 150–200 msec before the act" (123–24). The conscious awareness of an intention to act arose, then, approximately 350 milliseconds after the brain had already initiated it.

Libet rejects, however, the inference others were quick to draw that freedom is an illusion. Although "conscious free will does not initiate our freely voluntary acts," he argues, "it can control the outcome or actual performance of the act" through a kind of "veto" (139). This is different from instances of automatic or uncontrollable behavior, as in Tourette's syndrome where subjects "spontaneously shout obscenities" (142). Libet found experimentally that such automatic responses entail "a quick reaction to an unwarned stimulus" for which there is no readiness potential (142). That is, there is no temporal lag in such cases between an unconscious initiatory activity in the brain (the readiness potential his experiments measured) and subsequent awareness (after the time lag necessary for consciousness), and without this disjunction there is no possibility of retrospective intervention (the "veto power" of freedom). Once again homogeneity is disabling. The gap between a readiness potential and our awareness of an intention is what allows retrospective readjustment. Rather than evidence of our lack of autonomy, as Massumi (2002) claims, this lag is one foundation of our ability to exercise free will.

A temporal gap similarly characterizes many common experiences of action in the world that are free and intentional not because they are fully conscious and transparent but because they are capable of being recursively reoriented. As James J. Gibson (1979, 225) observes, "Locomotion and manipulation are neither triggered nor commanded but controlled. They are constrained, guided, or steered, and only in this sense are they ruled or governed." Motor control is a process of ongoing prospective and retrospective adjustment, and this steering or guiding is made possible by the subliminal temporal disjunctions that Libet has identified (see Gallagher 2012, 109).[11] "Motor perception is predictive," as Ivar Hagendoorn (2004, 83) explains, as it must be to compensate for these lags. Hagendoorn notes that it takes 50–100 milliseconds to process visual signals after they first reach the retina, followed by further delays in coordinating these signals with various embodied motor processes. We steer and guide our actions by anticipating how these visual and motor patterns will come together. In order to catch a ball, for example, we need to predict and anticipate its arrival subliminally—and if we think about what we are doing and try to intend the action deliberately, we are going to drop it—but we are of course free to act differently (jumping out of the way or batting the ball down). We can also improve our skills through learning and instruction (improving our predictions and our anticipatory coordination of perception and action) as we could not if these behaviors were outside the realm of freedom. Citing a study that "compared the performance of astronauts catching a ball on earth and under zero gravity," Hagendoorn suggests that "the brain uses an internal model of gravity-induced acceleration when predicting the trajectory of a falling ball" (83). When gravity is missing, the predictive processes underlying the coordination of action become visible because they don't work and need to be adjusted—which we can do because of the temporal disjunctions that allow the brain to construct various kinds of subjective referrals.

As Buzsáki (2006, vii) observes, "Brains are foretelling devices," and their "predictive powers emerge from the various rhythms they perpetually generate." These rhythms give rise, according to Marcus Raichle (2001, 8), to "changes in brain activity preceding the appearance of a to-be-attended sensory stimulus," cortical variations that are the neural correlates of anticipation. The brain's ongoing fluctuations allow interactions at the neuronal level to produce the signals that steer our embodied responses to the world, making subliminal predictions about how patterns will come together in perceptual experience and then retrospectively tuning these invisible, unnoticed guesses in a never-ending, to-and-fro, recursive process. Free will is not an illusion, then, but the story we tell ourselves of being freely choosing, fully conscious agents may be easier to understand than these back-and-forth processes of fluctuation and synchronization at various levels of awareness.

Reciprocal processes of pattern formation are fundamental to the brain's operation as a to-and-fro ensemble of neuronal assemblies that are constantly coming and going, waxing and waning. The technical term for this back-and-forth reciprocal processing is "reentry," a term coined by Edelman and Tononi (2000, 48, 49) to describe "the ongoing, recursive interchange of parallel signals between reciprocally connected areas of the brain, an interchange that continually coordinates the activities of these areas' maps to each other in space and time." As they explain, "re-entry allows for a unity of perception and behavior that would otherwise be impossible, given the absence in the brain of a unique, computer-like central processor." Varela and colleagues (Varela et al. 2001) call this decentered, interactive structure the "brain web." As Stanislas Dehaene (2014, 137, 156) observes, such a structure requires "long-distance communication and a massive exchange of reciprocal signals"—what he calls "recurrent processing" through "short local loops" within particular areas of neural anatomy (like the different specialized regions of the rear visual cortex dedicated to orientation, motion, color, etc.) and long-distance "global loops" for more complicated cognitive activities like reading or listening to stories that necessitate interactions between far-flung regions of the brain (including, for example, the visual, auditory, and motor cortices, the areas connected to emotions like the insula and the amygdala, the memory functions associated with the hippocampus, and interactions across the brain-body divide through the thalamus and the brain stem). "Consciousness lives in the loops," Dehaene memorably declares; "reverberating neuronal activity, circulating in the web of our cortical connections, causes our conscious experiences" (156). The processes of configuration, refiguration, and transfiguration that constitute narrative also characterize the interactions of the brain web, and that is one reason why stories can have such deep and lasting effects on the workings of our brains.

Some of these effects may occur subliminally, priming us to expect certain configurations that conform to our habitually established patterns of response. Narrative understanding often occurs beneath and before awareness, especially when the repetition of well-known stories draws on and reinforces familiar, expected configurations. Richard Gerrig (2012, 50) has shown (perhaps not surprisingly) that "preferences with respect to potential outcomes . . . affect the ease with which readers accept outcomes when they ultimately arrive." His laboratory demonstrated experimentally, for example, that readers took "longer to read sentences that were inconsistent with their preferences" and didn't align with what they expected or desired. This finding is consistent with experimental evidence that "we always perceive a predictable stimulus sooner than an unpredictable one" (Dehaene 2014, 127). Processing speeds up when "anticipation compensates" for the time lag of consciousness and facilitates the subjective referral of temporal attribution (Dehaene 2014, 127). Whether with stories or in life, we perceive faster what our habitual experiences have accustomed us to anticipate. But structuring unpredictability into a narrative pattern of suspense can counteract this effect. Gerrig's collaborator and former student David Rapp (2008) found that readers took measurably longer to read factually inaccurate statements (like "Shirley Temple starred in *The Wizard of Oz*") than sentences they knew to be true, but he also found that offering readers counterfactual information in the form of a suspenseful story significantly reduced these reaction times. Configuring counterintuitive, anomalous statements into predictable narrative patterns (the buildup and resolution of suspense) made it easier to assimilate discordant information.

This may be why Aristotle famously prefers probable if impossible plots to ones that are possible but improbable. Configuration matters for comprehension, as when the reversals in a story seem "right" because, as Ricoeur (1984a, 43) puts it, "strokes of chance . . . seem to arrive by design." Hence the surprising sense of inevitability that Pip reports when the revelation of the identity of his benefactor causes him to reconfigure the patterns through which he understood his life—refigurations that we readers duplicate on our parallel track of anticipatory and retrospective pattern formation as we form and reform our understanding of the story offered by the narrator's discourse. All of the connections Dickens weaves together, some defying probability—how unlikely, after all, that Magwitch would turn out to be Estella's father and that his daughter would happen to end up as a ward of a foster parent in Pip's hometown!—are acceptable and may even seem aesthetically inevitable because of how they fit together (although I have skeptical students every semester who find these links preposterous, despite my trying to convince them that they demonstrate Dickens's artistry and testify to his moral sense of the hidden interconnections binding the human community). Such experiences of discord that are resolved into new structures of concord can teach us to recognize and accept new configurative patterns, whether aesthetically or morally or epistemologically, introducing us to new ways of grasping together or following events. The plot of a bildungsroman like *Great Expectations* can offer an education not only to its protagonist but also to its readers through these kinds of reconfiguration.

Plots please and instruct through their manipulation of probability and improbability, familiarity and unfamiliarity, novelty and surprise. Reversals like these are not only entertaining but also potentially cognitively formative because the narrative work of configuring beginning, middle, and end manipulates temporal processes that govern the brain's perpetual balancing act as it revises its habitual syntheses and adjusts to novel, unexpected situations. As Nancy Easterlin (2015, 614) observes, "If our predilection for the new and for the knowledge that it can provide is tempered by a contrary disposition to avoid the unfamiliar, reading a literary work offers the experience of encountering novelty without imminent threat." By playing with the time lags built into cognition, narratives can reinforce established patterns through the pleasures of recognition, providing reinforcement for the structures that build coherence across our temporal experience, or they can disrupt the expectations through which we build consistency and offer new possibilities of recurrent processing, new patterns of reentry. Or, most typically, narratives can do both in varying degrees and in different ways that constitute the temporal art of emplotment.

If the conjunctions that smooth over temporal discordances can facilitate configurative activity, the disjunctions inherent in these time lags can also be productive. This is the case both with everyday cognition and with narrative. That is not only because these disjunctions may give rise to reconfigurations in cognitive patterns of the sort that the surprising twists and turns in a good plot enact. The temporal discrepancies that require subjective referrals to correct for the time lag of consciousness also allow consciousness to duplicate itself and thereby give rise to self-consciousness. What Dehaene (2014, 253) calls our "unique faculty for thinking nested thoughts" is made possible by the recursive operations of the brain web, the to-and-fro doubling of top-down and bottom-up assemblies that continually, reciprocally interact with one another.

Doubling of this kind is fundamental to consciousness and self-consciousness and also to narrative. The most basic narrative correlative of this capacity for nesting is, of course, the relation between discourse and story—the sometimes concordant, sometimes discordant interplay between the order of events in the telling and their sequence in the told. Narratives are essentially double structures because of narrative anachronies, "the various types of discordance between the two orderings" of story and narration that are fundamental to narrative (Genette 1980, 35–36). Even the classic formula "Once upon a time" has the basic temporal structure of doubling one time over against another, nesting the time of the story in the time of its telling. A doubling of temporalities is also fundamental to the recursive operation of reentry in the looping operations through which subjective referrals antedate and organize the timing of conscious experience. Cognitive processes that were temporally homogeneous and globally hypersynchronized could not give rise to the doublings that make possible nested thought or the interaction of discourse and story.

These doublings can take a variety of forms and have a range of different consequences in cognitive experience and in narrative. When discourse and story reinforce each other, the process of subjective referral is facilitated; when they veer off and diverge, the possibility emerges of interruptions and disjunctions through which the ordinarily invisible temporal operations of recursive pattern formation can come into view. The discourse-story opposition has within it the potential of either promoting the construction of narrative syntheses or supporting metafictional reflection because the temporal gaps that begin at the neuronal level can either be smoothed over through subjective referrals or give rise to the recursive nesting of cognitive operations that is responsible for self-consciousness, the doubling of living forward and understanding backward.

The temporal disjunctions typical of modern fiction expose this doubling in ways that may provoke reflection about the cognitive paradoxes of time. What Joseph Frank (1991 [1945, 1977]) famously calls the "spatial form" characteristic of much modern literature experiments with the temporality of narrative configuration in order to lay bare recursive, to-and-fro cognitive processes that ordinarily pass unnoticed. Frank recalls Lessing's classic argument in *Laocoön* (1962 [1766], 78) that painting and sculpture are spatial arts that should depict "only a single moment of an action" by juxtaposing parts in a simultaneous whole ("signs existing in space can express only objects whose wholes or parts coexist," Lessing argues), whereas the temporal art of narrative should depict the sequential unfolding of an action ("signs that follow one another can express only objects whose wholes or parts are consecutive"). According to Frank, the disjunctions of *Ulysses* and other modern novels that interrupt sequential, temporal coherence are "based on a space-logic" that turns Lessing upside down: "The meaning-relationship is completed only by the simultaneous perception in space of word-groups that have no comprehensible relation to each other when read consecutively in time" (15). Spatial juxtaposition replaces temporal sequence as the principle of narrative organization: "Joyce cannot be read—he can only be reread" because "a knowledge of the whole is essential to an understanding of any part," and "such knowledge can be obtained only after the book has been read, when all the references are fitted into their proper places and grasped as a unity" (21).

Frank's argument unleashed a fury of responses by critics and theorists who pointed out (among other things) that temporal processes of construal underlie our apprehension of the pictorial arts and that the retrospective construction of meaningful patterns prompted by modernist juxtaposition is itself a temporal activity.[12] These objections are of course valid. As neuroscientist Arthur P. Shimamura observes, even seemingly spatial works of art like a painting or a sculpture are comprehended temporally: "It takes time to experience art, as we cannot appreciate an artwork fully within a single eye fixation. We therefore *interpret* an artwork by successive glances, and this storyboard of experiences takes some time, about three fixations per second" (2013a, 125; original emphasis). Our cognitive habits for processing temporal and spatial works—how we "read" literature and the visual arts—are consequently capable of interacting and affecting one another. For example, although ordinarily "we seem to scan paintings from left to right, perhaps with an upward glance, thus starting from the bottom left and moving to the top right," Shimamura points out that "such biases appear to be guided by reading behavior," inasmuch as "Israeli and Arabic readers adopt a right-left scanning bias during picture viewing and show the opposite aesthetic preferences than those who read from left to right" (91, 92).

What was often missed in the controversy, however, are Frank's many acknowledgments that spatial form strains the reader's cognitive capacities and works against our natural, habitual practices of sensemaking, and that this is precisely because of the fundamental temporality of those processes. The disorientation and bewilderment that modernist formal experiments may cause are evidence that sensemaking entails temporal configuration, and so the question is not whether these works ever achieve "spatiality" but what purposes might be served by the incoherences produced by such an impossible quest. At least one answer is that they call attention to the processes of patternmaking that are impeded, interrupted, and blocked, promoting reflection by thwarting immersion in a coherent, self-consistent world. Spatial form does not escape or transcend time, then, but makes its otherwise invisible workings visible for inspection and contemplation—and one might even observe that the insistence of Frank's critics on the omnipresence of temporality is evidence that it has quite effectively done so.

This, then, is the cognitive takeaway from the spatial form debate: the back-and-forth construction of coherence through subjective referral and temporal antedating ordinarily goes without notice (as it does in conventionally realistic fiction), but the doublings, nestings, and shiftings of the brain's balancing act become visible when its recursive processes are interfered with (as in the experiments of modernism), and then the tension between stability and instability may come into view. In Faulkner's *Sound and the Fury*, for example, the disjunctions between the four nonconsecutive sections of the novel, compounded by the temporal leaps that Benjy's and Quentin's minds repeatedly make, unsettle the reader's sense of temporal coherence and expose the contingency and instability of our interpretive constructions. This unease may surprisingly if understandably make the reader feel relieved when the certainty of the bigoted, misogynist Jason announces itself: "Once a bitch always a bitch, what I say" (1994 [1929], 113). We finally know where we are, but the fixity of this self-certainty is unsettling not only because it is morally repulsive but also because it belies the contingency of pattern formation that the temporal disjunctions of the narrative expose. The sometimes incoherent fluidity of Benjy's and Quentin's narratives takes to disabling extremes the instabilities of the brain's balancing act between pattern and openness, but the rigid prejudice and self-defeating, paralyzing resentment of Jason's viewpoint give readers a visceral experience of the straightjacket of entrenched, immovable habit. The temporal disjunctions of Faulkner's narrative may make the reader long for coherence and dramatize the cognitive need for pattern, but once we have it, we don't want it, because it is presented in so debilitating a manner. The experiments of other great modernists may foreground different aspects of temporality—the malleability of subjective time as the years pass in Thomas Mann's epic *The Magic Mountain*, for example, or the horizonality of past and present in Virginia Woolf's elegiac *To the Lighthouse*—but a defining characteristic of spatial form is that it blocks temporal processes of cognitive pattern formation, not to overcome them, but to play with them and expose them to view.

Temporalities of Integration in Cognition, Narrative, and Reading

One of the paradoxes of time is that it combines both segmentation and integration. Time passes as a series of identifiable perceptual windows that flow into each other and are seamlessly joined together. The now is a perceptual gestalt, different from the past and the future, even as it is inextricably linked to what was and what will be across its retentional and protentional horizons. Narratives are similarly a paradoxical combination of separate segments that are integrated into an overall pattern. What Ricoeur (1980b, 169, 171) calls "the illusion of sequence" requires the construction of an "intelligible whole that governs a succession of events in any story," but this whole only does its configurative work if the elements it binds retain their distinctiveness. As Ricoeur (1980b, 178) notes, there is a fundamental, necessary tension between "the episodic dimension" of a narrative (the events of a story) and "the configurational dimension": "the plot construes significant wholes out of scattered events," but "the configurational dimension cannot overcome the episodic dimension without suppressing the narrative structure itself." In a circular manner (the narrative equivalent of the hermeneutic circle), the parts of a narrative constitute a whole even as the whole configures the parts. The tension that holds together these two dimensions (the episodic and the configurational) without collapsing them into each other is one aspect of the concordant discordance that characterizes narrative.

Basic tensions between the elements of any narrative and their organization occur across different temporalities of integration and segmentation, different scales at which binding and framing happen, from the sentence level up through the construction of the work as a whole. These interactions take advantage of what Buonomano calls "the brain's exquisite ability to process complex temporal patterns" (2014, 330). As Sylvie Droit-Volet (2014, 482) points out, "The mechanisms for processing short and long durations are different." These mechanisms interact in complex, reciprocal ways in ordinary cognitive activity and in our processing of narratives—a pattern of "upward and downward causation" on "multiple spatial and temporal scales where on one hand, activity on a lower scale gives rise to an emergent phenomenon and on the other hand, the large-scale patterns have the potential to re-influence the small-scale interactions that generated them" (Bagdasaryian and Le Van Quyen 2013, 4). Merlin Donald (2012, 40–41) distinguishes between "three levels of temporal integration": "local binding" that occurs "from fractions of a second to a few seconds"; the short-term "working memory range" that lasts "a few seconds or tens of seconds," and "longer lasting neural activity" like "conversations that last for many hours and organized games of various kinds"—or, of course, telling and following stories. Each of these levels of cognitive processing combines segmentation and integration at a different temporal scale, and what happens at each level and scale interacts upward and downward with the others. This is similar to (and the condition of possibility for) the way different timescales play off of each other in narrative.

At the most basic level of cognitive processing, the tension between segmentation and integration is evident first of all in the temporal binding that occurs at the microsecond scale, beneath conscious awareness. As Niko Busch and Rufin VanRullen (2014, 163, 166, 161) observe, our sense of time as "a pseudo-continuous stream . . . is actually made up from a series of discrete snapshots"—"a continuously moving temporal integration window" that, like a camera, "integrates and fuses information for as long as the shutter is open." A panel in a graphic novel is a similar "snapshot" of time passing. As Scott McCloud points out (1993, 95), "Each panel of a comic [that] shows a single moment in time" actually includes various not necessarily simultaneous events within a window of duration, a window that can be broadened or narrowed to varying temporal widths just as a comic panel can be elongated or compressed.

This framing begins in units of integration much smaller than a comic panel can register. What Ernst Pöppel (Pöppel and Bao 2014, 247) calls the "elementary integration unit" that is the smallest temporal window where "the before-and-after relationship of stimuli . . . is not defined or definable" has been experimentally "observed in the time domain of 30 to 60 ms [milliseconds]." For example, he reports, when "experimental subjects are asked to indicate in which temporal order stimuli have been presented, such as which ear was stimulated first when both ears are stimulated by acoustic signals with a short temporal delay," the differences between these stimuli are invisible within a "temporal order threshold . . . of some tens of milliseconds," and this holds equally "for the visual, auditory, and tactile modalities" (248). As Marc Wittman (2104, 512–13) explains, "These thresholds are indicative of elementary temporal building blocks of perception, because below such a temporal threshold a succession of events, their temporal order, is not perceived." Varela (1991, 73, 75) similarly describes effects of perceptual framing that produce "a natural parsing" of visual stimuli, whereby "everything that falls within a frame will be treated by the subject as if it were within one time span." For example, he points out, two lights flashing within a span of less than 50 milliseconds appear simultaneous but then seem sequential beyond a 100-millisecond threshold, and between 50–100 milliseconds they "appear to move" from one spot to another.[13]

The paradox however, as Wittman observes, is that "our experience is not temporally punctual, a static snapshot," and "we do not perceive the world as a sequence of individual events, but as a temporally integrated whole" (513). Microsecond units of temporal framing are integrated into consciousness first at the level of half a second, the window of integration in which a sense of the subjective present begins to be available to awareness. Another level of what Wittman calls "temporal grouping" seems to occur at 2–3 seconds. As he explains, "effortless and automatic synchronization" of the repeated beats of a metronome is possible from "a lower limit of around 250 ms" to "an upper limit of approximately two seconds," but "beat perception and subjective rhythmization" break down at longer intervals (514).

According to Pöppel, whose experimental research on these questions is foundational, "It is easy to impose a subjective structure" on "click sounds [that] follow each other with[in] an interstimulus interval" of two to three seconds, but this process of automatic figuration breaks down if "the temporal interval between the stimuli becomes too long (for instance, five seconds)" and "they fall into successive integration windows" (251). The familiar temporal gestalts of Morse code, for example, exploit the mechanisms of integration at this timescale, but there also are upper and lower limits to synchronization here owing to how the dots and dashes must be grouped for them to be intelligible (an operator clicking too fast or too slow would be incomprehensible).

Ambiguous figures like the famous rabbit-duck gestalt provide further experimental evidence of automatic grouping at the 2–3 second level. For example, Pöppel observes that "if stimuli can be perceived with two perspectives (like the Necker cube, or a vase that can also be seen as two faces looking at each other) there is an automatic shift of perceptual content after an average of approximately 3 seconds" (251). This "perceptual shift also occurs with ambiguous auditory material, such as the phoneme sequence KU-BA-KU, where one hears either KUBA or BAKU; one can subjectively not avoid that after approximately 3 seconds the alternative percept takes possession of conscious content" (251). As he concludes, "Metaphorically speaking, every 2 to 3 seconds, an endogenously generated question arises regarding 'what is new'" (251).

The neurobiological basis of this formation, dissolution, and re-formation of windows of perception at different temporal levels is what Varela and colleagues (2001, 235, 229) describe as an "alternation or balance between phase synchronization and phase scattering" of "neural assemblies" that are "transiently linked by dynamic connections." As Evan Thompson (2007, 335) explains, there is "suggestive evidence that long-distance phase synchronization and desynchronization may subserve the temporal parsing of cognition into coherent and momentary acts." This synchronization and scattering, fundamental to the brain's balancing act between stability and instability, happens in windows of temporal grouping at different timescales—at the 30–60 millisecond level, at the 500 millisecond interval for consciousness, and in larger gestalts at the 2–3 second range—as well as in a to-and-fro interaction between these different temporal integration units. These fluctuations between different timescales of segmentation and integration make possible what Marcus Raichle (2011, 9) calls "the dynamic interplay between the brain's ongoing rhythms and its ever-changing environment."

Windows of perception, attention, and awareness operate at different timescales, and these windows interact, forming and dissolving, in ongoing, ever-shifting patterns of synchronization and scattering. These interactions occur across the entire range of the brain's fluctuations, beginning with micro-scale neuronal spiking and the preconscious perceptual binding of stimuli and continuing up to the synchronization and dissolution of long-range assemblies across various sensory regions and between the brain and the body—all of the different interlocking, reciprocally formative, to-and-fro movements of what György Buzsáki (2006) memorably calls the "rhythms of the brain." That neuroscientists would resort to a musical analogy to describe these interactions is not accidental. The temporalities of segmentation and integration in the brain's fluctuations are less like the linear steps of a computer algorithm than the shifting, reciprocally interacting relations between musicians in an orchestra who all play different parts that resonate together in patterns that form, dissolve, and re-form over the course of a performance.

The patterns of segmentation and integration that characterize these rhythms are the neural basis of the episodic and configurational dimensions of narrative, which similarly entail reciprocally formative windows that group events at different interlocking, interacting timescales. Narrative, like other temporal arts, is what Tim van Gelder (1999, 252) calls "a dynamical system," which, unlike a linear computational model, "is a set of quantities evolving interdependently over time," bounded segments interacting as they become integrated into larger patterns of figuration at different temporal levels. As van Gelder observes: "Here's the puzzle: if at any given time I am just aware of the part of the song playing now, how can I ever be aware of the song as an integrated piece that takes place over time?" (245). We temporally bind the unit of the melody that we hear at the moment (on the 2–3 second scale) because the sounds form a temporal gestalt that we recognize (think, for example, of the memorable opening four notes of Beethoven's Fifth Symphony), but in and through these distinctive units we also perceive the melody as a whole: "When you listen to a melody, you do not have to wait around until the melody is finished in order to hear it as a melody" (247)—or to recognize the tune and change the channel on the radio or skip ahead on your playlist because it's not what you're in the mood to listen to.

Plots are similarly composed of subunits (events, episodes, conflicts) that horizonally project the larger configurations they suggest (a picaresque journey, a novel of education, a romance, a detective story, etc.), and these larger patterns, as they take shape, can in turn refigure our understanding of their components. This interaction of configurative patterns at different timescales enacts in narrative form the basic paradox of neurally based temporality—the inherent duality of segmentation and integration in the brain's rhythms, discontinuous "snapshots" that give rise to a continuous stream of experience. What Ricoeur calls the basic tension in narrative between its episodic and configurational dimensions is possible because the brain processes time in a contradictory manner both as distinct windows and as an integrated, rhythmic flow.

The duality of segmentation and integration in the temporality of cognitive processing undergirds the brain's perpetual balancing act between pattern and change—what Dehaene (2014, 189) calls its state of perpetually "unstable equilibrium." As he explains, this neurobiological balancing act is what makes possible "exploratory behavior" as spontaneously generated "fluctuating patterns of activity" synchronize, scatter, and re-form (189). At a variety of temporal levels, windows of structuration impose gestalts on the flux of stimuli only to give way to other syntheses that in turn are just temporary equilibria in an ongoing alternation between stability and instability, ever-changing phases of synchronization and scattering and resynchronization. If brain time were simply a continuous flow, we would not alternate between patterns of assembly and disassembly, but if temporal gestalts did not regularly, automatically fade and re-form, we would be stuck forever in one shape and be unable to explore, adapt, and change.

Narrative can be an effective instrument for organizing experience and exploring the world because it too plays stability and instability off each other at different levels of temporal organization. Temporal patterns of segmentation and integration characterize both the telling and the told. As James Phelan (2002, 211) points out, there are "two main kinds of instabilities" in narrative: "Those occurring within the story, instabilities between characters, created by situations, and resolved through actions," and "those created by the discourse, instabilities . . . of value, belief, opinion, knowledge, expectation" informing the pattern of narration and structuring the relation between the narrator and the recipient. In a plot, for example, a pattern is established only to be upset, overturned, and replaced by a new configuration in a temporary equilibrium that is open to subsequent dislodging. Todorov (1969, 75) has something like this in mind when he famously argues that "the minimal complete plot can be seen as the shift from one equilibrium to another, . . . two moments of equilibrium, similar and different, [that] are separated by a period of imbalance, which is composed of a process of degeneration and a process of improvement." This alternation between equilibrium and disequilibrium is not just a once-and-done effect of the overall course of the story but may happen over and over again as the plot sets up conflicts, resolves them, only to introduce new complications. A plot is constructed by the repeated creation, dissolution, and re-formation of temporal windows of integration.

Shifting patterns of equilibrium and disequilibrium characterize not only the story but also the discourse. Here too our cognitive ability to process alternating windows of integration may be put into play. An extreme case is unreliable narration, where readers may come to wonder whether the narrator is misleading them, either deliberately or unknowingly. Unreliable narration is only an especially visible instance of the different degrees of balance and imbalance that are possible in the interaction between the telling and the following of a story over the time course of the narrative. At the level of discourse, in the way a story is presented over time, a manner of telling proposes a pattern of organization or a mode of seeing that may then in turn be confirmed or challenged and questioned by what is told, as when we begin to doubt a questionably reliable narrator's version of events: is the supposition that ghosts are threatening to corrupt the children in *The Turn of the Screw* a more plausible configuration of the evidence, for example, than the suspicion that the governess who is telling us the story is beset by anxieties and unconscious desires that generate sexually charged fantasies? A shift in the reader's attitude toward the discourse (believing or doubting the narrator) may then refigure the pattern he or she sees in the events of the story.

The equilibrium between the story and the discourse is potentially unstable and open to alteration and re-formation as one window of the telling gives way to another and these perspectives blend (or do not). At what point do we shift from one gestalt (ghost story) to another (hysterical governess), or do we go back and forth between them? In *Lord Jim*, similarly, each time Marlow gets a different view of Jim from another of the many informants he consults (for example, the French lieutenant's take on Jim as a scoundrel who deserves condemnation for his breach of honor, or Stein's perspective on the young man as a romantic who merits sympathy), the narration offers a temporary window of integration that the recipient may accept or question, only to have it dislodged by the next window the narrator offers. Is Jim simply guilty of criminal conduct, or is he an example of the nobility and fragility of the capacity for dreaming and imagining that all of us share? Marlow's struggles to reconcile opposing interpretations of Jim in his narration are consequently as intriguing or disturbing (or both) as the story he is trying to tell. The shifting perspectives of the discourse challenge the reader's attempts to integrate them, and these disjunctions make Conrad's novel especially interesting for narrative theory by foregrounding what are usually invisible processes. Synthesis and scattering, segmentation and integration, units of interpretation and their interaction across the temporal unfolding of the narrative—these fundamental dualities of the temporality of cognitive processing characterize both the story and the discourse.

Just as the brain is constantly balancing the competing claims of stability and instability, pattern and change, so the shifting windows of integration in the tale and its telling entail an ongoing alternation between the imposition of patterns and their dissolution and reformation. According to Ellen Spolsky (2015, xxiv), stories and other "works of the imagination . . . help us keep our balance in a changing and often threatening world" and "contribute to the biological work of homeostasis. We are not stable in the way stones are stable, but we are evolved to maintain sufficient stability by sensing and repairing instabilities." This is, however, only half of the story of narratives and of cognitive life. Instabilities and imbalances that keep us open to changes in the world's patterns are also necessary as we adjust, explore, and create in an ever-varying environment. The temporality of cognition is characterized by ongoing rhythms of pattern formation, dissolution, and reformation, and these processes of stabilization and destabilization, synthesis and disruption, synchronization and scattering, are also integral to the construction of stories and their narration.

This necessary tension between equilibrium and disequilibrium is one reason why the endings of stories have received so much attention from narrative theory (see Kermode 1967 and Torgovnick 1981). As narratologists have often noted, closure in fiction is not a permanent imposition of stability because any ending is susceptible to reopening and may give rise to new beginnings. Closure may not necessarily be closed. Conversely, however, as Peter Rabinowitz (2002, 308) notes, "lack of closure does not mean lack of conclusion." An ending may establish a state of equilibrium at the level of the discourse ("That's all, folks") while leaving much unsettled in the story ("Did they live happily ever after or not?"). A classic case is the ending of *The Portrait of a Lady* where, as James himself acknowledged, the uncertain consequences of Isabel's decision to return to Rome leave him open to the "obvious criticism" that the novel "is not finished—that I have not seen the heroine to the end of her situation—that I have left her *en l'air*" (1987, 15). But as James memorably explained, "This is both true and false. The *whole* of anything is never told; you can only take what groups together" (15).

Ending is a temporal moment of integration that "groups together" elements in an inherently contingent, only seemingly stable equilibrium that is open to reorganization. This is why Phelan (2002, 214) distinguishes between "closure" and "completeness": "Closure . . . refers to the way in which a narrative signals its end, whereas completeness refers to the degree of resolution accompanying the closure." A narrative conclusion may be characterized by varying degrees of completeness, resolution, and openness, just as any temporal binding of a gestalt at whatever level of temporal organization is a more or less stable equilibrium in the ongoing alternation between segmentation and integration, more or less firmly fixed by previous cognitive activity and consequently more or less likely to give way to a different configuration. Similar tensions between equilibrium and disequilibrium characterize the different temporal structures of emplotment, narration, and ending because these are all ways in which narrative plays with the brain's perpetual balancing act between stability and instability, its fluctuations between synchronization and phase scattering at local and global levels of binding and everywhere in between.

The temporality of narrative piggybacks on processes of segmentation and integration that characterize cognition in general and the reading process in particular. As Genette (1980, 34) observes, "The narrative text, like every other text, has no other temporality than what it borrows, metonymically, from its own reading." The smallest units of temporal synthesis, from the microsecond level up to the 2–3 second integration window, correspond to the processing of letters and phonemes into words and words into sentences. Even at these levels of text processing, comprehension is configurative—a reciprocally formative grouping together of features into a gestalt. As Dehaene (2009, 49) explains, "Word decoding does not proceed in a strictly sequential manner, and the time needed to read a word is not related to the number of letters that it contains," as it would be if reading were a linear, additive process. According to linguist I. M. Schlesinger (1968, 42), "Decoding proceeds in 'chunks' rather than in units of single words, and . . . these 'chunks' correspond to the syntactic units of the sentence." Wolfgang Iser (1978, 110) points out, however, that these units in turn are not self-contained because "each sentence can achieve its end only by aiming at something beyond itself." Reading a narrative (or any text, for that matter) entails an ongoing alternation between what Iser calls "theme" and "horizon" that "actively involves the reader in the process of synthesizing an assembly of constantly shifting viewpoints," ever-changing perspectives that "not only modify one another but also influence past and future syntheses" (97).

This is not unlike ordinary, everyday perception where, as Gibson (1979, 66) notes, "a point of observation is never stationary, . . . and observation is typically made from a moving position." What Iser calls "the continual switching of perspectives during the time-flow" of reading (97) is a special case of the general rule that "observation implies movement" (Gibson 1979, 72), but this switching can also create unique effects characteristic of narrative. As Iser points out, "the wandering viewpoint" of the reader is "situated in a particular perspective during every moment of reading, but . . . it is not confined to that perspective" and "constantly shifts between" angles of observation in a "process of reciprocal spotlighting" that "offsets and relates" the shifting viewpoints that the reader occupies (114). In a mimetic fiction, for example, "the accumulation of views and combinations gives us the illusion of depth and breadth, so that we have the impression that we are actually present in a real world" characterized by an event-like happening as perspectives change and interact (97). Sometimes, as in a modernist text like *Ulysses* or a postmodern work like *Infinite Jest*, the "kaleidoscope of perspectives" (113) may multiply so variously and resist integration so playfully (or stubbornly and annoyingly, depending on your sensibility) that they become foregrounded in their own right, not merely serving as means to representational ends, and the temporality of integration may then emerge from invisibility, transformed from a passive process into an active topic for contemplation because its smooth flow has been interrupted. Or the temporal interplay of theme and horizon may give rise to various effects of ironic doubling as "two perspectives throw each other into distinct relief" (117) and disclose one another's defining limitations, whether for tragic or comic effect. Narrative irony is a temporal form that depends on the interaction between segmentation and integration as it sets alternative windows against each other in the time of reading.

These oft-discussed characteristics of narrative exploit the ability of the brain to form moments of integration of varying width and to relate them to one another in alternating patterns of synchronization and dispersal. A tension between segmentation and integration is pervasive in narrative, as it is fundamental to the temporality of cognitive life. The theme in focus at any given moment is a temporal gestalt (a window of integration), but it is then configuratively joined across its horizons to receding viewpoints immediately past and to perspectives anticipated ahead. What it would be like if these windows did not interact but instead existed in isolation is suggested by cases of motion agnosia, where the afflicted person "experiences the world as seemingly without motion, frozen in place, for several seconds. Things in the world may then suddenly seem to rearrange themselves in new positions" (Gallagher and Zahavi 2012, 78), making it difficult if not impossible to engage in routine acts like pouring a cup of coffee or crossing a street. Motion agnosia casts the segmentation of temporal windows into distressingly bold relief by disrupting their prereflective, ordinarily invisible integration.

The narrative equivalent of motion agnosia would produce disjointed episodes not connected by configurative emplotment or would offer up juxtaposed perspectives not organized by the discourse into coherent patterns. This kind of discordance without concordance is, of course, precisely the effect aimed for by the disjointed textual structures of many so-called unnatural narratives, disjunctions that subvert the reader's expectations of mimetic consistency (the surreal disconnections of Djuna Barnes' *Nightwood*, for example, or the shifting dreamscape of Calvino's *If on a Winter's Night a Traveler*). Just as motion agnosia is only understandable as a disturbance of ordinary processes of temporal integration, however, so the disruptions of unnatural narrative once again depend for their effect on the "natural" functions of cognitive patternmaking that they suspend, discordantly foregrounding the segmentation of narrative that is usually invisible because synthesized concordantly.

The Neuroscience of Memory and Forgetting

As narrative theorists have long recognized, the ability to follow a story depends on the connective glue of memory. Hence Aristotle's (1990 [355 BCE], 9) understandable if perhaps overly rigid assertion that "the length of a plot should be such as can be easily retained in memory." The cognitive intuition behind Aristotle's claim is that narrative integration requires the capacity to make and remember connections between temporally distributed segments. Although much narrative comprehension is subliminal and occurs beneath awareness, forging these connections, especially over longer timescales, would be impossible without explicit, conscious memories. As Dehaene (2014, 103) points out, "Subliminal thoughts last only for an instant," whereas "a temporally extended working memory requires consciousness." According to Dehaene, consequently, "we need to be conscious in order to rationally think through a problem" with multiple steps that have to be held in memory (108).

For example, solving a complicated problem in arithmetic (adding or subtracting a sequence of numbers) is something we can only do because we are conscious and can therefore remember its various steps. But this is also true of a story that is composed of different episodes and that, as it is told, passes through different phases of equilibrium and disequilibrium. Consciousness is consequently not an epiphenomenon irrelevant to the deep structures of narrative as some versions of structural narratology suggest (recall Ann Banfield's claim, for example, that we can understand stories only because of homologies at the level of "universal grammar" between narratives

and our preconscious minds). Although many of the effects of narrative occur subliminally, beneath awareness, it is also true that only a being en-
dowed with consciousness and the capacity it supports to hold together
multiple elements in memory would have the ability to tell and follow a
story. Without consciousness we would not have narratives at all. One answer to the oft-asked question, "Why have we evolved to have consciousness?" is that consciousness allows us to tell each other stories, and that is
something that gives our species all sorts of competitive advantages (see
Humphrey 2006 and Boyd 2009).

Perhaps paradoxically, the ability to forget is also essential to forging temporal syntheses in everyday cognition and in narrative. As Yadin Dudai
(2011, 36, 37) observes, "Memories too robust are a potential disadvantage,
as they may not fit anymore to guide the proper action and reaction in a
changing environment"; "too rigid a memory may lead to poor imagination,
one that plays scenarios of the future that are only similar to the past."
What Daniel Schacter (2002) famously calls "the seven sins of memory"—
"transience, absent-mindedness, blocking, misattribution, suggestibility,
bias, and persistence"—are not necessarily flaws but may be cognitively beneficial. His list of "sins" reflects the brain's never-ending balancing act between stability and instability—the recurrence of patterns from the past
("persistence," "bias") versus their contingency and susceptibility to variation ("transience," "absent-mindedness"). As Alcino J. Silva (2011, 49) argues, "Memory mechanisms are designed, not for accuracy and permanency,
but instead, for constant editing and fine-tuning of information with experience." The defects of memory may be functional and not maladaptive
because they support this "editing and fine-tuning." The temporality of the
brain once again reflects a double imperative. If memories did not preserve
cognitive configurations, we would be lost in the flux, but a perfect memory
would lock us into past patterns and make us resistant to change, whereas
our fallible, unstable recollections support cognitive flexibility.

The shifting patterns of equilibrium and disequilibrium characteristic of
narrative comprehension similarly require an ability not only to remember
but also to cast aside and revise previous configurations. Following a story
is a balancing act between memory and forgetting as patterns form and re-
form in shifting relations of stability and instability. In *Great Expectations*,
for example, Dickens relies on our forgetting Pip's youthful act of kindness
toward an escaped convict on the marshes in order to lull us into sharing his
hopes about his presumed benefactor Miss Havisham and her ward Estella—
but then our surprise when Magwitch announces himself as the true source
of Pip's fortune reminds us of what we may have forgotten. The snares we

fell for took advantage of our forgetfulness—otherwise we would not be surprised by Magwitch's revelations—but we can then edit and revise our understanding by recalling and readjusting our memories of Pip's past (just as he has had to do) and see how he (and we) had misled ourselves by unjustified expectations. The "sins" of memory make us vulnerable to the snares Dickens uses to misdirect our attention, but they also give us the flexibility to balance and rebalance shifting patterns of integration in response to changes in life and in stories, as we do when we revise and reedit our sense of the connections between events.

The usefulness of a fallible memory has led a growing number of cognitive scientists to recognize that our ability to remember the past is closely linked to our capacity to imagine the future. As Terence Cave (2016, 74) notes, experimental evidence convincingly shows that "memory and imagination are not, as earlier faculty psychologists believed, separate domains, but different aspects of the same cognitive processes." Schacter and Addis (2007, 773) observe, for example, that the liability of memory to "various kinds of errors and illusions" also allows it to support the imaginative simulation of future events, which "requires a system that can draw on the past in a manner that flexibly extracts and recombines elements of previous experiences." Citing lesion studies that show "an overlap between deficits of remembering and envisioning the future," Randy L. Buckner and David C. Carroll (2007, 51, 49) posit "a core brain network" or "common set of processes by which past experiences are used adaptively to imagine perspectives and events beyond those that emerge from the immediate environment." This has come to be called the "default mode network" (DMN) because it was first discovered by analyses of fMRI scans of the brain at rest, when it was not engaged in any specific attentive activity (its "default" condition). As Robert Stickgold (2011, 90) explains, the "resting or 'default' brain state" entails "envisioning the future, . . . remembering the past, . . . conceiving the viewpoint of others, . . . and spatial navigation." These interactions between remembering and imagining suggest, he argues, that "narrative construction is the default mode of the brain" (90).

The neuroscientists may have found these links surprising, but cognitive literary critics were quick to point out that they are not news to anyone familiar with the history of aesthetics. As cognitive theorist and historian of romanticism Alan Richardson (2011, 670, 665) was among the first to observe, the "Janus hypothesis" that sees "retrospection into the past and prospection into the future" as two sides of the same coin is widely attested by "centuries of literary scholarship on imagination." Ignoring this history, he argues, "has made for an impoverished scientific agenda" (665). Our ability to engage in what neuroscientists call "mental time travel" (Sudden-dorf and Corballis 2007)—our dual capacity to recall the past and imagine possible futures—will be familiar to anyone who has read "Tintern Abbey" (1798) or any of Wordsworth's many other poems about memory and imagination.

This coupling of retrospection and prospection extends across our cog-nitive life, from everyday daydreaming to aesthetic experiences of various kinds, and these connections suggest why it is a commonplace of discussions of literary imagination to relate daydreaming to creativity as Freud (1958 [1908]) does, for example, in his classic essay on the psychological sources of poetry. Indeed, neurobiologically trained literary theorist Gabrielle Starr (2013, 23), who has had an active collaboration with brain scientists at New York University, conducted experiments that showed measurable increases in the activity of the default mode network not only in internally-oriented acts of daydreaming but also in response to "intensely powerful aesthetic experiences" provoked by external stimuli (such as seeing a painting, hear-ing a musical composition, or reading a story). This stands in marked con-trast to the DMN's response to ordinary tasks requiring attention to exter-nal stimuli, during which its "activity generally decreases," and this evidence "suggests that powerful aesthetic experience calls on the brain to integrate external perceptions [our response to the artwork] with the inner senses" by drawing on the ordinarily inner-directed capacities of the DMN (Starr 2013, 23; for the original experiment, see Vessel, Starr, and Rubin 2012). Such in-tegration requires to-and-fro interactions between cortical areas devoted to memory and imagination and those involved in attention and perception.

Just as narrative comprehension occurs on various timescales, so memory itself is not uniform, either neurobiologically or experientially. As Shaun Gallagher and Dan Zahavi (2008, 70–71) point out, "Memory is not a single faculty of mind. Rather, it is composed of a variety of distinct and dissocia-ble properties," and fMRI scans show that "different parts of [the] brain appear to be particularly active depending on the type of memory task [we] are engaged in." Neuroscientists distinguish, for example, between short-term memories that may last from seconds to minutes to hours and long-term memories that may extend over days and weeks and may then become consolidated over a lifetime (see Baars and Gage 2010, 324–25). The differ-ences between short- and long-term memories have to do with how engrams, the anatomical basis of memories, are formed and reshaped and reinforced. Engrams are patterns of neuronal assembly that become established through repeated Hebbian firing and wiring—how neurons that fire together, wire together—in short-term processes of varying duration. These patterns may then become more enduring as they are reinforced through repetition and consolidated by various metabolic processes (during sleep, for example) and by specialized parts of the cortical anatomy like the hippocampus (see Bear, Connors, and Paradiso 2007, 725–59).

Cognitive scientists further distinguish between different kinds of memory based on the abilities they support—for example, between declarative memory, on the one hand, which can be semantic (that is, memory of facts) or episodic (memory of events), and nondeclarative memory, on the other, which is typically not fully available to consciousness, and that includes subliminal priming effects, emotional dispositions, habits, and procedural memories (skills like swimming, typing, or riding a bicycle) (see Baars and Gage 2010, 326). As well-known cases in the neuroscience literature attest, it is possible to lose one form of memory but retain others. A patient who suffers a stroke that blocks the retrieval of semantic or episodic memories, for example, may still be able to perform various skilled tasks that draw on procedural memories.[14]

These categories are somewhat fuzzy and the boundaries between them are fluid, and necessarily so. Memories pass from one form into another as different processes of integration and consolidation interact. For example, working memory is "a temporary form of information storage that is limited in capacity," usually encompassing five to seven items, but it can change from short- to long-term memory through repetition and rehearsal (Bear, Connor, and Paradiso 2007, 729). The distinction between episodic and semantic memories is similarly both fixed and fluid. Episodic memories typically "have a specific source in time, space, and life circumstances" and "are often autobiographical in nature," whereas semantic memories have to do with "facts about the world, about ourselves, and about other knowledge that we share with a community" (Baars and Gage 2010, 325–26). But these two kinds of memory are often related and combined. As Baars and Gage point out, for example, "semantic memories may be the neocortical residue of many episodic memories" (328) as particular instances are forgotten and "only the semantic knowledge remains." Experiments have also shown that "performance on semantic tests is better if the participant also has some episodic memory associated" with the question—an image of a celebrity from a film or a TV show one has seen, for example, as opposed to a famous name that evokes no particular episodic recollection (Baars and Gage 2010, 329; see Westmacott et al. 2004). Even though I can only remember a few of the tennis matches I played in my youth, those episodes inflect my semantic memory of tennis, and neurons in my motor cortex associated with the acts of hitting a tennis ball are also probably activated in response to viewing matches or even reading about the sport (see Jeannerod 2006, Rizzolatti and Craighero 2004, and Rizzolatti and Sinigaglia 2008). And so when I watch a Wimbledon final, my procedural, episodic, and semantic memories all interact.

One of the functions of narrative is to coordinate the different processes of memory and thereby to cultivate our ability to engage in processes of binding and integration across different timescales. Episodic, semantic, and procedural memories are all involved, for example, in the five narrative codes that Roland Barthes identifies in *S/Z* (1974), his classic structural analysis of Balzac's story "Sarrasine." For example, the code of actions (ACT) is intelligible only because our procedural memories interact with specific episodic recollections and learned semantic categories for various kinds of action. The deployment of enigmas and the revelation of "truth" in the hermeneutic code (HER) is primarily semantic, but it also requires an interaction between short-term and long-term memory across the ever-shifting boundaries of working memory, and these processes of integration will range from subliminal priming effects to explicit, conscious acts of episodic and semantic recollection. The three codes that Barthes claims are exempt from temporal sequence—the designation of "semes" (SEM), or signifiers of people, places, and things; the "cultural codes" of conventional wisdom (REF); and the antitheses (SYM) structuring the oppositions in the text—all draw on memories of different kinds and so are not really outside of the time of textual processing.

The "weaving of the codes," as Barthes describes it, that configures a particular text creates a temporal object that is a structure of memory and anticipation. Like a melody, a narrative consequently has a peculiar mode of existence that is neither completely reducible to the moments through which it passes nor entirely independent of them. Neither autonomous from its transient, ephemeral manifestations nor merely dependent on them, a narrative or a melody is a "heteronomous" object that we initially create in and through temporal experiences of anticipation and retrospection and that we are then able afterwards to recollect in various forms and from different perspectives (see Armstrong 1990, 20–43). This temporal heteronomy is especially visible, for example, in the paradoxical existence of a literary character like Isabel Archer or Marlow or Pip, whom we can designate and discuss without having to reproduce all of the sentences out of which they arose. These memorable characters would not exist without those sentences, but we can analyze them and talk about them without having to recite these word by word. Like a literary character, a narrative is a temporal object with a heteronomous existence because it is a construction of memory.

The ability to integrate temporal processes across various timescales—from microsecond binding at the neuronal level up through long-term declarative memories linking brain, body, and world—is necessary to create complex heteronomous objects like a narrative, a fictional character, or a symphony. Merlin Donald (2012, 39) argues that our species has developed a "slow process" of "intermediate-term governance" between the moment-to-moment binding of short-term working memory and the consolidations of long-term memory that uniquely equips us to produce and exchange such heteronomous objects. Longer than the moment-to-moment problem-solving of short-term working memory but more flexible and open-ended than long-term memory, this "slow process" of temporal integration, as he calls it, involves extended to-and-fro synthesizing activities that "can operate over long time frames" and require "a vastly extended working memory system" whose "prime function is to enable the mind to comprehend and navigate the multifaceted social-cognitive world that human beings inhabit" (38).

These mid-range powers of temporal integration undergird the human capacity for engaging in socially coordinated transactions like telling and following stories. Donald observes that "the capacity to achieve temporal integration on this scale seems to be absent in apes" (38) and our other close primate relatives, and he points out that it is necessary for "the comprehension of extended human social scenarios that engage several agents in interaction" (37) over hours at a time beyond what either short- or long-term memories typically entail—distributed, collaborative cognitive activities like exchanging stories, performing or listening to a symphony, or conducting a conversation. Activities like these require the coordination of "lengthy episodic experiences" that exceed the "pre-existing primate capacity for temporal integration" (36) in visual, aural, and haptic perception. According to Donald, "We have no good neural model of the activation or localization of such a long-lasting process" at an intermediate scale and (at least as yet) no firm empirical evidence of "a class of active neural traces that can last for hours on end governing decisions and maintaining the general direction of behavior and thought"—"yet this class of trace must exist," he argues, "given the overwhelming evidence of autonomous sustained imagination, thought, and planning in human social life" (39).

The limitations of available brain-scanning technologies make it impossible to map the locations and interactions that characterize these mid-range, transactional processes, and so this gap in the evidence is not surprising. The technologies would need to have more temporal sensitivity and precision than fMRI measures of changes of blood flow in the brain and more anatomical precision than EEG readings of intracranial electronic activity off of sensors attached to the skull. Scanning methods would also need to map longer durations than these instruments can easily accommodate (imagine spending hours on end in the noisy, claustrophobic confines of an fMRI machine) and, additionally, would have to be designed to compare and calibrate these processes not just within a single brain but across two or more participants in an interaction.[15]

Whether any measuring equipment can do complete justice to the brain-body-world interactions through which we create and exchange stories is doubtful because quantitative measures inherently miss "what it is like" to have an experience that the as-if quality of narrative figuration is uniquely able to convey (see chapter 4). Still, if the technology were ever to develop sufficient sensitivity and sophistication to overcome its current limitations, a heteronomous temporal object like narrative would be a promising candidate for studying the "slow process" of mid-range temporal integration. We can tell and follow stories because our species has evolved the cognitive capacity to pass back and forth between small-scale temporal binding and long-term memories in an intermediate range of sustained, intersubjectively coordinated temporal activity. The ability of narratives to cultivate and co-ordinate these "slow processes" is in turn fundamental to the social and distributed cognition that characterizes the life of our species. Stories facilitate processes of temporal integration along a range of timescales and across a distributed social network of interacting, embodied subjects, and this is an important source of their social power.

The Temporality of Intersubjectivity and Emotion

Our sense that we share time with others is integral to the lived experience of intersubjectivity, even as our inability to fully fathom someone else's passing moment is evidence of the solipsism we can never fully overcome because we cannot know what it is like to inhabit another embodied consciousness with its own perspective on the world. The paradoxes of social time embody and enact what Merleau-Ponty (2012 [1945], lxxvi) memorably calls "the paradox of the alter ego," the peculiar combination of indubitable community and insuperable isolation that characterizes our relations with others. As he explains:

Of course, another will never exist for us as we exist for ourselves: . . . we are never present at the thrust of temporalization in him as we are in ourselves. But unlike two consciousnesses, two temporalities are not mutually incompatible, . . . because they can intertwine. . . . Since my living present opens up to a past that I nevertheless no longer live and to a future that I do not yet live, ... it can also open up to temporalities that I do not live and can have a social horizon ... [and a] collective history that my private existence takes up and carries forward. (457)

As Heidegger (1927) similarly observes, being-in-time and being-with-others are correlative existential structures. The felt analogy in our experience between the horizons of the past and future and the horizons of other worlds allows these aspects of existence to intertwine, and these interactions are crucial to the social work of narratives.

Just as we experience the passing moment as a paradoxical structure of presence and absence where past and future intersect, so we experience other embodied subjectivities as horizonal to our world, simultaneously present and absent in ways that inform and are informed by our experience of time. Others are undeniably "there," present in our worlds, inextricably related to us, with a perspective complementary to what is open to our view. But the presence of others is also anticipatory, based on expectations about how their perspectives would probably complete what is disguised from our standpoint. The horizon of the past includes experiences with others that give rise to these expectations, but this future is inherently indeterminate, not yet completely specified, and our confidence in what it may hold is based on assumptions about what others experience that necessarily lie beyond what we can ever fully sense and know.

Narratives exploit the paradoxes of intersubjective time to various effects—drawing on and reinforcing or subverting and playing with our social experience of temporal horizonality. A multiple-plot novel like *Anna Karenina*, for example, relies on the reader's sense of the overlap and interconnection between the temporalities of different worlds in order to persuade us to coordinate the developments emplotted on implicitly correlated time lines. We assume that the development of Anna and Vronsky's adultery parallels in time the starts and stops of Levin and Kitty's courtship even though these stories actually cross only occasionally. Our assumption of the horizonal intertwining of these worlds and their temporalities is so compelling, indeed, that most readers do not notice that Tolstoy got it wrong. As critics who have carefully studied the structure of the novel point out, "the timeline of the Anna and Vronsky plot is out of sync with the Kitty and Levin plot by an entire year, while Dolly's story lags behind even more" (Auyoung 2018, 17; see Alexandrov 1982). When Anna and Levin finally meet toward the end of the novel, their encounter is strictly speaking impossible because of this temporal incongruity—but its absurdity is invisible to most readers because our immersion in a coherently developing illusion draws so effectively on our everyday assumption that the gears of time join worlds together. This assumption usually operates silently in Tolstoy's novel, but sometimes it becomes explicit, as in the well-known repetition of the steeplechase scene, first from Vronsky's perspective as a participant and then from Anna's as she observes the race from the stands, a repetition that makes visible the otherwise tacit workings of intersubjective temporal horizonality by separately depicting correlated experiences of the same sequence of events.

This is also the temporal principle on which *Ulysses* is structured, with Stephen and Bloom traversing separate paths over the course of a day (Bloom first briefly spotting the young man during the drive to the cemetery) until they meet at the maternity hospital. The coordinated horizonality of intersubjectivity and time is a principle the novel makes explicit and dramatizes in the "Wandering Rocks" chapter, which maps the interactions of various characters' intersecting worlds during the regal procession, and some critics consequently view this chapter as a small-scale model of the novel as a whole (see Blamires 1996). We do not hesitate as readers to make these temporal linkages because the horizonal parallels assumed by Tolstoy's and Joyce's narratives invoke our lived experience of time as an intersubjective intertwining of distinct but coordinated temporalities.

The temporal experiments of modern fiction dramatize and play with the paradoxes of social time, but these sometimes "unnatural" effects depend once again on the "natural" cognitive processes they invoke. For example, Virginia Woolf's representation in *Mrs. Dalloway* of urban life as an intersubjective intertwining of separate, opaque worlds is reinforced by the ringing of Big Ben and the other bells of London's clocks as the narrative passes from one world to another. This "natural" effect is echoed by the artificial poetic refrain "the leaden circles dissolved in the air," which the narrator repeats as the ripples of sound cross the horizons that paradoxically join but also separate the worlds of Clarissa, Peter, Septimus, and Rezia. This recurring metaphor is both unnatural and natural, rendering in textual, figurative terms how waves of interaction (like dissolving circles) connect passing moments and intersecting worlds. It is a poetic device, created and repeated by the narrator over the time of the discourse, that has the function of forging textual connections across the different stories joined in the narrative, but it is an artifice with a natural basis because it is an attempt to suggest a physical, embodied correlative for how the temporalities of disparate, otherwise unconnected worlds are joined in intersubjective experience.

Faulkner's games with time in *Sound and the Fury* are more disruptive and subversive, but they too are a metafictional staging of the interaction between social and temporal horizonality. The challenge of aligning the temporalities of this novel's different worlds begins with the disjunctions between the dates marking the four chapters, which are titled "April Seventh, 1928," "June Second, 1910," "April Sixth, 1928," and "April Eighth, 1928" (the last of which also happens to be Easter Sunday). Dates on a calendar coordinate the passing of time socially, and the intersubjective horizonality of time is especially marked on collectively celebrated holidays (even more so a holiday with symbolic resonances of death and rebirth). Because each of these chapters anchors the narrative present in a date, the reader assumes that the time they narrate is intersubjectively shared—but how these temporalities are linked is not only thrown into question by the fact that the dates are out of sequence but also (as the reader soon discovers in the initial pages of Benjy's narration) by the narrative's jumping back and forth across time without the guideposts provided by a clock or a calendar (in narrative terms Quentin's act of smashing his watch is a redundant joke). Making sense of this disjointed narrative requires coordinating the time shared by differently experienced events repeated across the various chapters (Caddy's muddy drawers, the older Quentin's suicide, the younger Quentin's absconding with Jason's stash, etc.).

This work of intersubjective and cross-temporal consistency building is, of course, a routine aspect of following even the most ordinary story. Such invisible, everyday cognitive processing, however, is precisely what Faulkner both invokes and subverts. These disruptions in turn call attention to the coordination of differently experienced moments in our intersubjective sense of time passing—horizonal intertwinings that we ordinarily do not notice in life or in mimetic narratives because they are so familiar, but that Faulkner denaturalizes and defamiliarizes and thereby brings into view.

There is a good deal of experimental evidence demonstrating that, as Sylvie Droit-Volet (2014, 496) points out, "people who interact with one another experience a more similar passage of time than people who do not interact in the same way." Shared emotions are one basis of such interactions. As William James (1950 [1890], 1:618) observes, our feeling of time "harmonize[s] with different mental moods." A primary example of the intertwining of temporality and intersubjectivity, our emotions attune us to one another by coordinating our sense of time. When stories invoke emotional responses, they intertwine us with each other by coordinating the temporal processes through which our experience of the narrative unfolds. The social power of narrative emotions derives from their ability to intertwine our experience of time.

Whether we perceive time to be passing faster or slower, for example, will vary according to the emotion we are experiencing, and this subjective phenomenon is intersubjectively shared. Experiments have shown that anger, fear, and other threatening situations cause time to be "judged longer than normal," producing a slowdown in our sense of time passing that enhances "the automatic preparation of the organism to act or to move" (Droit-Volet 2014, 488). Not all arousal affects our sense of time in the same way, however. For example, as Droit-Volet observes, "the perception of ashamed faces has been found to produce not an overestimation but rather an underestimation of time" (491). Some of these effects are odd and counterintuitive. For example, although disgust might seem to interfere with our sense of time, experiments show that viewing disgusted faces has no effect on the ability of subjects to report time spans accurately (see Droit-Volet).

The explanations psychologists give for why time seems to pass faster or slower in these experiments are speculative, but there is impressive evidence that variations in what is called "subjective time" are not merely phantoms. Experiments have demonstrated that the emotions generated by our embodied interactions with each other and our worlds have predictable effects on our sense of how time passes, and these subjective feelings are grounded on empirically measurable "changes in bodily states" (Droit-Volet 2014, 494; see Barsalou 1999). Someone experiencing anger, fear, or a threat will predictably report that a two-minute interval felt much longer, and someone undergoing shame or guilt will more often than not sense that a five-minute span was much shorter. These phenomena are not perfectly uniform across everyone (you may be reading this and saying to yourself "not me!"), but they are not random, and they are broadly shared. These similarities are compelling evidence of how subjectively felt experiences can intertwine in shared time.

There has been considerable debate about how to categorize emotions and about whether they are culturally variable or uniform across our species. Beneath these disputes, however, the scientific consensus is that emotions are embodied cognitive processes that guide our attitudes toward the world and that coordinate our relations with one another (see Barrett 2007, 2017). The ability of emotions to do this work depends on their power to orient us temporally, and that is why the future is the tense most frequently associated with emotions. Heidegger describes emotional attunement (our mood, or *Stimmung*) as fundamentally futural because it orients our anticipatory understanding of people, texts, and other states of affairs (on the fore-structure, or *Vor-Struktur*, of understanding, see Heidegger1962 [1927], 172–95). Emotions are configurative cognitive structures that attune us to our worlds, and this attunement is intersubjective and futural. Narrative emotions coordinate our reactions to the storyworld by orienting and manipulating our expectations.

Emotion and cognition are inseparable. As Lisa Feldman Barrett (2007, 390) observes, the "brain structures" and "neural circuitry" for emotion and cognition are interconnected, overlapping, and intertwined. Unlike, say, vision and hearing, which operate through distinct, anatomically identifiable neural systems (the visual cortex as opposed to the auditory cortex), the cortical structures supporting emotions are inextricably interwoven with other cognitive processes. Consequently, as Barrett observes, "No one would ever mistake seeing for hearing (although one sensory representation might trigger another), but the same cannot be said for feeling and thinking" (390). Not simply a private, internal state of affairs, "an experience of emotion is an intentional state—it is an affective state that is about something" (379)—attuning our attention and modulating our responses to situations we encounter. Emotions have meaning and value because of their intentionality—their directedness toward people, places, and things. This orientation is inherently temporal because, like other kinds of intentionality, it anticipates a certain kind of continuation of its perspective in experiences beyond our immediate horizon. Such horizonality characterizes the emotions we experience in life as well as those invoked by the stories we hear and read.

Consider, for example, the so-called basic emotions that Paul Ekman (1999) identified and that he controversially claimed are culturally universal: anger, sadness, fear, surprise, disgust, contempt, and happiness. Ekman compiled this list by showing pictures of facial expressions to members of a tribe in a remote region of Papua New Guinea whose exposure to outside cultures had been limited, and he found that faces expressing these emotions were immediately recognized—evidence, he concluded, that they must be biologically based universals, not cultural constructs, because they had not been learned from representations in external media. Recent research about the neurobiology of emotions has cast doubt on Ekman's claims that emotions are species-wide, neurobiologically based constants (see Colombetti 2014, 25–52; Barrett 2017). It turns out that there are no "neural signatures" that clearly demarcate different emotions, and there is considerable variability in the relation between particular emotions and the neuroanatomical structures on which they are based. Fear involves many parts of the brain and the body besides the amygdala, for example, and the amygdala is involved in a range of different emotions associated with novelty and uncertainty and not just responses to threats (see Lindquist et al. 2012).

Current research suggests that emotions are not products of universal characteristics of our neural anatomy but rather that emotional responses develop as our bodies interact with our worlds, and that it is consequently impossible to separate cleanly what is learned and what is biologically inherited (see Gross 2010, Colombetti 2014, and Barrett 2017). As Merleau-Ponty (2012 [1945], 195) argues, for human beings "everything is constructed and everything is natural, in the sense that there is no single word or behavior that does not owe something to mere biological being— and, at the same time, there is no word or behavior that does not break free from animal life." As evidence for this claim, Merleau-Ponty observes that "the gesticulations of anger or love are not the same for a Japanese person and a Western person. . . . When angry, the Japanese person smiles, whereas the Westerner turns red and stamps his foot, or even turns pale and speaks with a shrill voice" (194–95). Merleau-Ponty concludes: "Having the same organs and the same nervous system is not sufficient for the same emotions to take on the same signs in two different conscious subjects. What matters is the manner in which they make use of their body, the simultaneous articulation of their body and their world in the emotion" (195). As embodied expressions, emotions are biocultural hybrids.

If Ekman's "basic emotions" are indeed widely evident around the globe, they would have become established through a combination of biological and cultural mechanisms because, in a Darwinian manner, various comparative advantages were attached to them. These advantages could have accrued only because emotions are intentional structures—that is (recalling Barrett's description), "affective states about something" in the social and natural world. In an important critique of ideas about emotion that have been very influential in the humanities although they are scientifically dubious, Ruth Leys (2011, 437) notes that many so-called affect theorists have embraced Ekman's model because, in their view, it "assumes that affective processes occur independently of intention and meaning." As Leys explains, these theorists regard "affects" as "noncognitive, corporeal processes or states," intensities that are "capable of discharging themselves in a self-rewarding or self-punishing manner without regard to the objects that elicit them"—"rapid, phylogenetically old, automatic responses of the organism that have evolved for survival purposes and lack the cognitive characteristics of the higher-order mental processes" (437–38; also see Wehrs 2017, 34–41). If emotions were "noncognitive" intensities that lack "intention and meaning," however, they could not possibly have evolutionary value, and they would not have survived. Claims for the "autonomy of affect" (see Massumi 1995, 2002) are ill equipped to account for the social work of emotions, whether over the long duration of evolutionary history or for the shorter spans of narrative interactions through which we are made to feel together about a story.

Basic emotions could proliferate and endure only if they conferred a survival advantage by helping us respond to recurrent, typical problems or opportunities, and a powerful advantage would be how they helped us and our conspecifics coordinate our responses to states of affairs in our shared worlds. These states of affairs may be objects or situations about which we feel (say) fear, surprise, or disgust, or they may be other members of our species with whom we experience (citing Ekman's other categories) sadness or happiness or for whom we feel contempt. Such emotional responses are not only intersubjective and intentional (in the sense that they are directed toward something in the world); they are also temporal, because they predispose us to act one way or another in the future (different kinds of behavior would align, for example, with anger, happiness, disgust, etc.). By intertwining intersubjectivity and temporality, emotions may convey powerful survival benefits because they can facilitate collaborative interactions. The reverse side of this coin, of course, is that emotions can also fuel destructive conflicts through this same capacity for coordinating our attunement to the world and aligning aggressive and violent responses to rivals or perceived threats. The emotions evoked by narratives can similarly have either pro- or antisocial consequences because they can intertwine our worlds toward different ends, promoting compassion or stoking fears and anxieties about matters beyond the horizons of our worlds (see Armstrong 2013, 131–74).

Whether for good or for ill, emotions are embodied intersubjective structures that attune us to our worlds, and this attunement is a temporal phenomenon that orients us toward the future. This is the case not only with so-called basic emotions but also with what Suzanne Keen (2011, 6n) calls "complex emotions" that are indisputably (and even by definition) cultural constructs: "moral sentiments (empathy and compassion) and social emotions (shame, embarrassment, envy, guilt and hatred as well as the positive calm and *amae*, or comfort in belonging)." "Moral sentiments" and "social emotions" have intentionality because they are "affective states about something"—attitudes directed toward others whose experiences lie beyond what we can fully share but to whom we respond across our horizons. This attunement to others is also inherently futural, orienting us toward a horizon of anticipated interactions. Even the entries "calm" and "comfort" in Keen's list, which might seem to be about nothing other than themselves, project us in an anticipatory manner toward future involvements with others (as in the slogan "Keep Calm and Carry On"). Not purely subjective and internal, these emotions entail attitudes that respond to and configure our relations with others and the circumstances we find ourselves in. This capacity to respond to and configure situations we share with others is one reason why emotions of all kinds, whether "basic" or "complex," can be patterned into stories.

As intentional structures, emotions are characterized by the to-and-fro motions of recursivity that are fundamental to narrative. This is evident, for example, in the cycle that Jenefer Robinson (2005) describes between "non-cognitive affective appraisals" and subsequent "cognitive monitoring." Drawing on the work of Joseph LeDoux (1996), Robinson (2005, 45) describes affective appraisals as "swift and automatic" physiological responses, mediated through the amygdala and the thalamus, "without any conscious deliberation or awareness." According to Robinson's model, these intuitive, bodily-based reactions are then followed by "a slower, more discriminating processing system which operates through the cortex and figures out whether the thalamo-amygdala 'affective appraisal' is appropriate or not" (50). This model is better able to account for the social work of narrative emotions than theories that view affect as autonomous and outside the realms of in-tentionality and judgment. It is preferable not only to the affect theory that derives from Ekman but also to Hogan's [2011b, 46] influential account of "what literature teaches us about emotions" that wrongly claims that "emotions are not produced by the evaluation of situations or events in relation to goals."

Robinson's term "noncognitive appraisal" is an oxymoron, of course, because an appraisal necessarily entails cognition. She resorts to an oxymoron, however, in order to do justice to the nonsimultaneity of the brain's cognitive processes. Affective appraisals are part of the cognitive apparatus that makes it possible for us to respond to situations in the world before consciousness has a chance to form. The delay between prereflective percep-tion and the arrival of consciousness is not a "thought-o-genic lapse" (to recall Massumi) but an interval filled by affective appraisals. Emotions play an integral role in the to-and-fro processes that couple anticipatory attune-ment and retrospective revision as we review and rearrange what we have subliminally predicted across the gap that Libet identified in his "mind-time" experiments. This temporal doubling of reflection on unreflected experience is not a static, unbridgeable divide between affect on one side and meaning or cognition on the other. It is, rather, a temporal to-and-fro between two dif-ferent kinds of intentionality—between what Merleau-Ponty (following Husserl) calls "non-thetic, operative intentionality" at a primary perceptual level and "thetic, act intentionality" when we take up a posture of judgment or deliberation (see 2012 [1945], lxxxii). Whenever we reflect, as Merleau-Ponty points out, we discover not a meaningless, autonomous realm of impulses or intensities but rather a world of significations already there in our prereflective perceptual experience. Reflective monitoring may come after emotions have already projected preliminary attitudes, orientations, and assessments, but affect is (once again) not an autonomous system that operates apart from consciousness and evaluation.

The recursive interaction between anticipatory affective appraisals and retrospective, revisionary monitoring is the experiential correlate of neurobiological processes that are constantly forming and dissolving at different levels and rates. Recall, for example, Merlin Donald's tripartite description of different processes of integration: short-term and working memory in immediate experience, the consolidation of sequences of events in long-term memory, and the intermediate range interactions of conversations and narrative exchanges over longer durations. Similarly, Varela (1999, 300) proposes that we "distinguish three scales for affect," roughly corresponding to three different "scales of temporality," with specific terms for each level: "The first scale is *emotion*: the awareness of a tonal shift that is constitutive of the living present. The second is *affect*, a dispositional trend proper to a coherent sequence of embodied actions. The third is *mood*, which exists at the scale of narrative description over time." These scales are not exactly equivalent to Donald's levels or to other ways of marking the temporality of cognitive integration (recall the distinctions, for example, between the microsecond level of subliminal processing [100–150 milliseconds], the delayed emergence of conscious awareness [at 500 milliseconds], and the multisecond parsing of temporal windows [at 3–5 seconds]). But Varela's suggestion that a vocabulary for emotions might be based on temporal processing levels is intriguing because it follows from the recognition that emotions are temporal cognitive structures.

More than in most other experiential domains, however, coming to agreement about the definition of terms in emotion studies is difficult. Varela's distinctions are an interesting attempt to create order in an inherently fuzzy, ambiguous area, but his definitions themselves demonstrate why emotional categories are unstable. The processes of affective appraisal he is trying to pin down cross back and forth across the temporal boundaries he describes. His emotion categories blur into one another because of the recursivity and interconnectedness of the temporal processes on which they are based. For example, Heidegger's notion of mood (*Stimmung*) refers to the anticipatory attitude of attuned expectation that characterizes not only the third scale in Varela's scheme to which he assigns this term but the other two as well ("emotion" and "affect"). Gearing us toward the future is something emotion does across all of the various scales of temporal integration, even if this attunement may feel differently (if it is perceived at all) according to the level at which it operates (experiential differences that Varela's terms attempt to capture). The terms used by emotion researchers criss-cross these domains, as do the embodied, temporally fluid processes Varela's distinctions try to pin down. It may be useful and informative to ask what temporal level an emotion term refers to and what kind of attunement it describes, but agreement on a strict definitional taxonomy is unlikely, and fixed, clear-cut categories would reify and misrepresent this fluidity.

The play of emotions in reading and narrative enacts in different ways the basic temporal duality between affective appraisal and cognitive monitoring. For example, David Miall (2011, 330) has found considerable experimental evidence for "the role of emotion in initiating and directing cognitive processes while reading." Miall has attempted to measure what he calls "the anticipatory role of feeling" in the comprehension of stories, and he has reported that test subjects respond to the emotional valences of words "early in verbal response, around 250 msec after a word is first seen, or possibly earlier"—in any case before the processing of word meaning is complete (336, 327). There is also interesting experimental evidence that aligning our affective appraisals with the emotional valences of a text facilitates comprehension. Lawrence Barsalou (2008, 629) reports, for example, that "when facial emotion matched sentence emotion, comprehension was better than when they mismatched."

Text comprehension is not a static correspondence of affect and word meaning, however, but an interactive, temporally dynamic process of adjustment and readjustment. As Miall observes (2011, 327), "Several studies focused on the temporal unfolding of the first responses to verbal presentations" document a to-and-fro interaction between emotionally oriented anticipation and retrospective cognitive activity, consistent with the recursive cycle of affective appraisals and cognitive monitoring that Robinson describes. Emotions can set this loop in motion because they are configurative structures, projecting in their appraisals a part-whole gestalt that guides comprehension—a shape that is futural in orientation because it waits to be filled in, revised, refined, or overturned.

How a narrative invokes and manipulates the reader's or listener's emotional responses is integral to how it builds, breaks, and re-forms patterns of concordant discordance out of the events it configures. For example, Meir Sternberg's (1987) triad of affective attitudes fundamental to narrative—curiosity, suspense, and surprise—are all horizontal phenomena through which a story sets up expectations that it then confirms, revises, or overturns. Curiosity, suspense, and surprise are attitudes of affective appraisal that guide the configurative work of narrative comprehension by attuning us to future developments.

Emotions project a structured but open, incompletely determined horizon of expectations that orient the temporality of understanding. This horizon of expectations extends from the emotions invoked by a text's genre—will this be a comedy or a tragedy?—to the twists and turns of events in the plot—are we headed for a happy ending or a good cry? As Robinson explains, "Emotions focus attention" (126). This focus is both directed and open, oriented but not fully specified, in the manner of a horizon beyond which we anticipate certain kinds of continuation of the perspective available from our standpoint—but not all kinds. We can be surprised by some developments because they are not what we had expected, even if what we anticipated was not completely determined in advance (as when we react to the surprising ending of a novel or a film: "I couldn't tell you exactly what I thought would happen, but not that!").

A work's characters are obviously a primary focus of the emotions generated by a work. What we may feel about a particular character matters, however, because of how it may orient our attitudes toward much larger concerns. Our changing responses to a work's characters—the pity and fear we may feel for the tragic hero, for example—are central to our developing sense of the narrative's overall emotional tonality, and this tonality has broad hermeneutic implications. As Robinson explains:

> Emotional understanding "regestalts" the world in a global way: in responding emotionally to Anna Karenina, I see the whole world of the novel through the prism of that emotion. My feelings for her affect my feelings about the harshness of the marriage laws, the difficulties of Vronsky's professional position, the heartlessness of polite society, and so on and so on. Feeling compassion for Anna is not just a response to her but a response with wide implications for my understanding of the novel as a whole. (128)

Our changing emotional reactions to the fate of a particular character can have such broad ramifications because emotions entail affective appraisals that orient and attune our attitude toward what lies beyond our horizons. This will include the whole of the text of which the character is a part, but it need not stop there. The "beyond" of our emotional response to a character starts with the immediate future of our reading, and it may then extend across the horizon of our engagement with this particular story to other involvements that await us in our worlds. Because emotions are horizonal configurations that orient us to the future and to other people, manipulating our emotions is a powerful way for narratives to attune us toward the world at large—to "regestalt" our sense of the world's patterns far beyond the particular events, characters, and concerns in the story.

Narrative emotions intertwine temporality and intersubjectivity and connect us to other worlds by aligning our horizons toward what lies beyond our view. These emotions connect us not only to fictional characters whose desires and struggles we may sympathize with as we respond to their stories but also to other listeners and readers with whom we share narratives. The experience of telling and following stories coordinates subjectivities in time. As Hanne De Jaegher, Ezequiel Di Paolo, and Ralph Adolphs (2016, 5–6) explain, neuroscience has begun to acknowledge the importance of a range of phenomena that entail a kind of "inter-brain phase synchronization"— processes of "mutual coordination" and "participatory sense-making" that require "an interactive sharing of socio-cognitive processes" (also see De Jaegher, Di Paolo, and Gallagher 2010). What De Jaegher and her colleagues call the "interactive brain hypothesis" also pertains to the synchronization of teller and listener in the exchange of stories (see my discussion of brain-to-brain coupling in chapter 4). As Ian Cross (2003, 48) points out, these processes of intersubjective synchronization have their earliest instantiations in "the rhythmicity of caregiver-infant interaction" that in turn is "central to the development of human significative and communicative capacities." This to-and-fro coordination of subjectivities in a temporal rhythm of collaborative sensemaking carries over into adult experiences in music and dance and other instances of sharing patterned time and harmonizing emotionally with others.

As De Jaegher and her coauthors (2016, 8) explain, these kinds of "socially coupled interaction" give rise to "emergent dynamical patterns that do not reduce to the activity of" a single agent or brain. Hans-Georg Gadamer (1993 [1960], 101–10) has something of this sort in mind when he describes a game as a collaborative activity that seems to have a trans-subjective agency of its own that paradoxically arises from the activity of its players, even as it goes beyond what they can individually command. What Gadamer calls "the primacy of the game over the players engaged in it" is experientially evident in the control the game seems to have over the players' actions as they respond to movements generated by their agency but not entirely subject to their control. Games, music, dance, and the exchange of stories are all emergent intersubjective experiences of participatory sensemaking that would not come into being without the contributions of individual subjectivities who strangely but compellingly are not fully in charge of what they co-create but who find their responses guided and coordinated by these interactions. These kinds of experiences of mutual coordination are evidence of the emergent dynamical systems that the interactive brain hypothesis attempts to explain.

Exactly what is happening in the bodies and brains of participants in such interactions is not entirely clear because of the limitations of scanning technologies. But this kind of mutual entrainment of separate but linked dynamical systems is not unusual in the physical world. Karl Friston and Christopher Frith (2015, 391) compare it to the synchrony of swinging pendulums, a well-known instance of "the action at a distance among coupled dynamical systems." Two or more swinging pendulums miraculously seem to coordinate their movements, but this "emergence of generalized synchronization" is a common phenomenon that occurs whenever two oscillatory systems "are coupled to each other through action" (391). Experiences of rhythmical, temporal coordination between people suggest that this kind of coupling also takes place when two embodied brains interact. The rhythms of an embodied brain—"the oscillatory dynamics associated with binding, attention, and dynamic coordination" through which neuronal assemblies are formed, dissolve, and re-form (391)—are not unlike the to-and-fro movements of a swinging pendulum.

The capacity of these oscillations to become synchronized across two or more embodied brains is the neurobiological basis of the temporal coordination of collaborative meaning making processes in music, dance, or stories. These coupled oscillations are what make it possible for embodied brains to intertwine intersubjectively in time, and they are the neurobiological means by which aesthetic experiences synchronize the temporalities of different worlds. We have the ability to share rhythms and emotions in time because the oscillatory processes of our horizonal interactions with each other can synchronize. Coupling the dynamical systems through which cognitive patterns are formed and dissolved in narrative interactions, waves of synchronization can join the worlds of readers not only with the worlds projected by stories but also with the worlds of other readers, listeners, and storytellers through the to-and-fro rhythms of narrative exchange.

The bodily resonances preserved and transmitted through these rhythms of concord and discord, synchronization and desynchronization, give stories the power to align worlds across the horizons of history. As Gallagher and Zahavi (2012, 95) observe, "human time is the time of our life stories," and "the story of any individual life is not only interwoven with those of others (parents, siblings, friends, etc.); it is always embedded in a larger historical and communal meaning-giving structure." Our sense of embeddedness in communal time comes in large part from the stories we are told and learn to tell and that circulate in our culture. As members of historical communities, we inherit, preserve, transform, and pass on stories and other artifacts of our shared culture, and this is how our lives intertwine intersubjectively with others beyond our horizons. We participate in history by passing these stories on to those who come after us, some whom we know but many others whom we will never directly encounter. As Ricoeur (1980b, 188) argues, "Narrativity . . . open[s] any meditation on time to another horizon than that of death, to the problem of communication not just between living beings, but between contemporaries, predecessors, and successors." In this sense, he contends, "narrative time [is] a time that continues beyond the death of each of its protagonists" inasmuch as the exchange of stories enables "transmission between generations" (188). These processes of temporal transmission are horizonal and intersubjective, an intertwining of my time with the time of others beyond the limits of my life.

The temporal asynchrony of the embodied brain means that our horizons are always shifting and that we are never at one with ourselves for as long as we live, but the horizonality of temporal experience also makes possible the intertwining of my temporality with the time of others, and these open-ended interactions may reverberate long after we are no longer there to experience them ourselves. Death is not necessarily the end of the story, then, because we can live on beyond the horizons of our own mortal lives by the stories that we learn, create, and exchange in collaborative processes of cultural meaning making. There is life after death in the stories we pass on, and the neurobiological basis of this capacity for generativity is the asynchronous temporality of the embodied brain.

CHAPTER THREE

Action, Embodied Cognition, and the As-If of Narrative Figuration

THE TEMPORALITY of the decentered brain makes mimesis possible because imitation is not a static correspondence of a sign to a thing but a dynamic configuration of an action. Mimesis is a kind of action (a linguistic making) that produces an organization of events (an emplotment of actions) that the reader or listener follows and reconstructs (the activity of comprehension). Action is central not only to mimesis but also more broadly to cognitive life. This is why the building and breaking of narrative patterns can powerfully affect the formation and disruption of patterns across many different cognitive domains. The paradox of concordant discordance in narrative traverses the circuit of action that joins narration, story comprehension, and everyday embodied cognition. The ever-shifting balance and tension between concord and discord within, across, and between these modes of action is what allows stories to play with the brain's competing requirements for order and flexibility, organization and openness to change.

Recent work on enactive narratology by so-called second-generation cognitive literary theorists has brought renewed attention to the relation between action and narrative, but this has been a central topic of narrative theory since its beginnings.[1] Aristotle (1990 [335 BCE], 7; original emphasis) famously claims that "tragedy is an imitation not of men but of *action*" and, further, that "performers *act* not in order to imitate character; they take on character for the sake of [imitating] actions."[2] This priority placed on action, according to Ricoeur (1984a, 34), "excludes any interpretation of Aristotle's mimesis in terms of a copy or identical replica. Imitating or representing is mimetic activity inasmuch as it produces something, namely the organization of events by emplotment." Because narrative and action are inextricably intertwined, Ricoeur argues that "there is no structural analysis of narrative that does not borrow from an explicit or an implicit phenomenology of 'doing something'" (56). As he explains, "the composition of the plot is grounded in a pre-understanding of the world of action, its meaningful structures, its symbolic resources, and its temporal character" (54). Understanding narrative consequently requires understanding the role of action in our cognitive lives.

The Action-Perception Circuit and the Figurations of Narrative

Contemporary neuroscience suggests that an action-perception circuit makes action fundamental to many cognitive processes that might seem remote from motor control. In Andy Clark's (2016, 7) evocative words, "Perception and action are . . . locked in a kind of endless circular embrace." There is a growing consensus among neuroscientists that "action is rich in cognitive resources" (Schulkin and Heelan 2012, 224) and, even more, that "action influences perception at its very source" (Berthoz and Petit 2008, 46). As Alain Berthoz and Jean-Luc Petit (2008, 49) explain, it is impossible to demarcate "a frontier between sensation and motoricity, because action is already to be found in perception." Recent experimental evidence on the responsiveness of the brain to imagined action and even to action words suggests that the brain is primed to respond to linguistically staged configurations of action and that these can have a profound effect on our cognitive processes because perception in many different modalities (vision, hearing, smell, touch) depends on embodied action. Plots can play a central role in structuring our understanding of the world because action is thoroughly implicated in perception.

Perception and action are interdependent in many ways. According to Alva Noë (2004, 8), the neurophilosopher who has studied this interdependence most thoroughly, "the basis of perception . . . is implicit practical knowledge of the ways movement gives rise to changes in stimulation." As he points out, "the world makes itself available to the perceiver through physical movement and interaction" (1). The classic statement of this view is James J. Gibson's *Ecological Approach to Visual Perception* (1979, 66): "A point of observation is never stationary, except as a limiting case. Observers move about in the environment, and observation is typically made from a moving position." For all modes of perception, exploratory activity provides ever-changing information about regularities and irregularities in the environment, and it is these differences to which the organism responds. Noë consequently claims that "all perception is . . . touch-like," even vision: "As in touch, the content of visual experience is not given all at once. We gain content by looking around just as we gain tactile content by moving our hands" (17, 73). As he notes, for example, "in normal perceivers, the eyes are in nearly constant motion, engaging in saccades (sharp, ballistic movements) and microsaccades several times a second. If the eyes were to cease moving, they'd lose their receptive power" because "optic flow contains information that is not available in single retinal images" (13, 20). It has long been experimentally established, for example, that fixed images on the retina gradually weaken and vanish, just as we don't notice the clothes we wear, constant background noise, or other unchanging stimuli to which we become habituated.[3]

Seeing, hearing, and touching are all active processes that are especially attuned to difference and change. In vision, for example, the workings of opponency make the retina more sensitive to changes in light than to a uniform, constant illumination. As Margaret Livingstone (2002, 54–55) explains, retinal neurons have a center/surround organization that "respond[s] best to sharp changes," which set off an opposition between these two parts of the cell, "rather than to gradual shifts in luminance" or to "the overall level of the illuminant," which do not much if at all perturb the center-surround balance. As she notes, "it is much more efficient to encode . . . changes or discontinuities than to encode the entire image" because "the most information in an image is in its discontinuities" (also see Armstrong 2013, 65–66). Similarly, as Mark Bear and his colleagues (2007, 420) observe, the responsiveness of "warm and cold receptors" on the skin is "greatest during, and shortly after, temperature changes"; "with thermoreception, as with most other sensory systems, it is the sudden change in the quality of a stimulus that generates the most intense neural and perceptual responses." In all modalities of sensation, the organism's changing relation to its world produces differences to which our sensory equipment responds, even as changes in how we direct that equipment toward the world (moving our eyes or hands or the direction of our ears) can generate differences that are rich in information. A circuit joins action and perception because perception is an exploratory activity that produces and responds to differences.

There is perhaps no more vivid dramatization of the connections between action and perception than the opening of James Joyce's novel *Portrait of the Artist as a Young Man*, where the infant Stephen Dedalus is depicted as coming to consciousness through various kinds of exploratory activity that register sensory differences and attempt to configure them into meaningful patterns. Joyce portrays the dawning of an aesthetic sensibility by calling attention to the circuit between action and perception and shows how their intertwining is fundamental to embodied consciousness. The novel famously opens with words Stephen hears from a story about "a nicens little boy named baby tuckoo" (2007 [1916], 5). This story stages a configuration of actions and relationships ("a moocow coming down along the road" [5] to meet the boy) that in turn initiates a series of attempts by Stephen to organize perceptual differences by acting in the world. First he listens, then he sings ("He sang that song. That was his song" [5]), and then he dances to a "sailor's hornpipe" (5) that his mother plays on the piano. These modalities of action parallel a series of perceptual differences that he notices and tries to align. Moving from sound to vision, he first responds to the words he hears by looking at the speaker and noticing distinguishing facial features ("his father looked at him through a glass" and "had a hairy face" [5]), differences between speaker and listener that lead Stephen to identify himself: "He was baby tuckoo." The relation between self and other is figured to Stephen through the relation of different perceptual modalities (what he hears, what he sees) that then move from sound and vision to touch ("When you wet the bed first it is warm then it gets cold" [5]) and even to smell (the oilsheet had a "queer smell" but "his mother had a nicer smell than his father" [5]). Stephen comes to consciousness of his world by experimenting with different kinds of action (listening, seeing, singing, dancing) and exploring the relations between perceptual differences (sight, sound, touch, and smell).

Action is meaningful and can be a resource for perception because it is figurative. Marc Jeannerod (2008, 103), a leading authority on motor cognition, points out that "human infants as young as three months old are visually sensitive to the difference between the biological motion of dots produced by a walking person and the random, artificially produced, non-biological motion of similar dots." Infants understand biological movements as meaningful actions because they perceive them as a gestalt, a figurative arrangement of elements in a pattern. As Shaun Gallagher (2012, 175–76) observes, however, "the meaning of any action is not purely intrinsic to its motoric aspects." Gregory Hickok (2014, 136) similarly notes that "the meanings simply aren't in the movements," inasmuch as "the very same motor program . . . could mean" any number of things depending on the context and purpose of the action (is a raised hand a vote, a request to speak, a signal to attack, or simply a stretching motion?).[4] Context and purpose matter because an action is figurative. To perceive a movement as an action is to understand the pattern of part-whole relations that form its gestalt, its configuration as a means directed toward an end in a particular situation.

The idea that all consciousness is consciousness *of* something—phenomenology's classic definition of intentionality (see Armstrong 2012)—also applies to action. As Gallagher explains, "Actions have intentionality because they are directed at some goal or project, and this is something that we can see in the actions of others" (77). Our actions are not empty and random but are aimed at states of affairs we engage with and point toward ends we anticipate. This does not mean that we are always aware of this directedness—intentionality is not the same as intention—but rather that an action is meaningful because it has what Heidegger (1962 [1927], 188–95) calls an "as-structure" and a "fore-structure." We understand action X *as* signifying Y because it is projected *toward* Z.[5] What a raised hand means depends on what we perceive it as directed toward—the pattern to which it belongs and the ends it projects and aims to produce.

The gestalt processes at work in understanding and producing action are evident in oft-cited fMRI experiments that measured the brain activity of dancers observing a dance style they have or have not learned to do (classical ballet, for example, versus capoeira) and that then compared these scans to novices and choreographers. Dance lays bare the configurative structure of action that ordinarily goes unnoticed in our everyday lives but that allows us to interpret actions differently according to our familiarity (or unfamiliarity) with their underlying patterns, the as-relations that shape them into meaningful gestalts (see Sheets-Johnstone 1966, 2011). As Catherine Stevens and Shirley McKechnie (2005, 247) point out, in these experiments "brain activity was affected by whether observers could do the action or not," and these differences turned up not only in the motor cortex but also "in middle temporal areas suggesting semantic categorization of dance movement by experts" into the "vocabularies of 'steps' that constitute classical ballet and capoeira repertoires" (also see Calvo-Merino et al. 2004).

The brains of dancers responded differently to actions they could perform as opposed to those they could not because the dancers interpreted these movements as a configuration that is either familiar or strange. These patterns of response show up not only in the motor cortex but also in other areas of the brain because the steps have meanings that are not reducible to our physiological equipment for generating bodily movements. For the same reasons, scans comparing dancers to novices and choreographers showed that these steps are invisible to novices, whose brains do not respond to them, and that they have a different significance to choreographers, who imagine and create the patterns that dancers must then assimilate and reproduce and whose fMRI images differ accordingly, with more activity in cortical areas involved with planning and reflection. Not simply a one-to-one mirroring process, these experiments show that understanding actions entails configuring movements *as* something according to our past experiences and future expectations about their purpose, shape, and direction.

Both action and perception consequently have a virtual dimension that makes them a paradoxical combination of presence and absence, immanence and transcendence—a duality that Merleau-Ponty describes as the "intertwining" of the "visible and invisible" (see 1968 [1964], 3–49, 130–55). Any situation of perception is riven with absence, according to Merleau-Ponty, because its perspective is partial and incomplete, with invisible sides and undisclosed dimensions that we anticipate could be filled in by future experiences or by other, differently positioned observers. These indeterminacies make perception horizonal not only spatially (the hidden sides of an object) but also temporally (the not yet evident aspects we anticipate experiencing) and intersubjectively (our assumption that we inhabit a shared world with others whose perspectives disclose aspects concealed from us and who could confirm our hypotheses about what lies beyond our view). Action is similarly horizonal, defined both by presence and absence—not only by its immanent, embodied engagement with objects, instruments, and other actors but also by its transcendence, its directedness toward goals, purposes, and future events that lie beyond its immediate situation. Actions and perceptions are anticipatory in structure, projected toward states of affairs beyond their immediate horizons, and this virtuality is part and parcel of their "of-ness" and "as-ness" as patterned, intentional gestalts. There can be a circuit between action and perception because they share this as- and fore-structure.

Because actions and perceptions have an intrinsic virtual dimension, they are ready to be rendered into fictions—as-if narrative structures through which the imaginary transfigures and transforms the real. As Wolfgang Iser argues in his monumental and underappreciated late work *The Fictive and the Imaginary* (1993, 12–13), in fictional narratives "the incorporated 'real' world is, so to speak, placed in brackets to indicate that it is not something given but is merely to be understood *as if* it were given." This is a process of doubling that "turns the whole of the world organized in the text into an 'as if' construction" (13). As Iser explains, "every staging lives on what it is not" (301), and this is true not only of mimetic but also of nonmimetic and even (or especially) antimimetic texts of the sort foregrounded by proponents of "unnatural narrative" (see Alber, Nielsen, and Richardson 2013 and Richardson 2015). The capacity to tell stories and project fictional stagings of ourselves and our worlds is made possible by the virtuality of action and perception because their dual structures of immanence and transcendence can be refigured fictionally into what Ricoeur calls patterns of "split reference" (1977, 265–302)—narrative doublings of absence and presence classically rendered by fairy tales that begin "It was and it was not." We can double ourselves in stories that stage versions of ourselves because embodied action is already configurative and projective, characterized by both presence and absence, immanence and transcendence.

Fictionality and figuration go hand in hand because they are as-structures. The virtuality of the as if, according to Iser, allows the fictional world to "be taken to figure something other than itself" (19–20). The figurative processes of fictionality and narrative can take different forms across history and in different cultures because the as is variable and can set up any number of relationships. Indeed, Iser claims, "staging in literature makes conceivable the extraordinary plasticity of human beings, who, precisely because they do not seem to have a determinable nature, can expand into an almost unlimited range of culture-bound patternings" (297). As an evolved species with constraints on our cognitive and bodily potentialities that derive from our inherited biological makeup, we are perhaps more limited in how we can configure ourselves than Iser suggests here (see Armstrong 2013, 35–39, Boyd 2009, and Easterlin 2012). Human beings are biocultural hybrids, however, whose nature it is to experiment with and explore different versions of ourselves. This "almost unlimited" plasticity is an anthropological constant across historical and cultural variation and one of the defining characteristics of our species (see Malabou 2008 and Armstrong 2018). Our capacity to emplot actions into narrative configurations is both biologically based and culturally open ended, and this paradox is an important example of our biocultural hybridity.[6]

This hybridity is also on display in the opening of *Portrait of the Artist*. The virtual dimension of the actions and perceptions through which Stephen configures his world enables them to stand for meanings other than themselves. The split reference of doubling is evident in the juxtaposition of the time of the story—"and a very good time it was" (2007 [1916], 5)—and the time of Stephen's hearing of it (which soon turns out to be not such an ideal time after all), and this doubling allows him to take on a role that he also was not ("He was baby tuckoo," an identity that he can assume only because it is not who he is). Sensations similarly have a virtual dimension that allows them to be doubled and configured into as-relations, with differences in smell signaling mother versus father (supplementing visual differences like the father's glasses and "hairy face"). Singing and dancing similarly set up family relations (father reciting the song, mother playing the piano, Uncle Charles and Dante clapping) that are biologically based (including age differences: "Charles was older than Dante" [5]) and also culturally charged. The political resonances of the perceptual landscape emerge as Stephen visualizes the colors of Dante's two brushes and understands their references (maroon for one figure in Irish politics and green for another). The political problems of Ireland that will become crucial for Stephen's (and Joyce's) struggles to find an artistic voice are already signaled by his early response to colors as he configures perceptual differences into meaningful relations and imagines what various sensations might stand for. Actions and perceptions can take on these semiotic functions only because they have a virtual dimension and an as- and fore-structure that can be molded into patterns suggestive of aims, purposes, and directions beyond young Stephen's immediate horizons.

As this scene suggests, the many links between action and perception are crucial for language acquisition. Stephen hears words and reproduces them in song, using rhythmic patterns that are reinforced by music and dance. These intertwinings of action, perception, and language arise from cortical connections that have been documented experimentally. Citing extensive evidence from brain-imaging studies, Friedemann Pulvermüller and Luciano Fadiga (2010, 358) report that "language processing is based on neuronal circuits that reciprocally connect action systems of the brain with perceptual circuits." As they explain, "Rich links between articulatory and auditory neurons are required to learn the precise mapping between acoustic patterns and the motor programmes necessary for successful word repetition" (352). They point out that "these connections are strong only in humans and are weak in non-human primates," which may in part "explain why language has not emerged" in those species (352). Speech sounds elicit responses in the motor cortex according to their phonetic qualities, with tongue- and lip-produced phonemes generating measurable reactions in the corresponding topographical areas of the brain that control the tongue and the lips (353). Although the evidence is mixed (as I explain), Pulvermüller and Fadiga note that lesions affecting the "frontal and premotor areas" and interrupting the action-perception circuit have been shown to "compromise the patients' ability to comprehend meaningful words" (354).

Action, sensation, and perception are richly linked in language comprehension, just as they are in everyday experience. Brain-imaging studies have shown that word recognition is extensively and exquisitely connected to the cortical areas associated with different perceptions of sensation; "words related to odours (for example 'cinnamon') activate olfactory brain areas more strongly than do control words," and "words that are semantically related to sounds (for example 'telephone') . . . strongly activate superior temporal auditory areas even if presented in written form" (Pulvermüller and Fadiga 2010, 355). Similarly, words referring to a particular action (for example, kicking or throwing) activate motor areas of the cortex associated with them, so much so that left- and right-handed subjects evince responses in opposite sides of their brains (see Hauk and Pulvermüller 2004, Boulenger et al. 2006, Willems et al. 2010). There is also evidence that tool words, which entail action, produce responses in the motor cortex, whereas animal words do not (Puvermüller and Fadiga 2010, 355).

The linguistic resonances between action words and real actions are part of a more general association between real and imagined action. As Jeannerod (2006, 28, 39) points out, many different experiments have shown that "imagining a movement relies on the same mechanisms as actually performing it," and that is because "imagined actions are indeed actions in their own right: they involve a kinematic content, they activate motor areas almost to the same extent as executed actions, they involve the autonomic system as if a real action was under way." Imagining an action stimulates both the brain and the body in a manner very similar to real action, even down to the level of muscular response. For example, Jeannerod notes, measurements of "the changes in . . . the motor pathways during various forms" of imagined action have shown the presence of excitability "in the muscular groups involved in the simulated action"; ample experimental evidence demonstrates that, "during motor imagery, motor commands to muscles are only partially blocked, and . . . motoneurons are close to the firing threshold" (31).

Although imagining an action is not by itself sufficient to master it, many studies have shown that "mental training" by athletes and musicians can improve actual motor performance, enhancing speed, accuracy, consistency, and even "strength of muscular contraction" (41). These findings are consistent with brain-imaging studies that have disclosed that "learning a motor task by using motor imagery induces a pattern of dynamic changes in cortical activation similar to that occurring during physical practice" (41). These results have had important consequences not only for athletic training and observational learning but also for the rehabilitation of stroke patients suffering from motor impairments. Because of the physiological links between real and imagined movement, mental rehearsal of an action can have demonstrable effects on the ability of athletes, musicians, or patients with lesions to actually perform the action.

It consequently stands to reason that reading or listening to a narrative that imitates an action would have practical effects on the brains and bodies of the recipients and on their capacities for acting in the world. If the motor cortex and even muscle tissue can be excited by mental rehearsal of an action, that should also be true of linguistic simulations of actions, and there is experimental evidence that this is so. Lawrence Barsalou (2008, 628) reports, for example, that "when reading about a sport, such as hockey, experts produce motor simulations absent in novices." This is consistent with an fMRI study by Nicole Speer and her group (2009, 989) that showed correlations between six different kinds of changes represented in stories and the brain regions activated by "analogous activities in the real world" (changes in the location, cause, goal, character, timing, or the object involved in an action). "Different brain regions track different aspects of a story," Speer and her colleagues conclude, "such as a character's physical location or current goals," and "some of these regions mirror those involved when people perform, imagine, or observe similar real-world activities" (989).

There is also evidence that actions and sensations figured in metaphorical language evoke embodied, cortical responses correlated to literal, real-world perceptual experiences. A brain-imaging study conducted by Krish Sathian's group (Lacey, Stilla, and Sathian 2012, 417, 416) demonstrated that areas of the brain "previously shown to be texture-selective during haptic perception" were also "activated when processing sentences containing textural metaphors" from the same sensory domains. Even very familiar, unsurprising metaphors like "a rough day" or "a slimy person" that "have negative connotations because they refer to attributes that may be particularly unpleasant to touch" evoked responses in the somatosensory cortex associated with these bodily experiences (418). These and many other similar studies point to some of the neurobiological processes set in motion by the feigned figuration of action and sensation in narrative, brain-body interactions in response to imitation that could have the power to reinforce or reshape the recipient's embodied, configured experience of the world.

Action performs a fundamental role in coordinating different modalities of cognition, and this organizing role is crucial not only for language but also for narrative and our ability to construct and follow plots. The anatomical region of the brain central to these interactions is Broca's area, a region of the inferior frontal cortex adjacent to the sections of the motor cortex that control the mouth and the lips (see Bear, Connors, and Paradiso 2007, 620–23). According to Pulvermüller and Fadiga (2010, 351), "Studies have shown this area to be active in human action observation, action imagery and language understanding." Impairments in Broca's area have long been known to result in difficulties producing and comprehending grammatical sentences. Patients with lesions in this part of the brain can understand and pronounce single words, "but they have great difficulty in aligning scrambled words into a sentence or in understanding complex sentences," and these deficiencies are "paralleled in non-linguistic modalities" (357). A number of brain-imaging studies have shown, for example, that musical syntax is processed in Broca's area and that listening to musical rhythms activates the motor cortex (Maess et al. 2001, Chen, Penhune, and Zatorre 2008, Patel 2008).

This region of the brain is also apparently crucial for narrative. An intriguing experiment by Patrik Fazio and his group (2009, 1987) revealed that "a lesion affecting Broca's area impairs the ability to sequence actions in a task with no explicit linguistic requirements." His laboratory showed patients with Broca's aphasia "short movies of human actions or of physical events," and they were then asked to order, "in a temporal sequence, four pictures taken from each movie and randomly presented on the computer screen" (1980). Curiously, although these patients could still recognize before-after relations between physical events, they had a harder time reconstructing the order of human actions. Their ability to remember and compose a sequence of represented actions was impaired. This result suggests that the patients in Fazio's study suffered a deficiency in the capacity for emplotment, the ability to produce and follow configurations of action. Such an inference is consistent with Fazio's claim that "the complex pattern of abilities associated with Broca's area might have evolved from its premotor function of assembling individual motor acts into goal-directed actions" (1987). This capacity for organizing action into meaningful sequences makes the brain ready for language, but it also prepares the brain for narrative.[7]

Action has a fundamental coordinating role not only in perception but also in our response to imagery of various kinds. Neuroscientifically trained literary critic Gabrielle Starr (2013, 75) claims that motor imagery and motor processes are involved in the aesthetic pleasures offered by all three of the so-called sister arts. As she explains, embodied action underlies and coordinates imagery and perception in the different sensory domains on which literature, painting, and music draw. After observing that "investigations of imagery" offer "very good evidence that across sensory modes, when people experience perceptual imagery, areas of the brain involved in actual perception are active and function in similar patterns for imagined sensation as during actual perception," Starr points out that action underlies imagery across different sensory domains and that "imagery of motion" is "at the heart of our capacities for both simulation and aesthetic experience" (75, 81). For example, visual imagery typically has an implicit proprioceptive dimension, Starr observes, because "people imagine motion along with sight—the experience of moving one's body is, for sighted persons, both visual and kinetic" (82). Auditory imagery similarly has fundamental connections to movement because the perception of sound depends on patterns of repetition and variation. For imagery related to music and sound, Starr observes, action matters because "timing is everything and the tension between what is new and what is expected is ever present" (128). Multisensory imagery that invokes and interrelates all of these different perceptual areas can associate vision, sound, touch, and even smell, she argues, because of their bases in embodied action. If narrative as the emplotment of action similarly has the power to coordinate processes of configuration in different sensory domains, that is due in no small measure to the underlying organizing role of motor processes in perception.

Following a story, whether by listening or by reading, is not passive absorption or one-to-one mirroring. Here too action is fundamental to cognition. Making sense of a narrative involves an interaction between different kinds of action—the organization of story elements in patterns of discordant concordance (mimesis$_2$) and the work of pattern formation, gap filling, and illusion building in the process of reception (mimesis$_3$). The comprehension of a story requires active participation by the recipient, who must project relations between the parts that are told and their probable configuration in the whole that seems to be forming—this entails a to-and-fro work of anticipation and retrospection through which illusions are built and then broken, consistent patterns formed and then disturbed, disrupted, and reassembled as expectations are invoked, disappointed, modified, and fulfilled.

Reciprocal, to-and-fro pattern formation is involved in all cognitive processes, whether visual, auditory, or haptic, and across the multiple sensory domains that are bound together in embodied experiences of cognition. The construction of narrative, story comprehension, and embodied cognition are mutually formative because they all entail to-and-fro, reciprocal processes of configurative activity. The activity of construing a text or understanding a story has the power to change the way our brains and bodies respond to the world because the processes of configuration across these domains are not separate but congruent, mutually formative, and reciprocally interactive. This is why the interchange between the emplotment of action in narrative (mimesis$_2$) and the recognition and reconstruction of a plot in story comprehension (mimesis$_3$) can interact with the action-perception circuit in cognition (mimesis$_1$) in a potentially transformative manner.

These interactions play an important role in the brain's incessant balancing act between pattern and change, the tension between the need for order and the requirement for flexibility and openness to variation that is fundamental to successful mental functioning. Repeated patterns of activity form into habits, and the process of making and breaking habits is crucial to emplotment, story comprehension, and embodied cognition. It is a widely acknowledged paradox of cognitive life that habits are both good and bad, and necessarily so—habits are indispensable to skillful coping and efficient functioning but at the same time also an obstacle to innovation and adaptation to novelty, change, and unexpected irregularities (James 1890, 1:104–27; Noë 2009, 99–128). Habit formation is basic to cognitive life, even at the neuronal level, as Hebb's law (2002 [1949]) famously observes: "Neurons that fire together, wire together." The capacity of repeated neuronal activity to establish enduring cortical connections prevents the recursive interactions of "reentry" (Edelman and Tononi 2000) from being purely random, chaotic, and accidental, and this in turn allows learning to occur. The usefulness of habit is similarly evident in the conventions of storytelling and the repetitions of narrative patterns that facilitate the construction and recognition of plots.

But a brain locked forever in repeated patterns of neuronal assembly would lack the capacity to respond to changing stimuli, to explore an unpredictable environment, or to try out new cortical configurations that might eventually develop into new cognitive capacities (the joining up of the motor cortex to auditory, visual, and sensory areas of the brain, for example, that occurred as our species developed the capacity for language and reading). Similarly, although there is pleasure in recognizing a familiar story, even the retelling of a well-known tale typically varies the received patterns it deploys in order to keep the listener interested. Excessive homogeneity is once again bad for the brain. If the value of concord in repeated stories is to reinforce and teach habitual, socially shared cognitive patterns, the value of disruption, irregularity, and surprise in the concordant discordance of emplotment is to preserve and enhance cognitive flexibility, our openness to change, variation, and novelty. By invoking and disrupting the habits through which we pattern the world, the experience of telling and following stories has the power to bring about potentially transformative exchanges between different modalities of figuration. The neurobiological source of this power is the coordinated interaction between far-flung areas of the brain and the body that join together action, perception, and cognition.

Grounded Cognition, Graded Grounding, and the Paradoxes of Simulation

The many experimental findings on the links between cognition and embodied experiences of perception, sensation, and action have given support to the theory of grounded cognition most notably propounded by Barsalou. This theory rejects the view that "knowledge is represented in abstract codes, distinct from the sensory modalities through which the knowledge was acquired" (Lacey, Stilla, and Sathian 2012, 416). "The idea that the conceptual system draws on sensory and motor systems," Rutvik Desai and company note, "has received considerable experimental support in recent years" (2013, 862). And as Michael L. Anderson (2010, 257) observes, "It is quite easy to find studies reporting that the neural implementations of higher cognitive functions overlap with those of the sensorimotor system"; as proof he points to the twenty-seven-essay volume *Sensorimotor Foundations of Higher Cognition* (Haggard, Rossetti, and Kawato 2008).

So overwhelming is this evidence that the debate has recently turned and the question has become, how do we think abstractly? Warning against "some of the hyperbolic rhetoric used by supporters of embodied cognition," Guy Dove (2011, 3, 5) argues that "what we need to explain is our ability to go beyond embodied experience." As he observes, "Sensorimotor simulations seem ill-suited for representing conceptual content that is not closely tied to particular experience," and "some concepts appear to require what we might call ungrounded representations" (5). Similarly worried that "a quick acceptance of embodied accounts runs the danger of ignoring alternate hypotheses and not scrutinizing neuroscience data critically," Anjan Chatterjee (2010, 79) suggests that "the question of whether or not cognition is grounded is more fruitfully replaced by questions about gradations in this grounding. A focus on disembodying cognition, or on graded grounding, opens the way to think about how humans abstract." How narratives stage figurative versions of experience similarly requires an understanding of the relation between the abstract and the concrete. We can tell each other stories that reconfigure embodied experience and transform it into narrative patterns because action and perception have a virtual dimension and are both grounded and ungrounded, embodied and disembodied.

In ways that are not always recognized and understood, this duality is already evident in the key term "simulation" in Barsalou's theory: "Grounded cognition proposes that modal simulations, bodily states, and situated action underlie cognition" (2008, 617). According to Barsalou, "Simulation is the reenactment of perceptual, motor, and introspective states acquired during experience with the world, body, and mind" (618). Simulation is often a bit of a black box in cognitive and psychological theories, however (see Mumper and Gerrig 2019), and it is frequently invoked in ways that misleadingly imply causation or one-to-one correspondences. To a literary critic or theorist, however, this term is almost self-evidently an as-structure.

By definition, after all, a reenactment both *is* and *is not* what it reproduces. In terms familiar to literary theory, the equivalences established in a simulation are of the paradoxical Nietzschean variety—"das Gleichsetzen des Nicht-Gleichen," or "the setting equal" of things that are not the same (see Nietzsche 2015 [1873]). In a simulation, an as-if rendering reproduces a state of affairs as something that it is not, and this entails a doubling of the like and the not like (*Gleich* and *Nicht-Gleich*). The as and the as-if enable conceptual and narrative reenactments of perceptual and sensory experiences in simulations that both are and are not what they reproduce. The virtuality of the as and the as-if also makes possible graded transitions from the concrete to the abstract.

Barsalou's explanations of simulation again and again presume its as-structure without ever naming it as such or fully recognizing the complications it introduces to the model of grounded cognition. Barsalou acknowledges, for example, that "simulations rarely, if ever, recreate full experiences" but instead are "typically partial recreations of experience that can contain bias and error" (620). Because cognitive simulations are partial and incomplete, they necessarily entail what he calls "a pattern-completion inference mechanism" (622). As the very term "mechanism" itself implies, sometimes Barsalou unfortunately uses causal language to explain how this process works. For example, he states that "bodily states are not simply effects of social cognition; they also cause it" (630). An inference is not a causal mechanism, however, but a hypothesis about a pattern and a guess about how an incomplete perspective should be filled out.[8] Simulations entail variable, open-ended processes of pattern formation and gap filling because they are not straightforward, mechanical productions based on cause and effect but as-relations that make connections based on inference and association.

Simulations are products of selection and combination that can use the materials they draw on in a variety of ways. As partial re-creations, they do not retain all of the original experience, only traces of it or some aspects rather than others. These selections can then be combined differently as new situations arise, which is why past sensorimotor experiences can be used to configure new cognitive situations. Grounded cognition can only respond to unprecedented and unpredictable states of affairs because its simulations are not completely identical to the experiences these simulations draw on. New perceptions can be "grounded" in past cognitive experiences because of this variability—because, that is, they are not mechanical, one-to-one repetitions of previous sensations but as-relations, both like and not like the experiences they reenact, partial and incomplete in ways that make possible bias and error but that also enable novelty and creativity. The processes of selection and recombination in a cognitive simulation are much more variable and open ended than the language of mechanism and cause suggests, and that is a good thing because it makes cognition more flexible and more open to new and unexpected situations than it would be if grounding were seamless and ungraded. The paradox of grounded cognition is that its simulations work only because they are to some extent ungrounded.

The interpretive activity of figurative pattern construction and gap filling is evident in many of Barsalou's examples of how inference and simulation work even when he invokes a mechanical model. Here is a typical instance: "Representations of familiar situations that contain embodiments become established in memory (e.g., receiving a gift, feeling positive affect, and smiling). When part of this situation occurs (e.g., receiving a gift), it activates the remainder of the situational pattern, producing associated embodiments (e.g., smiling)" (630). This is a classic example of what Richard Gerrig (2010, 2012) calls "memory-based processing," which is evidence of the brain's recursive work of constructing cognitive patterns of seeing-as—here, seeing a new situation as associated with learned conventions from previous interactions. Traces of those associations may be embodied, but this is not a case where a bodily state simply causes a social cognition.

Not a cause-effect mechanism, this is an interpretive situation in which signs must be read as standing for something that must be construed. As Umberto Eco (1976, 6–7) memorably notes, one can tell signs are at work whenever there is the possibility of lying. Here, it is possible to feign a polite smile at a gift one hadn't really wanted—or that one knew was well intentioned but misfired—and the neurobiological basis of this possibility is that the reactivations of a simulation are partial and can be configured in different ways. For example, one can smile with a wink and a nod that suggests to someone in the know an ironic response ("Thanks a lot!" can be intoned in a lot of different ways). It is not always possible to tell whether someone is smiling sincerely or simply politely because they are following a social convention, and the as-if of simulation is responsible for this ambiguity. A polite smile is a biocultural hybrid, a bodily response and a conventional expression, and this duality is possible because simulations are both grounded and ungrounded.

A process of doubling characterizes the as-if of simulation because it is a reenactment of an experience that both is and is not like the original it reinvokes. The role of the as-if is evident, for example, in a prominent article in *Science* on "Embodying Emotion" by Paula Niedenthal (2007) which is based on Barsalou's model. Her account is couched in the language of mechanical causation, but her terminology interestingly and subtly shifts in ways that reveal the variability of simulative as-relations: "The embodiment of emotion, when induced in human participants by manipulations of facial expression and posture in the laboratory, *causally affects* how emotional information is processed. Congruence between the recipient's bodily expression of emotion and the sender's emotional tone of language, for instance, *facilitates* comprehension of the communication, whereas incongruence *can impair* comprehension" (1002, emphasis added). The slippage between "causally affects" and "facilitates" and "can impair" is telling, moving from billiard-ball mechanical certainty to the language of probability and contingency. The result may occur—but maybe not—because a simulation is both like and not like the original experience it reenacts.

In the reported experiment, subjects who were made to smile by holding a pen in their teeth (thus simulating smiling) rated cartoons as funnier than subjects holding a pen "between their lips," which "prevented them from smiling" (1005). Niedenthal explains that "using knowledge—as in recalling memories, drawing inferences, and making plans—is thus called 'embodied' because an *admittedly incomplete but cognitively useful reexperience* is produced in the originally implicated sensory-motor systems, *as if* the individual were there in the very situation, the very emotional state, or with the very object of thought" (1003; emphasis added). Note the as-if quality of this reexperiencing, which is incomplete in that only a subset of the neurons fire that were originally active, setting in motion only partial traces of the original physiological processes in the sensory-motor system that is reactivated by the simulation. The placement of the pen (between the teeth or the lips) recreates an embodied experience as if one were smiling or frowning. This simulation (which both is and is not like actual smiling or frowning) has associations (happy or sad, funny or not funny) that connect and fill out what is missing (how to evaluate the comedy of the cartoon, itself a blank not contained in any of its features, which is why it can be evaluated differently whether one is smiling or frowning).

This response is not a causal mechanism but an inference that completes a pattern and fills in a blank. This experiment illustrates the fore-structure of grounded cognition, in line with Heidegger's claim (1962 [1927], 172–88) that mood (*Stimmung*) provides an anticipatory understanding of a state of affairs.[9] A simulated smile or frown can prime a response, making one more or less likely to perceive something as funny, because it orients the perceiver's attitude toward a situation. As an as- and fore-structure, an embodied simulation is a hermeneutic figuration *of* something *as* something depending on how we are directed *toward* its various unspecified horizons (patterns that our inferences complete). Grounded cognitions are structures of intentionality, not deterministic processes.

Similar doublings and ambiguities are evident in well-known disputes about the relation between embodied experience and our ability to understand another's actions and gestures. The basis of these disputes is the much-discussed discovery by Giacomo Rizzolatti and his Parma group of "mirror neurons" in the motor cortex of macaque monkeys that fired not only when the animals performed an action but also when they observed the same action or even an object (like a cup) associated with the action.[10] The existence of mirror neurons, also subsequently found in humans, seemed to provide a straightforward neurobiological explanation for the grounding of cognition on embodied experiences and the relation between action and perception. But this explanation soon raised further questions. Mirror-neuron skeptic Gregory Hickok (2014, 43, 49) observes, for example, that "we don't need to be able to perform an action to understand it," and he also notes that "deficits in the control of action [because of lesions or physical impairments] do not uniformly result in deficits in understanding of action." These counterexamples cast doubt on the claim that we understand an action by reenacting (simulating) its performance.

The clinical and experimental evidence about the relation between performance deficits and cognitive ability is indeed mixed. On the one hand, some studies have shown that lesions in the motor and somatosensory cortices "can lead to the loss of multiple categories that share perceptual properties"; for example, "a selective deficit in action word processing has been found in patients with motor neuron disease" (Dove 2011, 3; see Bak et al. 2001). On the other hand, Gilles Vannuscorps and Alfonso Caramazza (2016, 86–87) have demonstrated that "individuals born without upper limbs can perceive, anticipate, predict, comprehend, and memorize observed actions with the same accuracy and speed as the controls," and they consequently conclude that "efficient perception and interpretation of actions can be achieved without motor simulation." Jeannerod (2006, 16) summarizes this ambiguous state of affairs: although apraxic patients who cannot perform a particular action "fail in action representation tasks," they "usually remain unimpaired in tasks evaluating their conceptual knowledge about objects or tools. . . . This dissociation between 'actions' and 'objects' stresses the limitation of theories based on motor simulation to explain conceptual knowledge." Despite his skepticism about mirror neurons, Hickok (2014, 153) offers a sensible compromise view: "We should not confuse the fact that action is an important part of perception with the idea that motor representations alone are the basis of perceptual understanding." As he explains, "This is not to say that the ability to act in the world doesn't make *some* contribution to perceiving and therefore understanding. On the contrary, action contributes a great deal" (152; original emphasis)—but it is not the whole story because cognition is both grounded and ungrounded, embodied and disembodied.[11]

These contradictions are based on a fundamental paradox of cortical functioning. Cognition is both anatomically localized and a function of network connections across the "brain web." On the one hand, some functions depend on specific parts of the brain that are active during a particular cognitive experience, and these abilities therefore get knocked out when these areas are damaged (as when, for example, impairments in various regions of the rear visual cortex may cause particular kinds of blindness to motion, colors, or faces). On the other hand, many cognitive functions set in motion reciprocal, cross-cortical interactions between different anatomical locations and assemble neurons into particular patterns that may even change what a specific area does (so that the visual cortex of a blind person can be repurposed to support touch in reading braille). Some localized somatosensory and motor areas would consequently be expected to fire in response to words, cognitive experiences, or even imaginings that trigger them (as happens, for example, when action words set off particular parts of the motor cortex). But other cognitive functions depend on network interactions that are not reducible to any anatomical location (as when we understand actions we have not experienced or that our bodies cannot perform). Someone who has not had a particular experience might not be able to understand it as completely as someone whose brain and body would be able to simulate and reenact a somatosensory, embodied cognitive act (recall that novices do not register reactions to the steps of ballet or capoeira that the brains of experts resonate to), but by combining various cortical areas across the brain web, we can understand actions outside our particular motor repertoire (and appreciate a dance performance of which we are ourselves incapable).

Cognition is not simply a linear, cause-effect, bottom-up mechanism of stimulus and response. It is, rather, a reciprocal, to-and-fro process of assembling cortical regions into patterns that may stabilize through repeated Hebbian firing but that can also shift and change and that can, in a top-down manner, mold and shape our understanding of what is "out there" in the world. As Hickok (2014, 238) observes, "There are more top-down neural connections (from higher to lower levels) than bottom-up connections (from lower to higher levels), about an order of magnitude difference (10:1 ratio)." This is anatomical evidence of the ability of network interactions to produce cognitive experiences that go beyond those generated by receptor neurons in local somatosensory regions. Noting that "action understanding is the interaction of many things," Hickok consequently proposes "a hybrid model of conceptual knowledge" that is based on network connections between motoric and somatosensory areas (180, 168; see 159–81).

Anderson (2010, 246) found similar empirical evidence for a network model: "An empirical review of 1,469 subtraction-based fMRI experiments in eleven task domains," including "action execution, action inhibition, action observation, vision, audition, attention, emotion, language, mathematics, memory, and reasoning," showed that "a typical cortical region is activated by tasks in nine different domains." What a particular anatomical region of the brain is doing depends not only on its own physiological characteristics, then, but also on the areas it is linked with. Anderson also found that "language tasks activate more and more broadly scattered regions than do visual perception and attention. This finding was corroborated by a larger study . . . which found that language was the most widely scattered domain of those tested, followed (in descending order) by reasoning, memory, emotion, mental imagery, visual perception, action, and attention" (247). These findings support Anderson's theory of neural reuse, which emphasizes the plasticity of the brain web and the ability of interactions between cortical regions to repurpose particular areas (as when, in an example he cites, an area of the visual cortex devoted to invariant object recognition is "recycled" into what Stanislas Dehaene [2009] calls a "visual word form area" that supports reading). As Anderson explains, "Modularity advocates are guided by an idealization of functional structure that is significantly at odds with the actual nature of the system. Instead of the decompose-and-localize approach to cognitive science that is advocated and exemplified by most modular accounts of the brain, neural reuse encourages 'network thinking'" (249). A dual model of cognition as both anatomically localized and a function of network connectivity has become widely accepted by the neuroscientific community.[12]

A combination of localization and network effects is necessary to explain the simulations of grounded cognition as well as the openness of grounding to various gradations. Simulations are partial, incomplete reactivations of particular cortical areas as well as reenactments of these experiences in new configurations. They are selections as well as combinations—partial traces of the original activity on which they are based, without the same fullness or intensity, that are then reassembled with different cortical areas in patterns that generate new inferences and that complete and fill out what is missing according to the demands of the new cognitive situation. This is the neurobiological basis of Barsalou's pattern-completion inference mechanism.

Because simulations are as-if re-creations that differ in the degree to which they activate a specific cortical area, they can be variously concrete and abstract. These degrees of grounding also depend on the interactions a simulation sets in motion across the brain web. Traces of sensory reactivation could be expected to occur in the most far-flung assemblies, as when specific motoric responses to action words are part of widely diverse, cross-cortical linguistic patterns (somatotopic reactions in the motor cortex to the words "kick" or "throw" in a narrative about football, for example), and these selections and combinations may result in different gradations of abstraction in the simulations they construct. Because the brain is a paradoxical web of local, anatomically based capacities and network connections that can activate and even repurpose particular areas in different ways, it can support simulations that are variously concrete and abstract, with gradations in how grounded they are in specific motoric and somatosensory regions and in how much these local reactions are transcended and transformed by the effects of cross-cortical interactions.

Embodied and Disembodied Metaphor

The paradoxes of simulation and graded grounding help to explain some of the contradictions and controversies related to the theory of embodied metaphor. As Raymond Gibbs and Teenie Matlock (2008, 162) explain, the theory that "many abstract concepts . . . are understood, at least partly, in embodied metaphorical terms" is based on simulation: "The recruitment of embodied metaphors . . . is done imaginatively as people re-create what it must be like to engage in similar actions. The key to this imaginative process is simulation, in this case the mental enactment of the very action referred to in the metaphor." As suggested by the title of George Lakoff and Mark Johnson's seminal text *Metaphors We Live By* (1980, 5), embodied metaphors like "affection is warmth," "important is big," or "happy is up" are as- and fore-structures that "understand . . . one kind of thing in terms of another." We "live by" these metaphors because they guide our engagements with the world according to the various patterns they project. Lakoff and Johnson's later formulation in *Philosophy in the Flesh* (1999, 47) of metaphors as "experientially grounded mappings" similarly implies both the as and the fore, inasmuch as a map establishes correlations and orients our expectations about pattern.

Rather than conceiving the relation between signifier and signified as purely arbitrary and conventional, as in Saussurean theory, proponents of embodied metaphor claim that our experiences of the world, constrained by our bodily-based abilities and dispositions, structure many, if not most (and the slippage here is where the controversy starts), of the relationships of similarity and difference through which we categorize states of affairs and (accordingly) reason, perceive, and act. As Lakoff and Johnson explain:

Experiencing the More Is Up correlation over and over should lead to the establishment of connections between those neural networks in the brain characterizing More in the domain of quantity and those networks characterizing Up in the domain of verticality. In the model, such neural connections would carry out the function of a conceptual mapping between More and Up and make it possible (though not necessary) for the words of verticality (such as *rise, fall, skyrocket, plummet, high, low, dip,* and *peak*) to be used conventionally to indicate quantity as well. (1999, 54)

It is not clear that there are specific regions or networks in the brain that encode More or Up or quantity or verticality as such, but otherwise the key claim here—that repeated correlations that "arise out of our embodied functioning in the world" establish "neural connections" that then become reactivated in simulations in new situations (54, 46)—matches up well with core principles of neuroscience. This is, after all, classic Hebbian wiring and firing.

As with simulations in general, however, a key question is how fixed or variable the connections established by the as-if might be. Here Lakoff and Johnson describe them as "possible (though not necessary)," although elsewhere they waffle between claiming that "the architecture of your brain's neural networks *determines* what concepts you have and hence the kind of reasoning you can do" and asserting merely that "the body and brain *shape* reason," or even less strictly that "our sense of what is real *begins with* and *depends crucially upon* our bodies" (16–17; emphasis added). These slippages are not surprising, however, because they reflect the contingencies of the as-structures that make possible gradations in grounding and variabilities in the concreteness and abstractness of our categories.

The experimental evidence on embodied metaphors is mixed, and its contradictions reflect these contingencies. Vittorio Gallese, a member of the Parma mirror-neuron group, joined up with Lakoff (2005, 456–57) to thresh out the connections between the theories of action understanding and embodied metaphor, based on their shared assumption that "imagining is a form of *simulation*—a mental simulation of action or perception, using many of the same neurons as actually acting or perceiving":

> For example, in the case of the concept of *grasping*, one would expect the parietal-premotor circuits that form functional clusters for grasping to be active not only when actually grasping, but also when understanding sentences involving the concept of *grasping*. . . . A further prediction of our theory of concepts is that such results should be obtained in fMRI studies, not only with literal sentences, but also with the corresponding metaphorical

sentences. Thus, the sentence *He grasped the idea* should activate the sensory-motor *grasping-related regions* of the brain. (472)

Interestingly, in fact, subsequent brain-scanning studies have not uniformly born out this prediction. Although some fMRI experiments have found sensory-motor resonances to nonliteral uses of action words *(*grasping an idea as opposed to grasping an object), others have not.

For example, a study by Shirley-Ann Rüschemeyer and her group (2007) comparing brain scans of responses to German action verbs like "grasp" ("greifen") and conceptual verbs based on them ("begreifen," "to understand") found premotor activation only for the action verb and not its conceptual derivative. This finding is in line with other experimental results that have shown responses in the premotor cortex to literal but not nonliteral uses of action verbs (for a summary, see Willems and Casasanto 2011, 7–8). In one case, an fMRI study by Lisa Aziz-Zadeh and associates in the Parma group (2006) found activation in the corresponding section of the premotor cortex in response to phrases describing literal hand, foot, and mouth actions like "grasping the scissors," "pressing the piano pedal," or "biting the peach" but not to nonliteral phrases that used action words in a conceptual or metaphorical manner ("handling the truth," "chewing over the details," "kicking off the year"). Similarly, a brain-scanning study by Ana Raposo's group (2009) documented motor cortex responses to individual action verbs like "kick" or action sentences like "kick the ball," but not to idiomatic phrases like "kick the bucket."

Still other experimental evidence has documented a gradual decline in sensory-motor activation along a continuum from literal to nonliteral usages, with metaphors sometimes eliciting responses, but less so as they become more abstract and conventional. For example, a study conducted by Cristina Cacciari and colleagues (2011, 149) showed greater "excitability of the motor system" when experimental subjects "were presented with literal, fictive, and metaphorical motion sentences than with idiomatic motion or mental sentences." Her experiment found gradations in somatosensory and motor response to linguistic simulations depending on the degree of the involvement of the original experience in the simulation. As she explains, "These results suggest that the excitability of the motor system is modulated by the motor component of the verb, which is preserved in fictive and metaphorical motion sentences" (149), but not in idiomatic expressions that have submerged the original action in a conventional expression or in an abstraction (like "begreifen" for grasping a concept ["Begriff"]) at a distance from the concrete motor act. An fMRI study by Rutvik Desai's laboratory (2013,

862) similarly "showed involvement of sensory-motor areas for literal and metaphoric action sentences, but not for idiomatic ones. A trend of increasing sensory-motor activation from abstract to idiomatic to metaphoric to literal sentences was seen," which suggests "a gradual abstraction process whereby the reliance on sensory-motor systems is reduced as the abstractness of meaning as well as conventionalization is increased."

These experiments do not support Gallese's strong prediction about the embodied grounding of nonliteral usages (literal versus conceptual grasping), but they are consistent with a graded view of grounding. These kinds of variations would indeed be predicted by a model of simulation as an as-if process of figuring relationships that can vary in their degree of abstractness and embodiment. According to such a model, as conventional associations take over and metaphors once alive become dead, traces of the bodily origins reenacted by a simulation would become less and less visible, dulled by repeated use in routine expressions because of the well-known desensitizing effects of habituation. The sensory-motor aspects of the simulation would consequently become less pronounced as the equivalences established by the as-relation become more customary and the abstract semantic elements come to the fore. Only an odd, unexpected use of the term—a defamiliarizing gesture that de- and recontextualizes it (as is typical, for example, in poetry)— might revivify those sensory-motor associations and reactivate the parts of the simulation that have gone dormant (see Armstrong 1990, 67–88). These variations are possible, however, only because a simulation is an as-relation that may activate local sensory-motor resonances in different and shifting degrees. Nonliteral usages may seem more or less abstract as they are more or less grounded in perceptual experiences, more or less a product of long-distance, cross-cortical network connections, more or less habitualized through repetition and conventionalization.

Narratives typically deploy metaphors to help organize the action they set in motion, and these figures similarly range along different gradations of grounding, from the concrete to the abstract. In a well-known passage from *Père Goriot*, Balzac's classic novel in the realist tradition, the proprietress Madame Vauquer figuratively embodies her boardinghouse:

The fat old face . . . , with the nose jutting from the middle of it like a parrot's beak; the podgy little hands; the body, plump as a churchgoer's; the flabby, uncontrollable bust—they are all of a piece with the reeking misery of the room, where all hope and eagerness have been extinguished and whose stifling, fetid air she alone can breathe without being sickened. Her face, with the bite of the first autumn frost in it; the wrinkles round her eyes; the expression in them that can quickly change from the set smile of a ballet dancer to the embittered scowl of a bill discounter—her whole person, in fact, explains the house, as the house implies her person. The prison cannot be run without a jailer; you can't imagine one without the other. The unwholesome corpulence of this little woman is the product of this life, as typhus is the product of a hospital. . . . When she is there, the exhibition is complete. (2004 [1834], 10–11)

As Erich Auerbach (2003 [1953], 470–71) explains in his famous analysis of this scene, "the motif of the harmony between Madame Vauquer's person on the one hand and the room in which she is present, the pension which she directs, and the life which she leads . . . is not established rationally but is presented as a striking and immediately apprehended state of things, purely suggestively, without any proof." Vividly embodied in Madame Vauquer's physical presence, the as-relations in this simulation seem so concrete and immediate as to be irrefutable even though they are purely figurative and metaphorical. The equivalences established by this configuration are offered as an intuitive demonstration of their truth, even as their hyperbolic strangeness and lingering discordance (how might one combine a ballet dancer, a bill discounter, a jailer, and typhus?) remind us of their rhetorical constructedness (a paradox consistent with Balzac's combination of melodramatic exaggeration and historical verisimilitude). The figurative coherence proposed by these embodied equivalences grounds this simulation in the concrete.

By contrast, the artificiality and even peculiarity of the equivalences at play in Henry James's typically elaborate metaphors are graded toward the abstract, so much so that many readers have complained that they are awkward and difficult to visualize. The best-known, most frequently commented example is perhaps Maggie Verver's invocation of a pagoda as a figure for her dawning intuition at the beginning of the second volume of *The Golden Bowl* that all might not be well in the arrangement that has thrust her husband and her best friend (and unbeknownst to her, his former lover) so much into each other's company while she and her father (now wed to this woman) cultivate the intimacy they enjoyed before their marriages:

This situation had been occupying for months and months the very centre of the garden of her life, but it had reared itself there like some strange tall tower of ivory, or perhaps rather some wonderful beautiful but outlandish pagoda, a structure plated with hard bright porcelain, coloured and figured and adorned at the overhanging eaves with silver bells that tinkled ever so charmingly when stirred by chance airs. She had walked round and round it—that was what she felt; she had carried on her existence in the space left her for circulation, a space that sometimes seemed ample and sometimes narrow: looking up all the while at the fair structure that spread itself so amply and rose so high, but never quite making out as yet where she might have entered had she wished. (2009 [1904], 327)

Concrete and embodied, this figure simulates Maggie's first faltering attempt to understand bewildering signs by rendering it as an exploratory stroll around a strange construction. At first glance the foursome seems not at all like a pagoda, however, and it is not surprising that many readers have found it a strained, unsuccessful figure.[13] This incongruity is nevertheless epistemologically appropriate because it is a sign of Maggie's groping effort to find new patterns of like and not like to make sense of her world. The very complication and ornateness of the pagoda image as James extends and elaborates it over several pages dramatize Maggie's inability to make her world cohere—her struggle to fit its parts into a consistent whole inasmuch their formerly familiar arrangement now seems incongruous and strange. Maggie's stroll around the garden is a concrete, embodied simulation whose disjunctions and abstractness call attention to the cognitive processes whereby she attempts to understand her world.

These discrepancies and complications also foreground the way in which metaphors construct patterns of relationship by joining the like and the not like. The very ornateness of the metaphor displays and plays with the as-if quality of a figurative simulation as an experiment with relations of equivalence (its as-structure). Rather than trying to submerge and naturalize these functions in an illusion of verisimilitude, James foregrounds and dramatizes them by elaborating the pagoda image with almost baroque complication. This unnatural, deliberately artificial display of the workings of figuration playfully exposes the as-relations set in motion by an as-if simulation instead of seeking, as Balzac does, to cover them up with a cloak of intuitive immediacy.

A further gradation in grounding, moving from the concrete to the abstract, characterizes the various figurations of embodiment in that most unnatural of narratives, James Joyce's *Finnegans Wake*. The most famous chapter in the novel, where washerwomen gossip about Anna Livia Plurabelle (ALP), is replete with bodily actions and bawdy figures, but the overall effect of Joyce's linguistic play is to foreground and call attention to the infinitely variable contingencies of "as if" simulations. Imagine the women talking (or Joyce reciting their speech in his Irish lilt in the remarkable recording he made of this section):

O
tell me all about
Anna Livia! I want to hear all
about Anna Livia. Well, you know Anna Livia? Yes, of course, we all know
Anna Livia. Tell me all. Tell me now. You'll die when you hear. Well, you
know, when the old cheb went futt and did what you know. Yes, I know, go
on. Wash quit and don't be dabbling. Tuck up your sleeves and loosen your
talk-tapes. And don't butt me—hike!—when you bend. Or whatever it was
they threed to make out he thried to two in the Fiendish Park. He's an awful
old reppe. Look at the shirt of him! Look at the dirt of it! He has all my
water black on me. (2012 [1939], 196)

These lines are very physical and corporeal—evocative back-and-forth exchanges spoken by women at work washing clothes by the riverside—but
abstract verbal play (not so visible when Joyce recites these lines) begins with
their inaugural typographical games, with the enunciated "O" also signifying
the dominance of the feminine in the chapter, an allegorical resonance reinforced by the inverted triangle it sits atop, which in turn is not only another
reference to the female anatomy but also the sigla (or hieroglyph) that Joyce
used during composition to identify ALP. A pun on the French word "eau,"
this letter also announces the chapter's preoccupation with water, a theme
suggestive again of the feminine (recalling Molly's flowing monologue in
Ulysses), and notoriously echoed by hundreds of indirect references to rivers
throughout the chapter (Roland McHugh [1991] finds allusions in this passage to the river Repe in Germany and the Blackwater River in Florida).[14]
    This is self-consciously both speech and writing, and that doubling is re-
iterated and reinforced in the further as-if games Joyce plays in this elaborate simulation. Even as the women talk and wash, their acts suggest the
sexual behavior ("don't butt me") that they avidly discuss, but these allusions come through portmanteau words and puns that are products of the
writer's games rather than their actual speech—"Fiendish Park" for Phoenix
Park, for example, where ALP's husband, HCE (the "chap" indicated by his
initials in "cheb"), is said to have "tried" to "do" whatever his notorious but
ambiguous crime was. The suggestive but indeterminate word-play here suggests yet another triangle ("threed," "thried," "two") where HCE was seen
by a third person trying to do some evil deed to a second—a sexual act of
some kind? The grime that befouls their washing water figures the foulness
of his sin as well as the dirt with which they enjoy besmirching their sup-
posed friend ALP. The physical rhythms of their speech give the language a
concreteness that the abstract allegorical references and the playful puns of

the writing counter with a lively virtuality. This juxtaposition in turn has a paradoxical effect, producing at one and the same time a very physical, natural, and bodily scene and a very artificial, abstract, and symbolic set of games, a duality that once again foregrounds the work of the as in as-if simulations.

The paradoxes and contradictions of graded grounding and as-if simulation are evident in the conflict over whether bodily-based metaphors are universal or culturally and historically variable. "When the embodied experiences in the world are universal," Lakoff and Johnson argue (1999, 56), "then the corresponding primary metaphors [those that derive from basic sensorimotor experiences] are universally acquired. This explains the widespread occurrence around the world of a great many primary metaphors." For example, a study by Benjamin Wilkowski and colleagues (2009) demonstrated that the metaphor of heat for anger is based on bodily experiences that transcend cultural differences. As they explain, "many parallels between heat and anger provide an embodied basis for anger-heat associations. . . . For example, just as boiling fluids expand and threaten to escape their container, anger threatens to erupt in the form of an aggressive 'explosion'" (475). Wilkowski's study concludes: "These conceptual parallels between anger and heat are embedded in the embodied experience of human existence and know no cultural boundaries" and, consequently, "are responsible for the robust cross-cultural belief that anger and bodily heat are systematically related" (475). These claims are supported by a series of experiments involving 438 participants that tested in various ways their tendency to associate anger and heat. Among the reported results: "visual depictions of heat facilitated the use of anger-related conceptual knowledge" (464), "priming anger-related thoughts led participants to judge unfamiliar cities and the actual room temperature as hotter in nature" (469), "participants were faster to categorize an angry facial expression when it was presented in a context suggestive of heat" (469), and "cues to heat led individuals to identify a greater degree of anger in blended emotional expressions" (475).

By contrast, however, a wide-ranging study by historian Joanna Bourke (2014, 484) provides compelling evidence that "the physiological body is not a culture-free object." As she observes, "Even a cursory look at the world's languages reveals a formidable number of non-universal metaphors" for even as fundamental an experience as pain—so much so that "the McGill Pain Questionnaire (an extensive list of pain-descriptors that was developed in America in the 1960s) could not always be translated straightforwardly into other European languages" (482). These discrepancies are even more acute, she points out, with non-European examples: "The Sakhalin Ainu of

Japan complain of 'bear headaches' that resemble the heavy steps of a bear; 'musk deer headaches,' like the lighter galloping of running deer; and 'woodpecker headaches,' as if pounding into the bark of a tree" (483). Similarly, comparing modern medical notions of homeostasis to eighteenth-century humoral theory that figured pain through "rich figurative languages of ebbs and flows," Bourke argues that what the opposition of balance versus imbalance means in these different systems is not identical: "Of course, the most basic schema survive: ones based on sensorimotor bodily experience of lying down and standing up (HAPPY IS UP and SAD IS DOWN), for instance, or those based on physical comportment relating to vigour versus infirmity (HEALTH/LIFE ARE UP and ILLNESS/DEATH ARE DOWN). But others take on such a different meaning in the humoural scheme of physiology [as] to be radically different" (486)—disequilibria or blockages, for example, involving "phlegm, black bile, yellow bile, and blood" that are connected to "personality types (sanguine and melancholic)" and "three kinds of spirits, which acted on the humours: the natural, the vital, and the animal" (485). "Eighteenth-century bodies-in-pain felt different to modern ones," Bourke concludes, because "the figurative languages of humoural bodies reveal different ways of being-in-the-world" (488).

Because different cultural worlds have a shared biological basis, however, they are not entirely opaque to each other. It is possible to translate these analogies into different as-relations, as Bourke herself does—explaining what these kinds of pain or imbalances resemble (or are like), with what sorts of as-if connotations. As-relations point both ways—toward the nonequivalence of the terms of an analogy that are not like each other, and also toward the equivalences that make the analogy meaningful and useful because of ways in which the terms are like. Metaphors configure bodily experience *as* something it is not (anger both is and is not heat, a headache is both like and not like the steps of a bear or the pounding of a woodpecker, pain is both similar to and different from a blockage of a fluid). We can understand and recognize the plausibility of these analogies (what it is like to experience pain through animal metaphors or humoral categories) even though they are not our own because our bodies are biocultural hybrids that are not totally disconnected from our Japanese conspecifics or our eighteenth-century forebears. We share some bodily experiences and associations (some "survive," as Bourke herself notes), but others are variable, and that combination allows commonalities as well as differences in what experiences of pain or anger or pleasure are figured as by different communities.

Figurative constructions like metaphors and narratives draw on as-relations that are prefigured in experience—analogies like these are deeply embedded in embodied cognition in its different degrees and kinds of grounding—and the as-if relations on which they are based can then be reconfigured in poems or narratives or other fictional forms in simulations that may reinforce or disrupt the configurations of the like and not like they draw on. The circuit between figuration and refiguration in the transformation of experience into narratives (the movement from mimesis$_1$ to mimesis$_2$) is possible because the connections posited by a cognitive or fictional simulation both are and are-not originally given in experience. This in turn is why the simulations of the as in the as-if of fictive reenactments can reshape the experiences of the recipients (as mimesis$_2$ is taken up in mimesis$_3$), which is how these culturally variable analogies get established and disseminated, through the stories that members of a community tell each other about what their anger, pain, or pleasure is like. The circuit of figuration (mimesis$_1$, mimesis$_2$, and mimesis$_3$) through which experience gets transformed and reshaped in fictional reenactments joins action and perception through the as of simulation. Narratives have the power to refigure our lives in these ways because we are biocultural hybrids who engage the world through configurations of action and perception that are constrained by our bodies but also open to wide variation.

Interactions of Action in Narrative and Narration

Narratives are constituted by the intertwining of different modalities of action, most basically by the interaction between discourse and story—that is, the relation between the act of telling and the actions and events emplotted in the told that is fundamental to our capacity to exchange and understand stories. The ability of narratives to bring into relation different kinds of action is grounded in (and can consequently have a powerful effect on) the role of action in coordinating different cognitive processes in our embodied engagements with our worlds. As Berthoz and Petit observe in their authoritative study of *The Physiology and Phenomenology of Action* (2008, 42–43), the synthesis of "multiple systems . . . of sense data" in the brain is accomplished through action: "The unity of the perceived world depends upon the extraordinary capacity of the brain which, in the first instance, breaks up the world into multiple components. The world of our lived experience is then the result of a synthesis of the activity of all these stations. . . . The *act* is an indispensable feature of this unity." For example, as Merleau-Ponty (2012 [1945], 151) points out, "What unites the 'tactile sensations' of the hand and links them to the visual perceptions of the same hand and to perceptions of other segments of the body is a certain style of hand gestures, which implies a certain style of finger movements and moreover contributes to a particular fashion in which my body moves." Because the felt unity of embodied experience is generated by the underlying "style" of these interactions, Merleau-Ponty famously declares that "the body cannot be compared to the physical object, but rather to the work of art" (152). Narratives are powerful cognitive and existential instruments because of their ability to organize and reorganize action of many different kinds, on different levels, across many perceptual and experiential modalities.

A particular style characterizes different modes of cognition because they are what Alva Noë (2015, 10) calls "organized activities." As he explains, "Our lives are one big complex nesting of organized activities at different levels and scales." These styles of organization are patterns integrating the differences registered by our perceptual equipment, the epistemological habits that develop over our lifetimes of embodied cognitive experience through Hebbian wiring and firing. The style that organizes these perceptual and cognitive modalities characterizes in turn our style of being-in-the-world, the characteristic intentionality (the directedness toward people, states of affairs, and the future) that comes to define our sense of self. Cognitive narrative theorist Guillemette Bolens's (2012, 22, 28) definition of gesture as "kinesic style" encapsulates these linkages: "Kinesic styles interconnect all degrees of expressivity. . . . A person's kinesic style is perceptible in her idiosyncratic movements and the singular way she negotiates social codes and physical constraints, while the kinesic style of a literary work is conveyed through its narrative dynamics." A person's distinctive kinesic style has to do with how her different ways of acting in the world are organized and interrelate, and the "dynamics" of a narrative are the ways in which it organizes the interaction of the different kinds of action it sets in motion.

The ability of linguistic narratives to coordinate embodied action depends on the relation between language, speech, and gesture. As Merleau-Ponty (2012 [1945], 187) argues, "The body is a natural power of expression." In his view, the expressive powers of language ultimately derive from an embodied capacity for communicative action that is evident in gesture: "Speech is a genuine gesture. . . . This is what makes communication possible" (189). According to this theory of the gestural basis of communication, the codes and conventions of language are secondary rather than primary. The rules of a language are "the depository and sedimentation of acts of speech" (202), abstract and socially encoded residues of expressive linguistic and bodily action.

Contemporary neuroscientific findings about the development of language confirm Merleau-Ponty's phenomenological intuition about the interdependence of language, speech, and gesture—the many deep connections between our ability to communicate with one another and our embodied capacities for expressive action. These connections pass through the motor cortex. As Pulvermüller (2018) explains, the motor cortex plays a key role in language development because it must bind with the auditory cortex in order to link the perception of speech sounds with the physical action of articulating speech through movements of the tongue and the lips. According to Marc Jeannerod (2006, 154–55), these developmental connections explain why, in adult communication, "speech perception . . . activates motor structures involved in speech production." When we listen to someone talk or even when we read a written text, the motor cortex is active even though our bodies may be totally still. As Michael Tomasello (2003) argues, these linkages are part of a broader network of connections between the motor cortex and various other areas of the brain (visual, auditory, haptic), cross-cortical connections that develop through the communicative exchanges that begin in infancy as parents and children imitate one another's expressions and otherwise gesture toward one another. These exchanges create links between the production and observation of actions of the kind registered in the mirror-neuron experiments (also see Armstrong 2013, 131–74). According to Tomasello (2003, 35), "It is gestures that for many children seem to be the first carriers of their communicative intentions. And it is gestures that seem to pave the way to early language." Kenneth Burke's (1966) memorable description of language as "symbolic action" is evocative and appropriate because it concisely encapsulates the diverse and profound connections between linguistic action and the bodily capacity for expressive communication evident in gesture.

As symbolic action, however, language both is and is not like other kinds of bodily action, and these differences also matter. The relation between linguistic and bodily action is paradoxical, as Shaun Gallagher (2005, 122–23) observes: "The thing that makes gesture more than movement is that gesture is language." At the same time, however, he cautions that "it would be wrong to lose track" of the fact that "gesture is nonetheless movement." The gestures that accompany speech often have communicative power, but not all of the gestures people make when they speak are expressive—some are just movements. By the same token, the expressive and instrumental dimensions of an action are related but not reducible to each other. Some movements that may seem expressive are primarily instrumental actions aimed at making changes in the world. Because actions have styles, an instrumental action may seem expressive, but not all actions are communicative gestures, and it is often possible to distinguish the communicative and instrumental aspects of an action. For one soccer commentator it is the beauty and grace of a goal that stand out, for example, while for another it's the tactical cunning and skill that matter.

Our bodily capacity to act makes it possible to communicate, but action and communication are different and (sometimes) separable. To recall an example I have already cited, people can lose the ability to act instrumentally through injuries to the motor cortex but still retain language and the capacity to produce and understand speech. Someone who is physically paralyzed may be able to understand and discuss actions which he or she cannot perform, and this would not be possible if action and communication were identical (see Hickok 2014). It is sometimes the case, however, that physical impairments result in deficits in language production and comprehension, and that is because the motor cortex is a hub that connects instrumental and expressive action. Physiologically as well as experientially, instrumental action and communicative action are inextricably linked, but they are not the same.

These distinctions are subtle and difficult to pin down, but they have important consequences. The relation between communicative and instrumental action is a paradoxical relation of equivalence and nonequivalence that is powerfully generative. For one thing, it helps to explain how we are able to organize actions into stories. The paradoxical relation of like and not like that holds between motoric and communicative action enables narratives to stage interactions between different levels and kinds of action. The fact that expressive movement and other modalities of cognitive and motoric action are at one and the same time like and not like one another—equivalent in many respects as styles and kinds of action, but nevertheless ultimately not reducible to each other—is what makes it possible for them to interact. Because of their many similarities and connections, their differences can resonate off each other and be shaped into meaningful configurations—as when dancers engage in expressive movements that can be read as steps in a choreographed performance or as when narratives emplot actions and communicate them in acts of narration. Similarly, the distinction between communicative action (gesture) and instrumental action (motoric and bodily capacities of various kinds, whether the movements of a dancer or the activities of characters in a story) makes possible the intertwining of discourse (the communicative act of telling) and story (emplotments of instrumental actions and events).

Keeping track of the differences between kinds of action is important for understanding how narratives perform various characteristic functions. For

example, the ability of narratives to coordinate and integrate different modalities of action helps to explain how a story can create an illusion of presence and facilitate immersion in a fictional world. As Anežka Kuzmičová
(2012, 25, 29) points out, narratives can produce "a higher degree of spatial vividness, arousing in the reader a sense of having physically entered a
tangible environment (presence) . . . when certain forms of human bodily
movement are rendered," and that is because "the motor and pre-motor areas of their cortices become somatotopically activated—the hand area of
the motor strip responding to hand-related action words, the feet area to
feet-related action words." Terence Cave (2016, 81) similarly explains that
"when fictional mimesis works, . . . that's not because it 'paints pictures' for
the imagination. It stimulates the neural areas that are involved when we
perform a given action or have a perceptual experience."

Anatomically based neuronal resonance is necessary but not sufficient,
however. The responses of particular neurons must also be organized into
action assemblies. This is what Tolstoy does with such mastery, according to
Elaine Auyoung (2018, 20–21). By directing the reader's "attention to ordinary physical actions, such as pulling on a loose button, stepping on a piece
of ice, or swallowing a piece of bread," she explains, Tolstoy activates the
reader's kinesthetic, procedural knowledge of how to perform everyday actions, and this integration of motor resonances into patterns of familiar instrumental activity "enables the text to evoke perceptual immediacy in a
surprisingly effective way" (and, as she shows by comparing various renderings of Russian phrases into English, in a manner that survives linguistic
translation). When Levin swings a scythe in the memorable mowing scene,
for example, the resonances activated by the descriptions of his actions in our
motor cortex become the basis for a vivid representation because they are
in turn organized into physical sequences of action (walking down the field,
pausing for a drink and a chat). Only when the motor resonances set off by
action words at the neuronal level are organized into recognizable bodily actions can they contribute to an illusion of presence—but a linguistic description alone without motor resonances would also lack the vividness Tolstoy achieves.

What matters is not just specific bodily references and neuronally based
motor resonances but the narrative recreation of patterns of action, and these
in turn must be readily synthesized in the act of reading. Here yet another
level and modality of action comes into play. As Auyoung explains (32), what
cognitive scientists call "fluency" in processing—"the subjective ease with
which we perform mental acts"—can make something that is strange and

even improbable seem familiar and acceptable. Her example is the wordless proposal scene in *Anna Karenina* that seems vivid and even moving although it is strictly speaking preposterous: "While the pleasure afforded by this miraculous exchange has many sources, one of them is how the scene, so utterly unique in the history of love, has been constructed from materials that are completely ordinary and ready to hand," with Kitty and Levin drawing letters on a tablecloth with a piece of chalk (33). Communicative action (telling and reading) interacts productively here with instrumental action as the ease of following the word game the lovestruck couple play makes their bodily interaction come alive.

As we read or listen to stories, the ability to fluently construct consistent patterns fosters the building of illusions (see Iser 1974, 282–90). Fluency in comprehension aids and abets the illusion of presence because mimesis is not simply a correspondence of sign and thing or a matter of motor resonance alone but a process of connecting modalities of action. The ease with which connections can be made at the level of communicative action facilitates the rendering of instrumental action because, borrowing a metaphor from neuroscience, it "mylenates" the circuit joining the three types of mimesis. Just as mylenation speeds the passage of an action potential down an axon (see Bear, Connors, and Paradiso 2007, 96–97), so fluency in communicative consistency building facilitates the interaction between a narrative's configuration of actions (mimesis$_2$), a reader's figurative reconstructions (mimesis$_3$), and patterns of activity from past embodied experience (mimesis$_1$). Fluent connections naturalize the strange and unfamiliar by facilitating the linkages through which narrative figuration passes.

The construction of patterns in reading or listening draws on our perceptual experiences with horizonal absences—the hidden and not yet in the situation of perception that Merleau-Ponty characterizes as the intertwining of the visible and the invisible. Recall how, as he explains, every act of perception has spatial, temporal, and intersubjective horizons across which it projects expectations about what is hidden from its perspective but available, we tacitly assume, to other perceivers or to us in the future. As Auyoung observes (2018, 21), "Literary artists who seek to evoke perceptual immediacy must contend with the fact that every sensory modality of the represented world—not just the visual modality but also the auditory, olfactory, haptic, spatial, and kinesthetic—is at all times absent from the text itself." These absences are not fatal, however, because gaps and indeterminacies are a familiar feature of perceptual experience. "We are accustomed," Auyoung explains, "to believing that more lies beyond the scope of our knowledge and perception," and it is "our readiness to contend with partial representational cues in everyday, nonliterary experience" that makes the mind alive to "what minimal cues imply" (2013, 69, 60, 66).

The action-perception circuit in cognition interacts productively here with the communicative action of following a story. Again what matters is the interaction between modalities of action that are different but that resonate and intertwine. Just as in everyday perception we integrate the partial perspectives through which people, places, and things present themselves in our experience and fill out what is hidden from our view, so in reading we are predisposed to take necessarily incomplete perspectives and, through what Iser calls "gap filling" and "consistency building," configure them into gestalts whose coherence encourages us to believe in them (see Iser 1978, 118–32, 165–79; also see Ingarden 1973 [1931], 217–84). As Iser argues, the eventfulness of the temporal act of reading contributes to and reinforces this illusion by re-creating the quality of happening that characterizes the represented events in the storyworld (see 1976, 118–51). Because we ourselves produce a narrative's configurations, we may feel a particular intimacy with them that further occludes their immateriality and endows them with a sense of immediacy. The coherence between these related modes of activity implies a completeness that a text's absences necessarily lack, and the ease with which readers can produce these patterns reinforces this illusion. The act of reading and the act of perception can interact in these ways because both involve processes of pattern completion that are facilitated by their fluency and coherence.

Reading is not the same as perception, however, and the concordant discordances of narrative rarely if ever leave these coherences unperturbed. Here again differences matter as much as the interactions they make possible. The illusion of presence in a storyworld is not the same as an hallucination but instead involves what Iser calls a "virtual dimension" (1974, 279–81). The virtuality of narrative immersion has an as-if quality that both is and is not like the perceptual experiences it draws on. If, as Iser (1974, 286) explains, "a consistent, configurative meaning is essential for . . . the process of illusion-building," nevertheless at the same time, this need for consistency leads readers to exclude many other possibilities. As a result, he argues, "the formation of illusions is constantly accompanied by 'alien associations,'" disturbances that make us "oscillate between involvement in and observation of those illusions" (286). These "alien associations" serve as reminders of the "quasi-ness" or virtuality of a fictional world.

The quasi quality of as-if states of affairs is often misunderstood. For example, Kendall Walton (1990, 244) misconstrues the paradoxical combination of equivalence and nonequivalence in as-if stagings of affect when he claims that "the emotions that audiences have in response to fictional works are not real emotions, but merely make-believe 'quasi-feelings.'" He is right, of course, that "when audiences experience fear and anxiety in response to ominous images on screen, they do not flee from the theater because their emotional response is part of the pretense" (244). But this does not make their feelings any less "real" (they may cry real tears and feel real sadness as the heroine sings her final aria and "dies" in *Carmen*, for example, or they may actually jump in reflexive fright at the sight of a snake in a movie). The bodily resonances evoked by as-if illusions have a virtual dimension because they are only traces of the original experience they simulate, but the pretense of immersive aesthetic experiences can have real effects on the bodies and brains of the recipient that make possible the illusion of presence. Not simply a quibble about terminological distinctions, this misunderstanding matters because the combination of like *and* not like in virtual experiences of the as-if is what allows fictional stagings of action to have real effects on our embodied habits of action in the world—it is how the quasi experiences of mimesis$_3$ in response to the as-if configurations of mimesis$_2$ can circle back and refigure our real, lived, everyday embodied cognitive practices (mimesis$_1$).

A similar failure to credit both the like and the not like undermines Roman Ingarden's (1973 [1931], 160–73) assertion that declarative statements in a work of art are only quasi judgments that do not make the same claim to truth as real judgments. Again, the fictional statements in a narrative may not be admissible in a court of law (no judge is going to convict Raskolnikov of murder), but the character Dostoevsky creates in *Crime and Punishment* may acquire a lifelike presence in what Ingarden calls the "concretization" of a text's potentialities that can affect a reader's real attitudes toward (and judgments about) states of affairs in her or his world (recall the discussion in chapter 2 of Jenefer Robinson's argument about the ways in which identifying with a character like Anna Karenina can affect moral and social appraisals of larger matters across the horizon of the fictional world). To dismiss fictional emotions or judgments as unreal because they are merely quasi is to misunderstand the real powers of as-if simulations. Sometimes quasi feelings and quasi judgments are just as real and true as the nonfictional states of affairs they simulate (and maybe even more so).

Narratives construct patterns of action that they then interrupt, reverse, and revise and that resonate off each other with different degrees of concord and discord, harmony and dissonance. As Iser argues, "The inherent non-achievement of balance" in the building and breaking of illusions "is a prerequisite for the very dynamism of the operation" (1974, 287). The imbalances of discordant concordance in narrative are inherently dynamic, and that makes them like other aspects of our cognitive lives. Shifting configurations of concord and discord create different possibilities of immersion in a storyworld and lead us as readers to alternate between participating in and critically reflecting about the illusions we create. This experience of back-and-forth movement between building and breaking illusions, between participating in and observing patterns of action that we produce as we read or follow a story, is why Cave (2016, 135) is right to declare that "it is a mistake to think that immersion and reflection are antithetical poles." They are, rather, interdependent products of the dynamic interaction of narrative concord and discord.

Narrative disjunctions interrupt immersion and prompt reflection by playing with a fundamental characteristic of embodied action—its habitual, natural "unthinkingness." As Jeannerod (2006, 59) notes, "We remain unaware of most of our actions, unless an unpredicted event interrupts their course and brings them to consciousness." For example, the surest way to make someone fumble in the execution of a routine behavior is to call attention to it and introduce self-consciousness into actions that are ordinarily automatic and habitual. Similarly, as Heidegger observes in his analysis of the ready-to-hand (*Zuhandenheit*), the tool is invisible as long as we can use it effectively. Only when the equipment breaks down do we notice its equipmentality—only when hammering fails do the act of hitting the nail and the characteristics of the hammer become available for thought (see 1962 [1927], 95–107). Our ability to act fluently, based on procedural memory and habitual skill, depends on not thinking about what we are doing—not noticing, for example, the time lags between execution and awareness that Libet measures in his mind-time experiments. Stage fright and performance anxiety are well-known examples. By the same token, as long as things fit together seamlessly while we follow a story, whether in the transitions between the events emplotted in the told or in the connections between different aspects of the telling, our deeply rooted tendency not to pay attention to the ordinary actions we are engaged in supports and reinforces our unthinking involvement in the states of affairs we produce. Only when this flow is interrupted does the illusion get broken and critical observation take over. What Vanessa Ryan (2012) calls "thinking without thinking" is a pervasive feature of lived cognitive experience and ordinary action, and it is a phenomenon that stories take advantage of in order to draw us in and keep us engaged—that is, until reversals in the told or disjunctions in the telling interrupt these involvements and make us reflect on what we had hitherto been processing unreflectively.

The characteristic unthinkingness of action supports and sustains what phenomenology calls the "natural attitude," our customary cognitive posture of unquestioned engagement with the world (see Armstrong 2012). As Merleau-Ponty points out, however, whenever we begin to reflect, we find a whole realm of unreflected meaning already there (see 2012 [1945], lxxiv–lxxxv). We may not have thought we were thinking, but we were. Reflection is consequently, in Merleau-Ponty's view, a perpetually incomplete, never-finished activity of reflecting on unreflected experience that always outstrips it.

As a systematic philosophical method, phenomenology *brackets* the natural attitude and suspends its engagements in order to bring to the fore various otherwise unnoticed aspects of lived experience. This technique is merely a formalization, however, of ordinary experiences of cognitive disruption and reframing. In our everyday lives, surprising interruptions and anomalies have a similar power to bring unthought thought processes into view. The ability of cognitive disturbances and anomalies to expose otherwise invisible epistemological processes is what makes optical illusions like the Necker cube or ambiguous figures like the oscillating rabbit-duck such favorites of philosophers and neuroscientists (see Armstrong 2013, 67–72). Narrative discontinuities have a similar ability to disrupt and suspend the natural attitude that typically characterizes the reception of stories. There is already a quality of metafictional self-display in narrative disruptions and reversals because they have the power to expose and cause us to reflect about cognitive processes whose smooth functioning ordinarily depends on their invisibility.

The various disruptions to narrative continuity for which Joseph Conrad is well known illustrate how interruption can suspend the natural attitude. In an oft-quoted passage from *Lord Jim*, Marlow remarks that "it's extraordinary how we go through life with eyes half shut, with dull ears, with dormant thoughts. Perhaps it's just as well; and it may be that it is this very dulness that makes life to the incalculable majority so supportable and so welcome" (1996 [1900], 87–88). As Conrad's fictions repeatedly show, however, the shock of baffling, unexpected events may intervene and produce "one of these rare moments of awakening when we see, hear, understand ever so much—everything—in a flash—before we fall back again into our agreeable somnolence" (88). Moments of bewilderment in his narratives again and again suspend unthinking involvement in the world and expose its tacit assumptions and operations to view (see Armstrong 1987)—for example: Jim's surprise that he had abandoned ship ("I had jumped . . . it seems" [67]) and that the bulging rusty bulkhead had not burst, Marlow's angry annoyance that a guilty young man should "look so sound" ("well, if this sort can go wrong like that" [29]), Gentleman Brown's violent destruction of the community of trust on Patusan, and the disillusioning impact of Jim's death on his supporters ("He passes away under a cloud, inscrutable at heart" [246]). These interruptions all disrupt patterns of consistency building that Jim, Marlow, and Patusan hadn't previously been aware of. As Marlow comments at one point, "It is always the unexpected that happens" (60)—and the unexpected can give rise to thought by exposing what we hadn't known we were thinking.

The revelatory power of narrative discontinuities—whether the twists and turns of traditional stories or the more radical disruptions of experimental, "unnatural" fictions—is parasitic on the habitual, automatic, unthinking everyday fluency of action and perception that they interrupt. In *Lord Jim*, at the level of the events of the story, discontinuities in the flow of the action in what would otherwise seem to be a tale of adventure or an imperial romance raise moral and existential questions about the contingency of our ethical norms and cultural codes that give Conrad's works an existential and metaphysical dimension usually absent from these genres whose conventions he subverts. In the discourse, Conrad deploys various strategies of narration that disrupt the presentation of events—the reversals of effect and cause, for example, that Ian Watt (1979) famously calls "delayed decoding" ("What had happened?" the narration asks when the accident occurs— "The wheezy thump of the engines went on. Had the earth been checked in her course?" (20)—only many pages later to identify the cause: "A floating derelict probably" [97]), or the many gaps that refuse to cohere in the perspectives through which the tale is offered as Marlow tries to piece together the contradictory views of the many different informants he consults. If fluency of action in the telling and the told facilitates immersion by drawing on the natural attitude, disruptions like these in the act of narration break the illusion in order to expose and call for reflection about processes of pattern construction that narratives otherwise tacitly exploit.

Narrative Affordances

The interaction of these modalities of narrative action calls to mind the well-known terminology of affordances introduced by Gibson's (1979) ecological theory of perception. According to Gibson, what we perceive in a scene are not the properties of objects but the possibilities of action they implicitly *afford*—that is, in his words, what "the environment . . . offers the animal, what it provides or furnishes, either for good or ill" (127).[15] According to this "'do-ability' theory," as Berthoz and Petit (2008, 66) explain, "we perceive primarily what has a practical bearing on our action." When we follow a story, we similarly respond in different ways and at different levels to the possibilities of action it offers. As Glenberg and Kaschak (2002, 559) explain, this entails a process of "meshing affordances":

> For example, one can judge that the sentence, "Hang the coat on the upright vacuum cleaner" is sensible, because one can derive from the perceptual symbol of the vacuum cleaner the affordances that allow it to be used as a coat rack. Similarly, one can judge that the sentence "Hang the coat on the upright cup" is not sensible in most contexts, because cups do not usually have the proper affordances to serve as coat racks. . . . If the meshed set of affordances corresponds to a doable action, the utterance is understood. If the affordances do not mesh in a way that can guide action (e.g., how could one hang a coat on a cup?), understanding is incomplete, or the sentence is judged nonsensical, even though all of the words and syntactic relations may be commonplace.

The consistency building that Iser describes is not only a matter of synthesizing the perspectives through which states of affairs unfold in a text but also a process of integrating (meshing) the affordances it offers—that is, of coordinating the possibilities of action held ready, for example, not only by the events emplotted in the story but also by the acts of interpretation and evaluation rendered by the discourse. As a structure of concordant discordance, however, the dynamics of a narrative will sometimes mesh these affordances and sometimes not, with various effects and for different purposes. Most competent readers of literature, for example, can readily imagine contexts in which the affordances of "Hang the coat on the cup" would be appropriate (think of Gertrude Stein's *Tender Buttons* or *Alice's Adventures in Wonderland*) precisely because the dissonances in their refusal to mesh in an ordinary, predictable way are resonant with new and interesting possibilities of response.

This is the kind of example Cave (2016, 46–62) has in mind when he proposes the concept of literary affordances. These refer not only to the possible actions associated with states of affairs represented in a novel or a poem but also to the responses held ready by its forms. The conventions of a genre, for example, afford more or less specific sets of action by writers and readers in their construction of and their responses to texts. These affordances are sometimes quite constrained, as with the sonnet, but they are never completely unbounded even in more open-ended genres like (to echo Henry James) "the big baggy monster" of the novel. There are affordances that have to do with the telling as well as with the told, and these are not the same, but the dynamics of the narrative are a matter of how these affordances intertwine—how the actions set in motion by the discourse mesh (or not) not only with each other but also with the actions afforded by the story. Discourse and story can have such interesting and unpredictable effects on each other because they are not inert forms with objective properties (as the reified taxonomies of structural narratology suggest); rather, they are modalities of action whose affordances we seek to mesh but that (thanks to the concordant discordances of narrative) settle into stable, coherent patterns only (if ever) at the end (and then only with texts where the possibilities of action afforded by both the telling and the told are finally closed).

As Cave points out, the affordances of literature typically invite improvisation: "What literature affords, indeed, is cognitive and cultural fluidity" (39). Affordances constrain but do not absolutely, completely determine our engagements with them. A chair affords sitting, for example, but it can also be used for a handstand or as a weapon in a bar brawl. With linguistic artifacts, according to Cave, this duality also reflects the fact that "all uses of language are highly underspecified" (25), manifesting the gaps and indeterminacies that Iser, Ingarden, and Auyoung emphasize. Literary texts take particular advantage of the underspecification of language and the capacity of these absences to make possible improvisatory, unpredictable responses. As Cave vividly explains, literature's "bold and highly precise modes of underspecification act like a prompt or a trampoline, creating unlimited possibilities for imaginative leaps into the blue—or into the minds of others" (27).

The duality of affordances in constraining response while inviting (and in the case of literary affordances even requiring) improvisation gives them a particular kind of historicity. In Cave's words, they are "Janus-faced: they point both back towards" the history of previous involvements that have established their current configurations and our inherited sense of their potentialities, even as they point "forward along time's arrow towards the present and future outgrowths of human cultural improvisation" (62) that may take them in unforeseen directions. Noting, for example, that "the essay had an afterlife that Montaigne could not possibly have imagined," Cave observes that "literary instruments are often defined and recognized retrospectively. Thinking of genres as affordance structures helpfully reorients attention forwards, towards the restless reworking of existing templates" (58) that writers and readers engage in by improvising in response to the possibilities of action that previous texts make possible.

In the case of narrative, the terminology of affordances is especially relevant to the much-discussed problem of probability.[16] Responses to the probabilities afforded by a narrative are, as Karin Kukkonen (2014b, 372) argues, a particular instance of the general rule that "embodied cognition is profoundly informed by sensing how actions are going to develop." Proposing a Bayesian model of cognition as predictive processing, Andy Clark (2016, 5) argues that "we see the world by . . . guessing the world." This is true of perception in general as well as in what Iser (1976, 108–18) describes as the anticipatory and retrospective to-and-fro processes of reading and following a story. According to Kukkonen (2016, 157), narratives have what she calls a "probability design": "As the plot arranges the sequence in which events are related in the narrative, it gives readers new observations about the fictional world, and these new observations can confirm or contradict their probabilistic, predictive model of what is likely to happen in the fictional world." These predictions about probability are not confined to the plot, Kukkonen points out, but interact in "feedback loops" with other modalities of action in the narrative that have an effect on readers' expectations—their predictions (typically nonthetic, unthinking, intuitive) about what will happen next in their experience of following the story, whether this is triggered by interactions among the characters and events in the plot or by a narrator's storytelling acts (what she holds back or reveals, how she judges, and whether we trust or are suspicious of those evaluations).

Not restricted to the level of the plot, predictions of probability in the unfolding of narrative action bring into dynamic relation all the levels of and interactions between the many various modalities of action in a narrative. As the narrative world unfolds in our experience in ways that either accord with or defy our expectations, Kukkonen (2014a, 724) observes, "it is not unusual that readers find different probabilistic models for the fictional world" in conflict or competition with one another, as when narratorial discourse comments ironically on plot events and leads readers to expect different things from what the characters may anticipate, or when our sense as readers, listeners, or viewers of what a genre typically affords (the rewards and punishments characteristic of a Greek tragedy or a Hollywood movie, for example) leads us to project probabilities not yet predictable from the events themselves. The probability design of a narrative is thus not a fixed structure but a dynamic, fluid, complex interaction between different modalities of action that sets off various predictive processes in the reader, feedback loops and "cascades of cognition" (as Kukkonen calls them), usually occurring beneath awareness through intuitive, prereflective assessments but sometimes breaking into self-consciousness in abstract, reflective judgments. These loops and cascades in response to narrative probabilities once again draw on and simulate perceptual processes at work in our everyday cognitive lives, where we are constantly comparing, synthesizing, and negotiating predictions about our worlds. And this (again) is why our experience with narrative probabilities can inform and refigure our predictive behavior in other aspects of experience.

The ways in which actions intertwine in a narrative are paradoxically both evidence of its social and historical particularity and evocative of resonances that enable stories to produce effects in listeners across temporal and cultural distance. This paradox is a consequence of our biocultural hybridity as embodied creatures whose capacities for action and cognition are shaped both by species-wide evolutionary processes and by our local, situated experiences as members of specific communities. As Kukkonen and Marco Caracciolo (2014, 267) point out, "Bodily experience shapes cultural practices" even as "cultural practices help the mind make sense of bodily experience." On the one hand, as they observe, "relatively stable bodily patterns" across history enable readers to respond emotionally and kinesthetically to texts from different cultural settings and historical periods (266). But on the other hand, as Bolens (2012, 42) notes, "the historical, cultural, and social context in which any kinesic signal is performed always bears on the gesture's sense, both for the person who emotes and for the person who perceives the emotional signal." The sedimentation of kinesic signals in linguistic signs, Bolens observes, can even result in perceptible cultural differences between the resonances of action words that embody "different ways of conceptualizing the dimensions of motion events" (38), differences evident in the English lexicon in the contrast between verbs with French or Latin as opposed to Anglo-Saxon roots.

Linguistic renderings of action may consequently at one and the same time demarcate and transcend historical distance. For example, quoting a passage from *The Adventures of Ferdinand Count Fathom*, a novel by Tobias Smollett published in 1753, Kukkonen (2014b, 368) claims that the "forceful kinesic language of the effects that fear has" on a character "give[s] the embodied reader a fairly precise idea of [his] state of mind, and this idea is replicable in the reader's own embodied resonances to the kinesic shape and directedness of the words she reads." The diction of the passage conveys these emotions, however, through phrases like "the brandishing of poignards," "every fresh filip of his fear," or "a new volley of imprecations" that are remote from the linguistic habits of most twenty-first century readers.[17] These linguistically coded kinesic signals, in all their strangeness, mark the historical and cultural boundaries that are being crossed if the passage succeeds in conveying an embodied sense of the character's anxieties—and it might not succeed in doing so if the unfamiliarity of the diction overwhelms the familiarity of the embodied emotion. As Bolens explains, "The kinesic style of the narrative, . . . its corporeal hermeneutics, . . . is shaped by the way the author stylizes language so as to create signifying gestures" (35). Because a style is an as-structure that conveys what an action is like through linguistic means that are also not like what it simulates, the kinesic style of a story will paradoxically signal its historical and cultural specificity in and through the very means (the linguistic action of the description) by which it transcends these horizons (in the embodied resonances the language produces in distant, future readers).

Stories can act as mediators between our different lives because they configure and refigure modalities of action that intertwine in our experience of the world. As biocultural hybrids, we share embodied motor capacities with other members of our species and engage the world through action-perception circuits that have evolved over a long shared history. As configurations of action, stories can put us in relation with other worlds that may seem familiar and strange because they draw on but also reorganize aspects of embodied experience we have in common with other conspecifics. Our biocultural hybridity makes it possible for us to resonate bodily to stories whose actions are far from our worlds, even as the way these resonances are styled may also make us feel how distant those worlds are from our own everyday experiences.

These differences in turn can be productive in all sorts of ways because of the further actions they can set in motion. Like other kinds of affordances, the stories we exchange with one another face in two directions. On the one hand, they bear traces of the experiential, cognitive worlds they draw from even as, on the other hand, they may reorganize these resonances into configurations of narrative action that offer possibilities of response to future generations of readers and listeners that are not entirely specified in advance. Human actions are intrinsically horizonal and future directed, characterized by both immanence and transcendence, as they project us beyond our present situation to the purposes and aims they are directed toward. The historical lives of stories as they get exchanged across cultural and generational horizons are made possible by the powers of transcendence embodied in the actions that narratives set in motion. The power of stories to act across cultural and historical distance may seem miraculous, but it is simply an example of the capacity of our species to engage in future-oriented, boundary-crossing actions. The act of telling stories can project us across the horizons of our worlds because actions transcend the situation from which they are launched as they aim toward ends not yet fully in sight.

CHAPTER FOUR

Neuroscience and the Social Powers of Narrative

O UR INTUITIVE, bodily-based ability to understand the actions of other people is fundamental to social relations, including the relation between storyteller, story, and audience. Stories have social powers because there is a circuit between the configured action emplotted in a narrative and our activity of following the story as readers or listeners as we assimilate its patterns into the figures that shape our worlds. Whether stories can inculcate positive moral attitudes and prosocial behaviors, however, is by no means a simple and straightforward matter. The power of narratives to promote interpersonal understanding, moral behavior, and social justice depends, among other things, on the ability of stories to change the brain-based processes of pattern formation through which we make sense of the other embodied minds with whom we share the world. If stories can promote empathy and otherwise facilitate the cointentionality required for the collaborative activity unique to our species, the power and limits of their capacity to do so depend on embodied processes of doubling self and other through mirroring, simulation, and identification that are basic to the operation of the social brain. The constraints and imperfections of these processes are reflected in the strengths and weaknesses of narratives as ethical and political instruments.

Philosophers and cognitive scientists often make broad claims about how stories can enhance our ability to understand and empathize with others that seem naively optimistic to literary critics and theorists who know that narratives can have a range of disparate, even contradictory effects. Martha Nussbaum and Steven Pinker are prominent examples of such naivete, and Suzanne Keen, one of the most astute theorists of narrative empathy, rightly takes them to task. As Keen (2007, xviii–xix) points out, a similar faith in the social and moral powers of stories informs Nussbaum's claim that reading novels may create "better world citizens capable of extending love and compassion to unknown others" and Pinker's assertion that storytelling is a "moral technology" that "has made the human species 'nicer'" by extending "the 'moral circle' to include 'other clans, other tribes, and other races'" (see Nussbaum 1997, Pinker 2011). "Well, it depends," Keen observes, noting many "examples of stigmatized characters who are held up for ridicule and humiliation, to the delight of protagonists and implied readers alike" (xix).

Specious, overly simplistic claims about the capacity of literature to improve social cognition unfortunately also abound in the psychological literature. The most notorious instance is the much-publicized study by David Comer Kidd and Emanuele Castano (2013) that purported to find that "reading literary fiction improves theory of mind"—a claim that led the *New York Times* to recommend reading "a little Chekhov" to "get ready for a blind date or a job interview" (Belluck 2013, A1). This claim has already become "accepted as conventional wisdom," as the authors of a less-publicized multi-institutional replication study observe (Panero et al. 2016, e47). A recent survey of the neurobiological bases of morality concludes, for example, with a ringing endorsement of this work: "Research indeed demonstrates that reading literary fiction can improve the capacity to identify and understand others' subjective affective and cognitive mental states (Kidd and Castano 2013)" (Decety and Cowell 2015, 295). Whether this is true and if so how fiction does this are not at all clear, however. For one thing, the replication study failed to verify Kidd and Castano's results: "In short, we found no support for any short-term causal effects of reading literary fiction on theory of mind" (Panero et al. 2016, e52; see Kidd and Castano 2017 for their reply). Not surprisingly, this finding did not make the *Times*.

In a similar vein, psychologists Keith Oatley and Raymond Mar have published several much-cited studies that purport to find a correlation between reading fiction and social competence. Claiming that "fiction is the simulation of social worlds," for example, Oatley proposes that "similar to people who improve their flying skills in a flight simulator, those who read fiction might improve their social skills" (Oatley 2016, 619). A study by Mar, Oatley, and colleagues even asserts that "bookworms" who are "frequent fiction readers" may perform better on various "empathy/social-acumen measures" than "nerds" who prefer nonfiction (Mar et al., 2006, 694). As I argued in the last chapter, however, simulation is an as-relation—a relation of like and not like—that is more variable and unpredictable than this assumption of straightforward cause-and-effect suggests. Widely respected cognitive scientist of reading Richard Gerrig rightly faults these studies for failing to explain in any detail how simulation works, and he calls for more specific analyses of the particular "processes of learning and memory" engaged by "readers' social cognition" (Mumper and Gerrig 2019, 453). The authors of the Kidd-Castano replication study similarly argue that "we should move from asking whether reading fiction increases theory-of-mind skills to asking under what circumstances reading may do this, and how, and for whom" (Panero et al. 2016, e52).

Analyzing in detail the neuroscientific and phenomenological processes entailed in telling and following stories is one way of meeting this need for a more specific, detailed account of the social powers (and limits) of narrative. Writers and readers activate their cognitive capacities for imagining other worlds when they exchange stories, but there is much evidence in literary and academic circles that this does not necessarily make them more caring or less aggressive and self-involved. Neuroscientific research won't change this, but it can help to explain the powers as well as the limits of stories to promote prosocial behavior, including empathy and mutually beneficial collaboration. What we need are not overly grand, simplistic assertions about the ability of narrative to facilitate empathy and social understanding but rather careful and detailed analyses of how the contradictory effects of stories relate to the complex, often paradoxical characteristics of embodied cognition.

Empathy, Identification, and the Doubling of Self and Other

In an illuminating analysis of the kinematics of narrative, Guillemette Bolens (2012, 1–3) distinguishes between kinesic intelligence and kinesthetic sensations—"our human capacity to discern and interpret body movements" as opposed to the motor sensations we may have of our own actions, whether voluntary or involuntary: "Kinesthetic sensations cannot be directly shared, whereas kinesic information may be communicated. I cannot feel the kinesthetic sensations in another person's arm. Yet I may infer his kinesthetic sensations on the basis of the kinesic signals I perceive in his movements. In an act of kinesthetic empathy, I may internally simulate what these inferred sensations possibly feel like via my own kinesthetic memory and knowledge." The ability to understand the actions represented in a story (what is told) as well as to follow the movements of the narration (the telling) requires both kinds of cognitive competence—the hermeneutic capacity to configure signals into meaningful patterns (kinesic intelligence) and the intuitive sense of how the structures emplotting the actions and the forms deployed in the narration fit with my own unreflective, habitual modes of figuring the world (embodied in my kinesthetic sensations).

The kinesic intelligence and kinesthetic empathy that we use to understand stories entail a kind of *doubling* of self and other that, according to Maurice Merleau-Ponty, makes the alter ego fundamentally paradoxical. As Merleau-Ponty explains, "The social world is already there when we come to know it or when we judge it" because the intersubjectivity of experience is primordially given with our perception of a common world—and yet, he continues, there is "a lived solipsism that cannot be transcended" because I am destined never to experience the presence of another person to herself (2012 [1945], 379, 374). The kinesthetic empathy Bolens describes is paradoxically both intersubjective and solipsistic, for example, inasmuch as I "internally simulate" what the other must be feeling as if her sensations were mine which, of course, they are not (otherwise I wouldn't need to infer them on the basis of my own). Following a story is similarly a paradoxical process, with both intersubjective and solipsistic dimensions, whereby my own resources for configuring the world are put to work to make sense of another, fictive, narrated world that may seem both familiar and strange because its figurations both are and are not analogous to mine. Narrative understanding is an as-relation whereby I think the thoughts of someone else but think them as if they were my own—a doubling of the "real me" I bring to the story and the "alien me" I produce by lending it my powers of consciousness (see Iser 1978, 152–59). This doubling overcomes the opposition between self and other (giving me access to another world with an immediacy that is impossible in everyday life) even as it reinscribes it (this other world is fascinating, after all, because it is not my own).[1]

The grammatical categories that dominate narratological analyses of so-called fictional minds cannot by themselves do justice to the inherent contradictions and complications that the paradox of the alter ego entails. For example, in her classic study of techniques for representing consciousness, Dorrit Cohn (1978, 5–6) wonders about the apparent, inexplicable absurdity that "the special life-likeness of narrative fiction . . . depends on what writers and readers know least in life: how another mind thinks, another body feels"—states of affairs "whose verisimilitude it is impossible to verify." From a phenomenological perspective, however, this paradox is indeed wonderful, but it is not mysterious. It is simply an instance of the everyday experience that we are able to intuit automatically what others are thinking and feeling even as their inner lives lie beyond our grasp. As Wittgenstein points out, "We *see* emotion. . . . We do not see facial contortions and *make the inference* that [someone] is feeling joy, grief, boredom. We describe a face immediately as sad, radiant, bored" (1980, ¶570; original emphasis). Others are primordially, originally present to us, but as Shaun Gallagher and Dan Zahavi (2012, 204) observe, "The givenness of the other is of a most peculiar kind. The otherness of the other is precisely manifest in his elusiveness and inaccessibility." As Merleau-Ponty explains, "My experience must present others to me in some way, since if it did not do so I would not even speak of solitude, and I would not even declare others to be inaccessible" (2012 [1945], 376). Solipsism is only a problem because we are intersubjectively attuned to one another. Intersubjectivity and solipsism may seem to be mutually exclusive categories, but they are inextricably and paradoxically linked in our lived experience of others.

These contradictions may seem illogical, but they are an existential fact of life. The paradoxical presence and absence of others is, Merleau-Ponty notes, an example of "how I can be open to phenomena that transcend me. . . . [J]ust as the instant of my death is an inaccessible future for me, I am certain to never live the presence of another to himself. And nevertheless, every other person exists for me as an irrecusable style or milieu of coexistence, and my life has a social atmosphere just as it has a flavor of mortality" (381–82). Our ability to share stories that transport us into other lives is evidence of this primary intersubjectivity—something so natural and automatic that we take it for granted—even as, like death, the worlds of others are an inalienable aspect of our lives only because they are always on the horizon, paradoxically present in their absence, immanent in their transcendence.

The paradox of the alter ego is evident in many of the contradictions of our social lives (and, consequently, of stories), one of which is the curious fact that I come to understand my self-for-myself by observing and interacting with others. As cognitive narratologist Alan Palmer (2004, 138) notes, "We cannot learn how to ascribe mental states to ourselves only from our own case: this ability depends on observing other people's behavior." This is a paradox, he observes, that stories often exploit: "While it is true that we have immediate access to some parts of our own current mental world, in other ways we have less access to our minds than other persons do," and the example he cites is *Great Expectations*, where "Biddy . . . knows the working of Pip's mind much better than Pip himself does" (128). Chris Frith (2012, 2216) interestingly observes that "there is [experimental] evidence that we are more accurate in recognizing the causes of the behaviour of others than we are at recognizing the causes of our own behaviour. . . . Therefore, our understanding of our own behaviour is likely to benefit from the comments of others"—even if, as the example of Pip also shows (and as we don't need science to predict), this is likely not to be appreciated.[2]

This is one of the many ways in which stories stage and explore the paradox of the alter ego that are better understood through phenomenological than grammatical categories. Paradoxically, as Gallagher and Zahavi (2012, 207) point out, "The language we learn for our mental states is a language that we learn to apply to others even as we learn to apply it to ourselves." By providing us with categories and terms for interpreting other lives, stories also give us tools for understanding ourselves. That is because others are both like and not like ourselves, and this as-relation allows differences to be configured in a vocabulary for understanding ourselves and others that would not otherwise exist. If folk psychology (the conventional wisdom about behavior circulating in a society) is a resource for making sense of others, it also gives us instruments for interpreting our own inner lives as both like and not like what we observe in the social world, and stories are an important source of those tools (see Hutto 2007).

Free indirect discourse is similarly a narratological technique whose contradictions and paradoxes are not reducible to its linguistic features but call out for phenomenological analysis. This double-voiced discourse is a kind of ventriloquism in which the text expresses thoughts of a character which only he or she knows in words that are the narrator's. Consider, for example, this famous complaint of Emma Bovary's about her husband's dullness: "Charles's conversation was as flat as any pavement, everyone's ideas trudging along it in their weekday clothes, rousing no emotion, no laughter, no reverie" (Flaubert 2003 [1857], 38). Voicing her private reflections in the language of the narrator, this both is and is not what Emma thinks. After all, the text has just announced a few lines earlier that "she didn't have the words" to "give voice to [her] elusive malaise" (38), which the narrator then does for her here and in doing so expresses her self-for-herself as she herself cannot—but again, in another twist, with an ironic undertone and through evocative metaphors that are identifiably the narrator's and not hers. Hence what Cohn (1978, 107, 105) calls the characteristic ambiguity of free indirect discourse, its baffling but intriguing "quality of now-you-see-it, now-you-don't that exerts a special fascination" by "superimposing two voices that are kept distinct" in other, less paradoxical techniques—such as when, for example, a narrative directly quotes a character's thoughts (" 'Charles's conversation was as flat as any pavement,' Emma thought") or paraphrases them with an explicit attribution ("Emma thought that her husband's conversation was as flat as any pavement").[3]

Cohn's narratological approach proposes various grammatical markers of tense and person to distinguish and define these techniques (see 104–5), but the epistemological and phenomenological ambiguities here cannot be explained by purely linguistic categories. The paradox of free indirect discourse is the paradox of the alter ego—namely, that the narrator thinks the thoughts of someone else but thinks them (or at least gives voice to them) as if they were his or her own, so that the discourse becomes double and split, with the me of the character's consciousness expressed by the me of the narrator's language. For the reader, the experience made available by this technique is similarly double and paradoxical, as we inhabit a character's interiority immediately but also at a distance, through the filter of the narrator's discourse. The reader consequently has a doubled experience of being both inside and outside a character's consciousness, participating in her thoughts even as we observe them, granting us privileged access to a self-for-herself whose inaccessibility is simultaneously made evident by the narrator's presence.

The doubleness of free indirect discourse is odd, elusive, and paradoxical—but also natural and familiar, so that readers automatically and intuitively know what to do with it and typically don't stumble over its interpretive challenges, even as narratological theorists struggle to pin it down. As Cohn remarks, "The device is irresistible precisely because it is apprehended almost unconsciously" (107), without the need for special instruction from a critic or the terminology of a narrative theorist. In a rare moment of uncertainty, after offering a series of fine-grained grammatical distinctions, Cohn confesses: "Purely linguistic criteria no longer provide reliable guidelines" for characterizing this technique, a device that "reveals itself even as it conceals itself, but not always without making demands on its reader's intelligence" (106). The double negative here ("not always without") is revealing because it suggests how paradoxically unnatural but also natural and familiar this technique seems. Its ambiguities may defy "purely linguistic" or grammatical demarcation, but readers are usually untroubled by them because our ordinary lived experience of the social world has accustomed us to doubled experiences of other minds as intersubjectively accessible and solipsistically opaque, simultaneously both accessible and inaccessible. We can effortlessly understand free indirect discourse because we are familiar with the paradox of the alter ego, but the complications and puzzles implicit in this technique can also seem bewildering and make us marvel when we stop to think about them—and the same is true of the strangely double presence and absence of the others with whom we share our worlds.

Cognitive scientists and psychologists have proposed three ways of explaining the paradox of the alter ego, and the emerging consensus is that all three probably work in combination in the brain's complicated, messy interactions with the social world (see Armstrong 2013, 131–74, and Gallagher and Zahavi 2012, 191–218). The first approach, known as theory of mind (ToM) or theory theory (TT), focuses on our capacity to attribute mental states to others—to engage in "mind reading" through which we theorize about the beliefs, desires, and intentions of others that we recognize may differ from our own. The second approach, simulation theory (ST), argues that we do not need theories to understand the simple, everyday behavior of others but that we instead automatically run "simulation routines" that put ourselves in their shoes by using our own thoughts and feelings as a model for what they must be experiencing. Critics of ST claim it begs the question of how the simulator senses what is going on in the other person, but one possible answer has been provided by mirror neurons that were first discovered in the motor cortex of the macaque monkey. As I explain in chapter 3's analysis of action understanding, these neurons fire not only when the animal performs a specific action but also when it observes the same action by another monkey or an experimenter—not only when the monkey grasps a piece of food, for example, but also when the scientist does the same thing. Although the mirror neuron research has been controversial and is still somewhat unsettled, experiments have conclusively shown that mirroring processes are evident not only in the motor cortex but also across the brain, in regions associated (for example) with emotion, pain, and disgust.[4] In different ways, all three of these theories—theory of mind, simulation theory, and mirror neurons—are attempts to explain the acts of doubling me and not me that human beings routinely, automatically engage in as they negotiate their way through a paradoxically intersubjective and solipsistic world.

All three processes are involved in the activity of following a story, and narratives differ from one another as they draw more or less and in various, distinctive ways on each of these modes of doubling self and other. Mind-reading skills emphasized by TT of the sort necessary to pass false-belief tests may be invoked by stories that depict characters who act in a surprising or suspicious manner and whose motives and desires we may speculate about or that are told by narrators whose reliability we may have reason to distrust, so that we feel compelled to oppose their versions of the story with counternarratives we invent. Other narratives that encourage immersion in the action of the story may set in motion the automatic, subliminal simulation routines of ST as we involve ourselves in the illusions we construct and get carried away by our vicarious participation in the characters' dramas, and the embodied, emotional reactions that these involvements may provoke (whether the sympathy of pity, the contagious excitement of represented conflict, or the fear of suspenseful threats) may trigger embodied resonances of the kind identified in the mirror neuron experiments.

Whether and how the activation of these processes in following a story might improve our social skills is unclear, however, because the acts of identification entailed in narrative understanding are instances of doubling that are inherently unpredictable and open to a wide range of variation. This is why the moral and social effects of empathy are notoriously ambiguous, as the scientific literature on the topic amply attests. It is widely acknowledged, for example, that the fellow feeling of empathy does not necessarily produce ethically beneficial, prosocial sympathy and compassion. Indeed, as Grit Hein and Tania Singer (2008, 154) point out, "empathy can have a dark side" because it can be deployed for Machiavellian purposes "to find the weakest spot of a person to make her or him suffer." Or, as Jean Decety and Claus Lamm (2009) observe, feeling another's emotional state may cause "personal distress" and result in aversion from the sufferer rather than sympathetic concern and involvement. Because identification is an act of doubling, its consequences are not foreordained, whether in literature or in life. Empathy may promote either pro- or antisocial behavior depending on how the as-relation of identification configures the relation between me and not me.

The doubleness of empathic understanding is evident in the classic definition of identification as *Einfühlung*, in which one "feels oneself into" the experience of another. Theodor Lipps's (1903) oft-cited example is the anxiety a spectator may feel while watching a circus acrobat on a high wire, where the thrill of the performance derives from the spectator's vicarious sense of the tightrope walker's danger. What Antonio Damasio (1994, 155–64) calls the "as-if body loop," whereby the brain simulates body states that are not caused by external stimuli, may indeed be set in motion by such a participatory experience. But an as-if re-creation of another's observed behavior may not produce the same kinesthetic sensations she or he is experiencing. In this case, the cool, calm, and collected professional performer probably does *not* experience the same fear, anxiety, and excitement as the spectator—otherwise he or she might become paralyzed and fall—even as the spectator's ability to enjoy the act depends on his or her not being in any real danger. Consider, for example, the famous tightrope walker Philippe Petit's report of his sensations when he walked between the Twin Towers of the World Trade Center in 1974: "After a few steps, I knew I was in my element [even though] I knew the wire was not well rigged[,] . . . but it was safe enough for me to carry on. And then, very slowly as I walked, I was overwhelmed by a sense of easiness, a sense of simplicity" (quoted in Nodjimbadem 2015). The thrill of the performance for the spectator is anything but this feeling of tranquility! As Adriano D'Aloia (2012, 94) explains, "The spectator's subjectivity is not 'one with' the acrobat's subjectivity, but only 'with'"—" side-by-side" in an adjacency that "implies a paradoxical proximity at a distance" (see Stein 1964 [1917]). Empathy entails "proximity at a distance" because identification is a doubling of me and not me and not a merger of subjectivities.

Similarly, when we read about a character's fictionally represented experiences or identify with a narrator's point of view, our self does not simply disappear in a merger of ego and alter ego. Rather, setting in motion a paradoxical doubleness that both joins and separates self and other, readers exercise their own powers of configurative comprehension so that another world, based on perhaps different pattern-making structures, can emerge. The result, as Wolfgang Iser (see 1978, 155–59) points out, is a paradoxical duplication of subjectivities, an interplay of the "alien me" whose thought patterns I recreate and inhabit, and the "real, virtual me" whose configurative powers of understanding cause this other world to take shape and, in the process, can find themselves transfigured and transformed. These unpredictable, dynamic, open-ended interactions can only take place because the act of following stories entails doublings of various kinds and is not a static correspondence between or a homogeneous merger of self and other.

The bodily feelings generated by following a story and vicariously, empathically participating in the actions it represents—whether Aristotle's classic examples of pity and fear or any other of the widely various emotional responses stories can evoke—are consequently double and split. They are as-if emotions that both are and are not the bodily, kinesthetic sensations we would have in an original experience unmediated by the interface of narrative. This doubling helps to explain, for example, why Dostoevsky's novel *Crime and Punishment* is so thrilling and disturbing. "Raskolnikov's waiting is *my* waiting which I lend to him," Jean-Paul Sartre (1965 [1947], 39; original emphasis) observes; "his hatred of the police magistrate who questions him is my hatred which has been solicited and wheedled out of me by signs." Our identification with the criminal is a peculiar doubling whereby I experience his anger and anxiety as if these emotions were my own because in a sense they are, even as they are also not mine because they are Raskolnikov's (and I am not an axe murderer). They are *my* emotions that I project onto him and feel *with* him, even though I never cease to be me, the reader, who is *not* the character I both identify with and observe (and the ability to do both is a consequence of the doubling of identification through which boundaries are simultaneously maintained and crossed). It is thrilling to identify with Raskolnikov because we experience the anxieties of an axe murderer—and disturbing, because this crosses boundaries between my everyday world and another, bizarre, and frightening world—but only as if that were happening, so that we can maintain the detachment of an observer even as we experience the emotions of a participant.

The as-if quality of embodied experiences of identification has been widely documented in experimental studies of an observer's vicarious participation in another's pain or disgust. Oft-cited experiments by William Hutchison (1999), Tania Singer (2004), and Yawei Cheng (2010), among others, have shown that neurons in the insula and the anterior cingulate cortex fire not only in response to a pinprick or an electric shock but also at the sight of someone else receiving the same painful stimulus—or even to a report that someone else would be poked or shocked. But the responses of observers are also sensitive to individual differences—more intense, for example, if a loved one is receiving the stimulus, or less intense if the witness is someone (like a nurse or an acupuncturist) conditioned to view pain and to regard it as potentially beneficial—and these variations suggest in turn that the "as-if body loop" set in motion by the brain's simulation routines is a doubling of self and other, not a simple one-to-one match. Similarly, well-known experiments by Bruno Wicker and his group (2003) have shown that the anterior insula responds not only during the experience of disgust prompted by an unpleasant smell but also during the observation of someone else's disgusted facial expression. But observing another person's disgust is not likely to result in actual vomiting because the experience both is and is not the same bodily sensation as the feeling it duplicates. Feeling with a character depicted in a story or adopting the attitudes suggested by a narrator would similarly entail a doubling process of simulation and inference as if we were experiencing embodied, kinesthetically original sensations. Our reenactment of these sensations in response to stories makes narrative identifications possible, but these simulations both are and are not like the experiences whose underlying biological mechanisms they draw on and (partially) duplicate.

This doubleness makes the consequences of our emotional responses to narrative more variable and unpredictable than Aristotle's theory of catharsis suggests. The doubling of the like and the not like in as-if simulations helps to explain the oft-observed paradox that emotions such as fear and terror that would otherwise cause discomfort or pain can instead give rise to pleasure in aesthetic reenactments. Our identification with the tragic hero both is and is not the same as his or her experience, and this makes all the difference. But this doubling also need not result in a purgation of the emotions it simulates because mirroring another's sensations can instead stimulate and spread them contagiously. As Paul Bloom (2010, 192) observes, experimental evidence shows that "watching a violent movie doesn't put one in a relaxed or pacifistic state of mind—it arouses the viewer." Marco Iacoboni (2008, 209, 206) similarly worries that "mirror neurons in our brain produce automatic imitative influences of which we are often unaware," which in turn may explain why "exposure to media violence has a strong effect on imitative violence." Representations of violence do not immediately and necessarily provoke aggressive behavior in the viewer, however, because responses depend on several factors that influence what psychologists call "observational learning"—for example, whether the behavior is rewarded and reinforced, whether the model is viewed positively and seen as similar to the observer, or whether the behavior is within the viewer's spectrum of abilities (see Gerrig and Zimbardo 2005, 199–200).

Aggression is not an automatic response to represented violence because the doubling of me and not me in empathic identification is an as-relation that can be variously configured and can have different outcomes depending on how the negation in the interplay of like and not like is staged and received. The patterns of emplotment that configure the conflictual relations between persons in a dramatized action are widely variable—some representing aggressive behavior as heroic, for example, and others foregrounding the suffering of its victims—and these different plots in turn will be transfigured and transformed in various ways according to the interpretive dispositions of the respondent, who may be thrilled or repulsed and will construct his or her own reading of the story accordingly (responding with sympathy or reacting with horror or with both in some unique combination). The interactions between these patterns of representation and response may result in the transformation of renderings of aggression and conflict into aesthetic pleasure, moral repulsion, or imitative violence depending on how the as is configured in the narrative and on how it is refigured in the listener's or reader's response. None of this is predetermined or foreordained.

All of these complications and contingencies are very difficult to measure with the instruments that psychologists like Kidd and Castano (2013) have at their disposal in attempting to assess whether "literary fiction improves theory of mind." Scientific ingenuity often entails figuring out how faulty, limited measuring instruments might be deployed to reveal states of affairs that would otherwise be inaccessible (as is the case, for example, with fMRI technology, which measures differential blood flow to construct visual images of neuronal activity in the brain). But sometimes the limitations of the instruments only call attention to the complexities that elude them (hence the joke cognitive scientists often tell about why someone who lost their wallet was looking for it under the lamppost—because that's where there's light, even though that's not where it went missing). The Kidd-Castano study takes one black box (literary fiction) and asks how it affects another black box (cognitive and affective theory of mind), and the authors' findings are vague and questionable because their instruments are blunt and crude. For example, as the authors of the replication study point out, by using "prestigious awards" as a measure of "literary fiction," Kidd and Castano create a "fuzzy" category (containing authors as diverse as DeLillo, Chekhov, and Louise Erdrich) so that "it remains unclear which aspects of literary fiction might be causally responsible" for the effects they identify (Panero et al. 2016, e47). As the replication study notes, "Other experiments . . . obtained effects on social cognition using popular fiction," not works regarded as "literary" (whatever that means), with some studies finding "higher levels of theory of mind in readers of romance than readers of domestic fiction and science fiction/fantasy" (e47).[5] What kinds of acts of doubling me and not me are set in motion by a story can vary widely according to its stylistic and generic features, and even some works of domestic fiction and science fiction or fantasy would no doubt challenge and extend a reader's abilities to interpret and identify with other minds. For example, Octavia Butler's *Parable of the Sower* (1993), in which a narrator afflicted with "hyperempathy" navigates the dangers of a violent, dystopian world, is as insightful an exploration of the ambiguities of identification as any modernist psychological novel or (for that matter) neuroscientific study. Literary fiction is too broad a category to register these contingencies.

What Kidd and Castano mean by "theory of mind" is similarly too vague to illuminate the paradoxical processes of doubling entailed in following a story. Their study employed two tests for ToM—one test for "cognitive theory of mind" that asked participants multiple-choice false-belief questions about what a cartoon figure Yoni was probably thinking in different circumstances, and another for "affective theory of mind" (the reading the mind in the eyes test) that required participants to choose one of four emotions that was likely expressed by a series of photographs of pairs of eyes. Both tests have demonstrated their usefulness as diagnostic tools to identify rudimentary difficulties with understanding others that someone afflicted with severe autism or Asperger's syndrome might have, but neither is sufficiently differentiated or complex to distinguish the various kinds of theory building (TT), simulation (ST), or mirroring that might be required to interpret the states of mind portrayed in a story. Answering false-belief questions about a cartoon character's preferences could involve theorizing or simulating his or her state of mind or even resonating at a sensory-motor level in response to imagined actions. Guessing the emotions suggested by a pair of eyes could similarly prompt theorizing, simulating, or emotional mirroring—and probably all three, in varying combinations, for different respondents. What is going on in the black boxes of cognitive and affective ToM here is unclear.

Understanding others who are paradoxically present and absent, intersubjectively accessible and solipsistically opaque, is a complicated process of theorizing, simulating, and resonating with other embodied consciousnesses, and the interactions of TT, ST, and mirroring mechanisms are more complex than the notion of a ToM module (even divided into cognitive and affective dimensions) encompasses. How these processes are then set in motion by following a story introduces further complications and contingencies that multiple-choice tests about general cognitive and affective competence cannot measure. Hence, perhaps, the confused array of not entirely consistent ways in which Kidd and Castano actually describe the effects of literary fiction, which they variously assert "hones," "recruits," "enhances" or simply "primes" ToM (378, 380). If all a story does is "recruit" or "prime" preexisting cognitive abilities, it doesn't necessarily "improve" them, and what kind of improvement is entailed by "honing" or "enhancing" is not at all clear. The complicated, paradoxical processes of doubling self and other in following a story are more variable and elusive than Kidd and Castano's instruments and categories can capture.

A similar insensitivity to the contingencies of doubling undermines Oatley and Mar's model of fiction as a simulation of social worlds (Oatley 2016; Mar et al. 2006) that, in their view, has a positive, univocal impact on our social abilities. Oatley's (2016, 618) claims are strikingly simple and straightforward: "Fiction is the simulation of selves in interaction. People who read it improve their understanding of others." Simulation is an as-relation, however, and not the one-directional mechanism linking cause and effect that this model posits. Simulating the "real" world through a "fictional" world is a process of doubling, with one world rendered *as* another world (a simulation is only revelatory, after all, if it is *not* identical with what it models). Fictional simulations set in motion doubled interactions between my world and another world, between like and not like, whose consequences cannot be predicted in advance and will vary according to what each party brings to the encounter. As the debates about the ambiguities of identification and empathy suggest, for example, these to-and-fro exchanges may "improve understanding" and increase compassion, or they may cause personal distress and revulsion. One kind of simulation (of, say, a tragic situation) for a certain recipient (like, say, Aristotle) might provoke pity and fear and result in catharsis, but for another it might set off mimetic violence and aggression (as Bloom and Iacoboni fear). To claim that fictional simulations of social interactions simply and straightforwardly improve interpersonal understanding is to ignore this variety of potential outcomes, and this blindness is a consequence of a model that views narrative understanding as a one-directional cause-and-effect mechanism rather than a recursive, reciprocal process of doubling.

Oatley's and Mar's studies are very prominent in the psychological literature, but they are based on assumptions about the relation between teller, tale, and audience that are crude and mechanical. According to Oatley, for example, "Fiction can be thought of as a form of consciousness of selves and others that can be passed from an author to a reader or spectator and can be internalized to augment everyday cognition" (2016, 618). This model reifies consciousness, regarding it as something that can be transferred unidirectionally from author to recipient, with predictable results (straightforward "augmentation" of preexisting capacities). Conceiving of consciousness as a transferrable object grossly simplifies and misrepresents the dynamic processes that intertwine and mutually transform each other in the recursive circuit of figuration (mimesis$_1$), configuration (mimesis$_2$), and refiguration (mimesis$_3$). On the rare occasion when Oatley does acknowledge that simulation entails doubling, he reduces and contains its effects: "Fiction is a set of simulations of social worlds that we can compare, as it were stereoscopically, with aspects of our everyday world, to suggest insights we might not achieve by looking with the single eye of ordinary perception" (618). The image of a "stereoscope" stabilizes doubling into a static juxtaposition of views that once again has only a single predictable outcome—a simple, positive instructional benefit. Stereoscopic effects can in fact be more peculiar and bewildering than this, but only if the oppositions they set in motion play out indeterminately, without freezing them into fixed form. The doubled effects of thinking another's thoughts and feeling another's emotions as we follow a story are potentially more productive—if also possibly more troubling and less benign—than Oatley's model suggests because the interactions between worlds that narrative understanding sets in motion are more unpredictable and open ended than a stereoscopic juxtaposition or a one-directional transfer of consciousness.

After observing that "simulation theory has emerged as the most common explanatory mechanism" in psychological accounts of the cognitive effects of narrative (they have the work of Mar and Oatley in mind), psychologists Micah Mumper and Richard Gerrig (2019, 453, 457) rightly complain that its workings are typically underspecified: "Although researchers frequently cite simulation as a causal mechanism, the concept has never been associated with concrete claims about what types of processes embody simulation and how those processes unfold over time." The corrections and refinements that

Mumper and Gerrig propose are noteworthy because they all attempt to register the contingencies of consistency building and doubling entailed in narrative understanding.

For example, Mumper and Gerrig argue that making sense of a story may involve what they call "inference making" and "memory-based processing," guesses about implications and hidden sides (what a character may be thinking or feeling, for example, or what motives or designs she may secretly harbor), and they correctly note that these cognitive processes are not causal mechanisms and do not necessarily require simulation (see 459–61). Similarly, they observe, the feelings represented by stories need not generate equivalent emotions in the reader, which is what the simulation model presumes. Instead, as Mumper and Gerrig point out, a narrative may provoke "emotional appraisals" that result in "mismatches" as well as "matches" between reader and storyworld (462–63). After all, how we may feel about a character or the fictional world may be quite different from (and even radically opposed to) the emotions and appraisals dramatized by the text. Such is the case, for example, when readers of *Lolita* respond to Humbert Humbert's rhapsodies about nymphets with disgust and moral repulsion.[6] Even when stories encourage "narrative participation," Mumper and Gerrig observe, this may not involve simulation because (think again about *Lolita*) there may be "circumstances in which readers' participation likely yields emotional responses that will be dissimilar to the character's responses" (464). As these amendments and corrections to the simulation model all recognize, fictional renderings of social worlds do not cause a univocal, linear transfer of social cognition but instead set in motion complex, multivalent, heterogeneous processes of doubling, recursion, and inferential pattern formation.

Interesting experimental findings have confirmed that experiences of doubling are triggered by stories. In a recent study that combined the quantitative instruments of psychology and the qualitative methods of phenomenology, an interdisciplinary team from the Hearing the Voice project at Durham University solicited responses from 1,566 participants through the *Guardian* newspaper and the Edinburgh International Book Festival and, employing a questionnaire that also provided for individual verbal descriptions, asked about their experiences hearing the voices of characters and narrators when reading a narrative (see Alderson-Day, Bernini, and Fernyhough 2017). The principal investigator Charles Fernyhough (2016) is a psychologist and a novelist, and his postdoctoral colleagues are a psychologist trained in quantitative methods (Ben Alderson-Day) and a phenomenologically oriented narratologist (Marco Bernini). The Durham team hypothesized that their survey would elicit reports of "auditory simulation of character's voices" (99), consistent with fMRI-based evidence that "voice-selective regions of auditory cortex" are activated more by linguistic representations of "direct speech" than by "indirect reference (e.g., 'He said, "I hate that cat"' vs. 'He said that he hates that cat')" (see Yao, Belin, and Scheepers 2011). Similarly, they speculated, stories that represent narrators or characters speaking might activate voice-like experiences if their speeches triggered cortical areas that also respond to real voices. And that is indeed what they found, with 79 percent of respondents reporting they heard voices more than occasionally in response to stories and 72 percent describing these as vivid: "Our results indicated that many readers have very vivid experiences of characters' voices when reading texts, and that this relates to both other vivid everyday experiences (inner speech) and more unusual experiences (auditory hallucination-proneness)" (106).[7]

These experiences were not identical for all readers, however: "The features and dynamics of readers' descriptions of their voices were varied and complex. . . . [F]or some participants this was an intentional, constructive process, for others an automatic immersion, and for others again an experience that appeared to seep out into other, non-reading contexts" (106). Just as "traits towards having unusually vivid and hallucination-like experiences are thought to exist along a continuum in the general population," Alderson-Day, Bernini, and Fernyhough suggest, so "participants with more vivid experiences of reading in general would also be more prone to hallucination-like experiences" (100). Understanding stories does seem to entail a doubling of me and not me, then, which for some readers may take the form of hearing characters' and narrators' voices, but the extent to which this occurs depends on their preexisting cognitive proclivities. That such a large number of people hear voices when they read but with different degrees of immediacy lines up well with the theory that a real me and an alien me interact in the doubling of my world with a storyworld (my auditory cortex triggered to produce another voice within me) but that this doubling will vary for different readers (as the coupling of real and alien me takes different shapes).

The variability and heterogeneity of doubling call into question Steven Pinker's much-discussed claims for the beneficial moral consequences of the expansion of literacy and the rise of the novel. Pinker's description of the reading experience is phenomenological but without an appreciation of its paradoxes. "When someone else's thoughts are in your head, you are observing the world from that person's vantage point," he declares; "not only are you taking in sights and sounds that you could not experience firsthand, but you have stepped inside that person's mind and are temporarily sharing his or her attitudes and reactions" (2011, 175). Endorsing the argument of historian Lynn Hunt (2007), Pinker attributes special moral efficacy to epistolary novels like Samuel Richardson's *Pamela* (1740) because of their power to produce beneficial experiences of identification: "In this genre the story unfolds in a character's own words, exposing the character's thoughts and feelings in real time rather than describing them from the distancing perspective of a disembodied narrator. . . . Grown men burst into tears while experiencing the forbidden loves, intolerable arranged marriages, and cruel twists of fate in the lives of undistinguished women (including servants) with whom they had nothing in common" (176).

This has not been the reaction of all readers, however. Hunt and Pinker oddly overlook the notorious controversies *Pamela* unleashed, which pitted readers who sympathized with her valiant and ultimately successful efforts to fend off the lecherous advances of her employer, against "anti-Pamelists" like (most notably) Henry Fielding who in *Shamela* sought to expose Richardson's heroine as a hypocrite whose real motives were mercenary and self-serving: "I thought once of making a little Fortune by my Person. I now intend to make a great one by my Vartue" (1961 [1741], 325). Other skeptical readers accused Pamelists of voyeurism and erotic titillation, debunking their claims of moral edification as a thin veil covering over the vicarious, quasi-pornographic pleasures of reading about repeated episodes of attempted seduction.[8]

Similar ambiguities afflicted the reception of other epistolary novels, as in the notorious case of Goethe's *Sorrows of Young Werther* (1775), which is reported to have spawned a series of copycat suicides across Europe as readers imitated the disappointed hero's romantic demise, resulting in bans on the novel in Leipzig, Denmark, and Italy (see Phillips 1974). This work also inspired a satiric counterversion by Friedrich Nicolai, *The Joys of Young Werther* (1775), in which the hero's suicide is thwarted by a friend who jams his pistol, and the woman who had refused his advances relents. The Werther crisis shows how the doubling of me and not me in acts of readerly identification may produce an unconscious replication of the feelings and actions staged by the story, recalling the concerns of many cognitive scientists that the mirroring processes of identification may not necessarily result in catharsis but may instead promote less beneficial mimetic effects. These doubling processes are not all conscious and self-conscious, contrary to Pinker's naively optimistic view, and they may consequently have darker effects than the increased ability to imagine another's perspective, with attendant improvements in insight and sympathy, that proponents of the moral benefits of epistolary novels celebrate. Pinker acknowledges that "'empathy' in the sense of adopt-ing someone's viewpoint is not the same as 'empathy' in the sense of feeling compassion toward the person," but he claims that "the first can lead to the second by a natural route" (175). This step is less straightforward and au-tomatic than he suggests, however, because the doubling of worlds that understanding stories brings about may also "naturally" result in conflict, suspicion, and mimetic acts of violence.[9]

Cognitive science cannot predict what the social consequences of narra-tive will be. The variabilities introduced by the as-if of narrative simulation and the as of doubling are too many and too uncontrollable to support simple, sweeping generalizations about the social powers of narrative. As Suzanne Keen (2015, 139–40) wryly observes, "The evidence for altruism induced by narrative empathy is scanty though the cultural faith in the ben-efits of narrative empathy is strong." Claims that stories make us better people by enhancing empathy and ToM or that narratives inherently pro-mote social progress should be met with skepticism because such assertions oversimplify the complex, paradoxical interactions involved in the exchange of stories.

The neuroscience of embodied action and self-other relations does sug-gest that narratives have social power, however, because of the brain- and body-based processes that they set in motion. And so it is not surprising that some psychological studies report improvement in performance on various empathy and ToM measures as a result of experiences of reading stories. For example, Bal and Veltkamp (2013) provide evidence that "emotional trans-port" in reading can produce empathy, while Hakemulder (2000) has con-ducted experiments that demonstrate the capacity of stories to promote rational, "ethical reflection." These studies need to be taken with several grains of salt, however, not only because of the difficulties of measuring such effects but also because of the variability and heterogeneity of the ways the doubling processes of narrative understanding can unfold. As I have argued, neither the experience of being carried away emotionally by a narrative that Bal and Veltkamp endorse nor the ability to reflect self-consciously about another's point of view that Hakemulder emphasizes need have morally ben-eficial effects, and both can have antisocial consequences.

The experimental evidence for the moral and social powers of stories is ambiguous. A meta-analysis conducted by Mumper and Gerrig (2019, 455) comparing multiple studies of the moral effects of stories showed that "life-time fiction reading had a small positive correlation with empathy and ToM measures. That is, across all the studies we analyzed, as the amount of fic-tion participants read increased, their empathy and ToM scores also tended to increase by a small amount. We also found nonfiction reading to be positively correlated with empathy and ToM, although the effects were numerically smaller." It is important to remember, however, that correlation is not causation. As the authors of the Kidd-Castano replication study point out, for example, one confounding factor in such studies is that people with high empathy and ToM may tend to read more fiction (and perhaps nonfiction as well), and so it may be difficult to sort out what is causing what (see Panero et al. 2016, e46). The Mumper-Gerrig meta-analysis could support either interpretation—that is, either reading improves ToM and empathy or the other way around. My cautionary comments about the moral and social effects of stories are not meant to suggest that they do not have beneficial social consequences—just that these effects are likely to be more variable and heterogeneous and harder to measure than the optimistic claims recognize. Simplistic generalizations do not help us understand what the social powers of narrative actually are or how they work, and the ends that those powers may serve are not predetermined by the workings of the brain.

Collaboration, Shared Intentionality, and Coupled Brains

The doubling of worlds in the exchange of stories is a fundamentally collaborative interaction that can promote shared intentionality, a unique human capability that other primates seem to lack. Michael Tomasello (2005, 676) calls "'we' intentionality" the capacity for "participating in collaborative activities involving shared goals and socially coordinated action plans (joint intentions)." "Human thinking is fundamentally cooperative," he points out (2014, ix). Apes and other nonhuman primates also have "complex skills of social cognition," but according to Tomasello (2014, 76), their readings of their conspecifics' intentions "are aimed mainly at competition (i.e., their intelligence is Machiavellian) . . . for food and mates." In our species, the ability to share intentionality is already evident in parent-infant "proto-conversations" that involve "turn-taking" and "exchange of emotions" (2005, 681, 675)—activities also entailed, of course, in telling and following stories—and such collaborative interactions culminate in what is known as the "ratchet effect" of "cumulative cultural evolution" (2014, 83). We can pass along cultural accomplishments (like, for example, literacy) and build on what previous generations have learned because we can collaborate and share intentionality.

The ability to collaborate is also crucial for language acquisition. Among other reasons, that is because both require a capacity for coordinating attention. As Tomasello (2003, 21) notes, "A number of studies have found that children's earliest skills of joint attentional engagement with their mothers correlate highly with their earliest skills of language comprehension and production." "This correlation," he explains, "derives from the simple fact that language is nothing more than another type—albeit a very special type—of joint attentional skill; people use language to influence and manipulate one another's attention" (21). This is also why they tell stories. Whether in everyday conversation or in exchanging narratives, communication requires joint attention.

Collaborating with other humans necessitates that I coordinate my perspective and your perspective, resulting in what Tomasello (2014, 43) calls a "dual-level structure of simultaneous sharedness and individuality," a double structure that combines "joint attention and individual perspectives." This duality is also characteristic of the doubling of me and not me in the collaborative work of narrative understanding. The joint intentionality that powers cultural collaboration does not produce a union of subjectivities—a merger that overcomes the opposition of self and other. It is, rather, a double structure that relates ego and alter ego, like and not like, without completely eradicating their differences.

This doubling can once again have both beneficial and deleterious consequences. For example, as Joshua Greene (2015, 210) argues, it is probably the case that "morality evolved, not as a device for universal cooperation, but as a competitive weapon, as a system for turning Me into Us, which in turn enables Us to outcompete Them." For better or worse (and it is both), this "ingroup/outgroup psychology . . . is, in all likelihood, unique to [our] species," according to Tomasello (2014, 84); "as far as we know, great apes do not have, and early humans did not have, this sense of group identity at all." The legacy of this development can be seen in oft-documented "implicit group preferences" which, as Jean Decety and Jason Cowell (2015, 280, 289–90) point out, "can directly conflict with moral behavior"; for example, they note, "children do not display empathy and concern toward all people equally" but "show a bias toward individuals and members of groups with which they identify," and these prejudices may continue on into adulthood. In a comprehensive review of the experimental evidence on ingroup bias and stereotyping by race, age, and gender, Mina Cikara and Jay J. Van Bavel (2014, 245) found that "the propensity to prefer one's in-group has been observed in every culture on earth and in children as young as five."[10] The ability to identify with a group makes cooperation and collaboration possible among like me's, establishing the uniquely human capacity for cumulative cultural development, but it does so by differentiating like me from not me, thereby setting the stage for conflicts between self and other and for distinctively human acts of violence.

Neuroscience has increasingly recognized the need to take into account the various effects of collaboration and joint intentionality that go beyond what is happening in a single brain, but its measuring instruments are extremely constrained in their ability to register these kinds of interactions. Instruments like an fMRI machine or an EEG recorder are designed, after all, for a single, immobile subject. Calling for a "second-person neuroscience," Leonhard Schilbach and colleagues (Schilbach et al. 2013, 405) consequently lament that "the state of the art in neuroimaging provides severe limitations to studying free-running interactions using the full range of verbal and nonverbal channels."[11] "The dominant focus on single individuals in cognitive neuroscience paradigms," Uri Hasson and his coauthors argue, "obscures the forces that operate between brains to shape behavior," and this blindness is unfortunate because "brain-to-brain coupling" may lead "to complex joint behaviors that could not have emerged in isolation" (2012, 114–15). Behaviors of this kind have long been observed in animals as well as humans. One oft-cited example is the production of songs by some species of birds that involves a complex "dance" between males and females, with performer and listener adjusting their behaviors in light of what the other does (see West and King 1988).[12] Humans also often attune their behaviors to what they observe in others. For example, as Uta and Chris Frith (2010, 167) point out, "When two people 'tune in' to each other, they tend unconsciously to imitate each other's movements and gestures" in a kind of "chameleon effect." Similarly, people sitting next to each other in rocking chairs soon start to rock in unison, as if somehow linked mechanically (Richardson et al. 2007).

So-called hyperscanning methods that employ innovative, mobile EEG technology to simultaneously record and compare the brain-wave patterns of participants in interactive experiments have begun to document the neural synchronization underlying such coupled behavior. For example, guitar players and pianists performing duets play with accuracy equaling or exceeding the precision of individual performers, and EEG measurements of their brain waves reveal patterns of synchronized oscillatory coupling (Keller 2008, Lindenberger et al. 2009). Similar brain-wave synchronization has been recorded in studies of people gesturing to each other, tapping fingers in rhythm, or playing cards (see Sänger et al. 2011).

The hyperscanning experiments provide interesting evidence that synchronization is not a merger that erases differences but a process of doubling that may vary according to the skills and attitudes of the participants.

For example, Chris Frith's laboratory (2012, 2217) has demonstrated that "two people working together to detect a subtle visual signal can do better than the best one working on his own." As Frith observes, however, "collaboration on the signal detection task is not always advantageous" because, "if partners have very different abilities, . . . the pair will perform worse than the better partner" would alone (2218). Another hyperscanning study showed that "interbrain synchrony is also dependent on the nature of attachment between team members. For example, during a cooperation task, dyads involving lovers showed larger prefrontal interbrain synchrony than dyads involving friends and strangers, which was also mirrored by their better task performance" (Bhattacharya 2017; see Pan et al. 2017).

Collaborative interactions entail a coupling of differences that sometimes produces better consequences than individuals working alone, but other times worse. Because of the benefits of "pooling information" and canceling out each other's prejudices, Dan Bang and Chris Frith observe that "groups have been shown to outperform individuals for many problems of probability and reasoning" (2017, 7). They also point out, however, that groups "have their own biases" and "often amplify the initial preference" of a "majority of its members"—and so, surveying the literature on "group decision-making," they reach the perhaps unsurprising "Goldilocks" conclusion that "individuals who are too similar" and "individuals who differ too much" are equally bad for group performance (10, 13). More like than not like does not always produce a superior interaction. What matters in a successful collaboration is not how differences are overcome but how they intertwine.

Productive synchronization is inherently paradoxical. As Karl Friston and Chris Frith (2015, 391) observe, "communication (i.e., a shared dynamical narrative) emerges when two dynamical systems try to predict each other," each adjusting its expectations about how the other is likely to behave and reacting accordingly. But this to-and-fro process of mutual prediction and accommodation, anticipation and adjustment, is a contradictory activity that also requires the suppression of activity. For example, taking turns is a practice that demands the skill of knowing when *not* to act. Similarly, as Friston and Frith point out, successful conversation necessitates that the participants recognize that "one can either talk or listen but not do both at the same time" (391). Reciprocal interaction requires the participants not only to act but also to know when they should *not* act in order to make the interaction reciprocal. Hence the finding of Ivana Konvalinka's group (2012, 215) that "when two people engage in a synchronization task, they do better when they both continuously and mutually adapt to one another's actions—in other words, when they become two followers, instead of adopting a leader-follower dynamic."

Cognitive scientists who study collaboration point out that reciprocity is both a natural and an unnatural phenomenon. Humans are apparently social animals whose reward systems encourage the risk taking involved in collaboration. Schilbach's group (2013, 410) notes that some experiments have documented "the involvement of reward-related neurocircuitry during congruent interactions." Our brains are wired to reward collaborative activity, he suggests, and "Humans appear to have a default expectation of reciprocation" (410). We are inclined to want to reciprocate because we are rewarded when collaboration succeeds. This brain-based predisposition to collaborate is consistent with other evidence that participating in group interactions is intrinsically rewarding (see Tabibnia and Lieberman 2007).

Our species may be predisposed to collaborate, but the to-and-fro of cooperative activity is also risky, fraught, and contradictory. As Frith (2012, 2218) notes, "Thinking about collaboration is essentially recursive: your partner will collaborate only if she is confident that you will collaborate"—and even that is not enough, because she must also be "confident that you are confident" about her—and, he observes, "absolute certainty can never be achieved in this situation." Because reciprocal interactions are paradoxical and precarious, the openness to others and the suppression of self-interest required to initiate and sustain them are tenuous and can easily break down or go wrong. Frith claims, perhaps correctly, that this uncertainty "does not cause problems in the many real-life situations requiring collaboration" (2218). But it has prompted many cognitive scientists and philosophers of mind to worry about the problem of "free riders" who take advantage of the trust of others without which cooperation fails (see Decety and Wheatley 2015). The natural thing to do, these theorists observe, would be to "ride free" and reap the benefits of the group without contributing. There is also a good deal of evidence, however, that people inherently tend to scorn such behavior—that they will go out of their way to punish free riders even when there is no need to do so (so-called altruistic punishment). Failing to behave reciprocally and collaboratively is perceived as unnatural, then, and is frowned upon by our conspecifics (see Delton and Krasnow 2015 and Flesch 2007).

The paradoxes and contradictions of we-intentionality characterize many forms of cultural production that involve collaboration. Music is a prime example. According to Ian Cross (2003, 48), music "enables the sharing of patterned time with others and facilitates harmonicity of affective state and interaction." The "communal experience of affect elicited by moving together rhythmically in music and dance," Cross argues, "could have enhanced cooperative survival strategies for early humans, for example, in hunting or in inter-group conflict" (50). Sandra Trehub (2003, 13–14) points out that an ability to share intentionality is already visible in the predisposition of infants "to attend to the melodic contour and rhythmic patterning of sound sequences" and in their attunement "to consonant patterns, melodic as well as harmonic, and to metric rhythms." This is early evidence of the ability to coordinate attention and to respond to other-generated patterns of action that is required for any kind of collaborative interaction, including the exchange of stories.

Cross and his colleagues (Rabinowitch, Cross, and Burnard 2012, 111) propose the term "musical group interaction" (MGI) to describe "the joint creation of music." MGI is interestingly contradictory in ways that foreground the double structure of we-intentionality: "At its simplest, each MGI participant may have an almost separate subjective experience of the musical encounter. At its richest, MGI may elicit a complex entanglement between individual players entailing a fluid sharing of intentions, emotions and cognitive processes." This sharing of intentionality is once again paradoxical, not a homogeneous merger or union of selves but a doubling that simultaneously overcomes and preserves the opposition between self and other: "As intense as [MGI] may become, individuals still feel themselves to be distinct subjects. However, under certain circumstances, this sense of distinction may be elided," so that "the boundaries separating self and other become blurred and players are led to experience the actions of their fellow players, at least in part, as their own," and in extreme cases, "one subject may regard another participating subject almost as himself, to the point that one may experience another's sensations as one's own" (111, 118). In such a paradoxical experience, the mutuality of coordinated, collaborative activity results in a synchronization of coupled subjectivities so harmonious and intense that borders seem to disappear as one is absorbed by something beyond oneself, even as the actions and interactions that give rise to this shared intentionality are undertaken by separate individuals.

As a to-and-fro interaction between coupled and collaborating but distinct subjectivities, this contradictory state of affairs is precarious and prone to disturbance and disintegration. As Cross and his colleagues point out, "There are many factors that can disrupt the harmony within the group, such as personal conflict, excessive competitiveness, unbalanced musical skills, lack of patience, unwillingness to cooperate and perhaps more than anything else, the great difficulty of stepping aside and accepting the group as a whole where no member dominates but rather all members embark on a joint project" (115). An inherently paradoxical phenomenon, MGI requires both the concentrated, expert application of individual ability and (at the same time) a surrender of will, a letting go of control, and this contradiction is a striking illustration of the double structure of collaborative activity.

The paradoxes of collaborative meaning making are not unique to music. As Hans-Georg Gadamer points out, similar contradictions characterize many kinds of games and play. The paradox of play, according to Gadamer (1993 [1960], 104, 106), is "the primacy of play over the consciousness of the player": "All playing is a being-played." The game would not exist without the acts of the participants who initiate and sustain it, even as, together, their collaborative activity creates something that seems to have its own agency, its we-intentionality directing, steering, and even controlling the individual intentionalities of the players. According to Gadamer, "the real subject of the game . . . is not the player but the game itself," which is "what holds the player in its spell, draws him into play, and keeps him there" (106). Similarly, as Merleau-Ponty (2012 [1945], 370) observes, "in the experience of dialogue, . . . my words and those of my interlocutor are called forth by the state of the discussion and are inserted into a shared operation of which neither of us is the creator. Here there is a being-shared-by-two, . . . our perspectives slip into each other, we coexist through a single world." Like a game or a musical performance, a conversation can sometimes seem to have a life of its own, guiding and eliciting the contributions of the participants, even as it only exists because of their acts and will break down as soon as one party declines to go along.

Games, music, and conversation are all what I have elsewhere (1990, 20–43) called "heteronomous" states of affairs that paradoxically would not exist without the meaning-making acts of individual agents, even as they then acquire a quasi-independent status, over and above and even (sometimes) against the participants, as when the game seems to compel a player to make a certain move, or a musician adjusts her performance to match the rhythm and tonality of the ensemble. Similar effects can be produced by the to-and-fro interactions set in motion by telling and following stories, as a reader or listener finds herself moved to tears by the emotions of a character constituted by her own acts of identification, feeling the feelings of this quasi person as if they were her own (which, to some extent, paradoxically, they are). In all of these cases, the collaborative interaction of coupled subjectivities makes possible the emergence of a shared intentionality that is more than the sum of its individual parts and that seems to have its own agency, even as it results from and would not exist without the activity of the participants who join together in its production.

The comparison of games and stories to music is instructive because rhythmically coordinated action beneath conscious awareness can be both enabling and disabling. The sensation of boundaries dissolving in experiences of rhythmic interaction and harmonic unification recalls Nietzsche's (1994 [1872]) famous analysis of the Dionysian power of music to overwhelm Apollonian line and form. Dionysian abandon may miraculously, even sublimely transport us outside of ourselves, but such experiences of merger and boundary loss can also result in well-documented contagion effects (the shared "thrills" of an audience response at a concert, for example, or the collective enthusiasm of a crowd at a sports event or a political rally) that disable cognitive capacities for criticism and evaluation (see Garrels 2011 and Lawtoo 2013). Although perhaps less sweepingly powerful, the experience of being carried away by a narrative may similarly transport the listener and seem to erase boundaries between worlds. If not as intoxicating as the Dionysian dissolution that Nietzsche describes, such a merger of subjectivities may facilitate the inculcation of patterns of feeling and perceiving and have a more powerful impact on habitual pattern formation than cooler, less absorbing, less transportive exchanges of signs and information.

The synchronization of coupled subjectivities that can produce experiences of self-transcendence can also be a force for habitualization and social control. For better or worse (and, again, it can be both), the power of stories to reshape or reinforce the listener's unreflective patterns of configuring the world may increase to the extent that the difference between self and other in collaborative experiences of we-intentionality is reduced, erased, or overcome. The ideological workings of narrative—its ability to inculcate, perpetuate, and naturalize embodied habits of cognition and emotion—are optimized as the not me in the doubling of real me and alien me diminishes or disappears. If stories ask us to suspend disbelief to immerse ourselves in the illusion they offer, this invitation may be a temptation to the dissolution of boundaries that the demystifying suspicions of ideology critique rightly resist in order to shake the hold on us of habits of thinking and feeling whose power we may not recognize because they are so deeply ingrained, familiarized, and naturalized. The capacity of stories to facilitate beneficial social collaboration and to habitualize ideological mystification are two sides of the same coin.

Distributed Cognition and the Social Life of Stories

These complications call for important caveats to the oft-heard claim that a culture's narratives constitute a valuable source of collective knowledge and social cohesion. Ricoeur (1987, 428) argues, for example, that stories offer "narrative intelligence," providing "practical wisdom" different from "the theoretical use of reason" in philosophy or science, a cultural reservoir of implicit ways of understanding that Jerome Bruner (1986, 69) identifies as a "major link between our own sense of self and our sense of others in the social world around us." These arguments have recently been reformulated in the terminology of distributed cognition based on Andy Clark's influential notion of the extended mind. Surveying the various tools and affordances (to recall Gibson's [1979] well-known term) provided by the environment that extend our cognitive capacities, Clark (2011, 226) observes that a "linguistic surround envelops us from birth"—a "sea of words . . . and external symbols [that] are thus paramount among the cognitive vortices which help constitute human thought." These include, of course, the stories we find circulating around us. David Herman (2013, 162, 192) consequently claims that "narrative's capacity to distribute intelligence—its ability to disseminate knowledge about or ways of engaging with the world—makes it . . . a key instrument of mind," with a culture's repository of stories constituting "a society of mind" through the "suprapersonal systems for sense-making" they offer.

Cognition is not limited to what happens inside the skull, then, but this does not mean (as some advocates of distributed cognition seem to think) that what occurs there is unimportant. Clark himself acknowledges, for example, that "the brain (or brain and body) comprises a package of basic, portable, cognitive resources that is of interest in its own right" (224).[13] Alva Noë (2009, xiii) is certainly correct that "you are not your brain"—"human experience is a dance that unfolds in the world and with others," as he explains, and "we are not locked up in a prison of our own ideas and sensations"—but the to-and-fro "dance" of we-intentionality depends on what the embodied consciousnesses of the participants bring to the interaction and how their configurative powers shape and are transformed by the doubling of their subjectivities with the subjectivities of various collaborators. The notion of distributed cognition should not replace brain-based analyses of the social powers of narrative, then, but it can usefully supplement them by clarifying the dynamics of the transaction between stories and the cognitive processes of their recipients.

These interactions are in some respects similar to but in other ways importantly different from our involvements with other kinds of external resources that extend our minds into the world. Cognition occurs, according to Clark, whenever "the human organism is linked with an external entity in a two-way interaction, creating a coupled system" between the brain and its extensions in which "all the components . . . play an active causal role" and "jointly govern behavior" (222). Like Clark's examples of a blind man's stick or a notebook with formulas or directions a user may consult, a culture's stories may provide navigational equipment or a set of tools that increase our individual mind's capacities to negotiate its way through the world. Like the resources for problem solving afforded by features of the environment, the preformed patterns that we find already circulating in our culture's stories offer readily available resources for thinking about commonly encountered situations that we do not have to invent from scratch. As participants in "two-way interactions" in a "coupled system," however, these extensions of the mind may not leave the user unchanged. The acquisition of language, for example, has powerfully and profoundly transformed the brain. By the same token, just as we need to learn how to use a tool or adapt our practices to the environment's affordances, so stories can only extend our minds if we let ourselves be shaped by them. We need to learn how to follow stories by acquiring competence in recognizing and responding to the patterns they deploy, and these ways of configuring narratives will only have cognitive power in other realms of our lives if they reshape our brain- and body-based habits of figuring the world.

A culture's narratives provide patterns of shared intentionality that we can take up by coupling our cognitive proclivities with the configurative patterns they hold ready for our use, and this doubling is a to-and-fro process that may reshape both parties to the interaction. This is not a linear or one-way process. Even learning to follow the instructions for using a particular tool or device can transform not only the user but also the instrument, whether through applications of its features to problems for which it may not have been initially intended or through discoveries that lead to improvements or alterations in its design. As Terence Cave (2016, 48) observes, "affordances are by definition open-ended, since someone or something may always come up with a new use for the most unlikely object." The responses made possible by what Cave calls "literary affordances" are, he notes, both constrained and "underspecified," inviting and facilitating particular uses but also leaving open unpredictable improvisations that can transform both the instrument and its users (see 51–62). Once again these interactions can take a variety of shapes depending on both the affordance and the respondent and on what happens in their encounter. The coupled, to-and-fro processes of doubling set in motion by these interactions are not necessarily under the exclusive direction or control of either party.

To follow a story is to engage in a two-way, back-and-forth interaction between the configured patterns of action emplotted in the narrative and the figures through which the recipient experiences the push and pull of the world. These exchanges can take a variety of forms, with different results. As in the experience of playing of a game, the to-and-fro of the interaction can be so absorbing that it may take over and submerge our sense of self in the communal operation of the exchange (offering the pleasure of immersion in a story or reinforcing the ideological power of customary cognitive patterns). Or the reciprocity between story and recipient can open up a space between them for innovative interactions neither partner alone controls but that may transform both—resulting in new interpretations of the narrative, new ways of configuring its elements, or new possibilities of pattern formation that break the recipient's past habits and reshape his or her world. Stories get reshaped through their transmission as they are refigured in their reception in ways that may then get passed on in their subsequent retelling and rehearing. This circuit in turn can be transformative for the audience—or, again, can inculcate and reinforce existing patterns. The shared intentionality produced through these interactions is heteronomous to the participants; it depends on the configurative patterns both parties bring to the encounter, but it results in the emergence of a state of affairs (the historically shifting and various "lives" of the narrative in and through its reception) that paradoxically transcends them even as it is created by them (see Armstrong 1990, 20–43).

This circuit is not unique to narratives. Skillful use of even a simple tool like a hammer can be such an absorbing experience that the boundary between worker, instrument, and task becomes blurred in the job at hand, and an instrument is susceptible to a wide range of unpredictable, transformative applications (a hammer can be used for building a house or committing murder, with unforeseeably ramifying consequences in both cases). There are differences here that matter, however. Stories are equipment for navigating the world and solving problems, but they are not entirely defined by their instrumental dimension. The as-if of aesthetic experience is potentially more playful and open ended than the use of tools for particular ends, even if those ends can lead to other unforeseeable consequences.

The transactions through which stories are received and transformed in the lives of recipients are to-and-fro interactions whose dynamics may become open ended, playful, and unpredictable to the extent that the narratives serve noninstrumental purposes and can dwell in the realm of the as-if—the realm in which fictions operate, as Ricoeur puts it, according to a double logic of "it was so and it was not" (see 1977, 265–305). If the to-and-fro of play between telling and following stories mobilizes the brain's habitual sense-making patterns and sets these against its need to test, revise, and change its customary ways of configuring the world, then the as-if of the aesthetic dimension opens up more room for experimentation, flexibility, and play than may be available in the instrumental use of patterns for problem solving (although here too the brain needs to be open to adjustments and realignments in its habitual gestalts when anomalies don't fit the figures it typically deploys). Paradoxically, perhaps, the pragmatic usefulness of stories for keeping our cognitive processes from congealing into rigid habitual patterns—for holding open their capacity to be reshaped and re-formed—may be enhanced by the noninstrumental play of the aesthetic. Exchanging stories for their own sake is cognitively useful, then, especially to the extent that the play of configuration and refiguration is able to loosen the habitual, ideological hold of any particular set of narrative patterns on our individual and social minds.

The social power of stories to defamiliarize, disrupt, and play with the cognitive patterns that hold us in their grip calls for a different "cognitive politics," however, than the program of "therapy" through repetitive "cognitive retraining" that Mark Bracher (2013) advocates. His pedagogical program proposes the use of social "protest novels" to expose and rectify "faulty cognitive schema" that result in injustice: "One must get people to repeatedly recognize, interrupt, and override the old, faulty schema elements when they are triggered, and to activate instead the elements of the new, more adequate schema" (25–26). This is a particularly egregious demonstration of the kind of mechanical, reductive thinking that schema theory can lead to.[14] One can agree with Bracher's criticism of what he calls "four key faulty assumptions about . . . human nature" (see 8)—the assumptions that people are fully "autonomous," defined by "essences," separated "atomistically" from each other, and "homogeneous" ("simply good or bad")—without endorsing any particular conception of justice or injustice. These assumptions are not a "faulty schema" that can be reversed and replaced by a "new, more adequate schema." The figurative processes of seeing-as are much more variable and pluralistic than this rigid dichotomy acknowledges (see Armstrong 1990). As Bracher's critique of essentialism itself suggests, humans are biocultural hybrids who can organize their social and cognitive lives in a variety of ways, and science cannot (and should not try to) prescribe any particular mode of interpretation or any specific moral or political order.

Bracher's reverse cognitive engineering through repetitive reinforcement of correct cognitive categories is not only a morally and politically questionable assertion of dominance and authority; it also fails to recognize the power of the as-if in narrative interactions to suspend and challenge the habits that hold sway over our sense of the world's patterns. The to-and-fro interactions through which we exchange stories can upend conventional, naturalized patterns of we-intentionality and open up different, perhaps more enlivening possibilities of collaborative interaction. Bracher's program of therapeutic, repetitive retraining would stomp out the very unpredictable, open-ended play that potentially gives our experience with stories emancipatory power (and what a dreary, Gradgrind-like place Bracher's classroom must be!).

Justice is a historically contingent, culturally variable, and essentially contestable concept that narratives can help to reshape and re-form through their play with our cognitive habits. The play of the as-if in aesthetic experiences and the unpredictable to-and-fro of narrative interactions can have political consequences by making possible the kind of negotiation and re-alignment of social and moral categories that Judith Shklar (1990) describes in her analysis of how the "sense of injustice" develops and changes in democratic societies. What counts as an "injustice" rather than a "misfortune," she argues—the kinds of things that a society regards as unfair and not merely unfortunate (the suffering caused by racial discrimination, for example, versus the harm and loss resulting from a natural disaster like a volcano or an earthquake) and that thus demand political remediation rather than charitable assistance—is a culturally and historically variable state of affairs that can change through argument and debate in democratic communities. How these boundaries get drawn and redrawn may be powerfully influenced by the stories we tell each other. These lines are necessarily fuzzy, but their contestability is precisely Shklar's point—"Yesterday's rock solid rule is today's folly and bigotry," she observes (8)—because questioning and readjusting these categories is, she argues, the crucial work of democratic exchange.[15] The kind of reconfiguration of injustice that Shklar describes is facilitated by the sort of open-ended, to-and-fro exchanges that the potentially transformative play of stories with our configurative habits can promote (see Armstrong 2005).

Cognitive science can help us analyze and understand the coupling processes of we-intentionality that these different political and pedagogical programs set in motion, but it cannot decide between them. The synchronization of coupled subjectivities can reinforce the cognitive habits of the participants—or, as in Bracher's program, restructure them through repetitive retraining. Or, as in the politics of play that I prefer, the to-and-fro of as-if interactions as we tell and follow stories may expose the limits and the contingency of our cognitive constructs and open them up to transformation through the noninstrumental effects of the aesthetic. Once again, neuroscience can help us understand the social powers of narrative, but these powers can serve various ends, and their consequences are not foreordained.

An interesting recent hyperscanning experiment has documented various kinds of brain-to-brain synchronization that different pedagogical activities may produce. Employing EEG skullcaps to record the brain-wave patterns of twelve high school seniors during eleven classes spread out over a semester, neuroscientist Suzanne Dikker and her colleagues (2017) found evidence of significant variations in brain coupling that led one commentator to conclude that "classroom engagement and neural coherence do go hand in hand" (Bhattacharya 2017, R347). Perhaps not surprisingly, brain-to-brain synchronization was greater when students were "watching videos and engaging in group discussions" than when "listening to the teacher reading aloud or lecturing" (Dikker et al. 2017, 1376). Even more, "students showed the highest pairwise synchrony during class with their face-to-face partner" compared to side-by-side or nonadjacent student pairings (1379). Although perhaps intuitively obvious (most students would probably agree that a discussion or a film is less likely to be boring than a lecture), these findings are important because they provide material evidence of the neural processes of brain-to-brain coupling that underlie collaborative interactions in the classroom and elsewhere.

Interpreting their evidence, the experimenters conclude that "students' neural entrainment to their surrounding sensory input"—that is, "the teacher, a video, or each other"—varies according to "joint attention." Or, in technical terms, "brain-to-brain synchrony increases as shared attention modulates entrainment by 'tuning' neural oscillations to the temporal structure of our surroundings" (1380). That is, oscillations of neuronal assemblies in my brain resonate in synchrony with your brain waves ("tuning" resulting in "entrainment") as we attend jointly to phenomena unfolding in time. Collaboration produces oscillatory brain-to-brain coupling (we-intentionality) as we coordinate our perspectives in temporally unfolding, to-and-fro interactions with each other and the world we share (the video we watch or the lecture we listen to or the discussion we participate in). Joint attention requires the ability to double me and not me in experiences of shared intentionality, and this doubling is the two-in-one cognitive structure underlying successful collaborative activity all the way down to oscillations at the neural level.

Exactly what was going on in the heads of these high school students can't be detected by an EEG apparatus, however, and the synchronization of their brain waves doesn't mean they were all thinking the same thoughts, any more than the members of an orchestra performing harmoniously by blending the sounds from their different instruments would have identical experiences or neural signatures. Synchrony, again, is not homogeneity but a harmonization of different processes and perspectives. If a film or a group discussion is more successful at inducing immersion in a collective activity than a reading or a lecture, that is probably because they encourage involvement through individual meaning making, creating more possibility for imagination, emotional resonance, and active contributions from participants in a joint enterprise. A didactic exercise may aim at getting a group to react in unison, and it may succeed if it can compel joint attention into patterns of synchronization that coordinate the intentionality of its members ("Repeat after me"). Joint attention can result in groupthink, but different group activities may produce synchronization with more or less uniformity among the participants (rooting for one's hometown sports team versus exchanging arguments in a lively debate would both produce brain-to-brain synchronization but with different degrees of homogeneity). In this experiment, curiously, the activities that were less coercive resulted in greater brain-wave synchronization, and that may be because they were more conducive to promoting the to-and-fro of shared intentionality, the paradoxical combination of active contribution and immersive letting go that characterizes collaboration.

How brains synchronize is crucial to understanding the to-and-fro interactions set in motion by the experience of telling and following stories, and another recent experiment has produced suggestive results about the intracortical patterns underlying these exchanges. Extending its innovative work on intersubject correlation analysis of fMRI images, Uri Hasson's laboratory (Silbert et al. 2014, e4687) analyzed the cortical activity generated by producing and understanding a narrative—first mapping "all areas that are reliably activated in the brains of [three] speakers telling a 15-minute-long narrative" and then comparing the time course of this activity with areas "activated in the brains of [eleven] listeners as they comprehended that same narrative." This study compared not only which cortical areas were activated by telling and hearing a story but also the temporal progression of this activity in both speakers and listeners—not only "the spatial overlap" of brain regions but also how "the neural activity is coupled . . . during production and comprehension" (e4687). Some regions didn't overlap (speaking and listening are different activities, after all), and some overlapping areas didn't respond similarly over time, but other parts of the brain that were activated by both the production and the comprehension of the story were temporally correlated—that is, their firing was coupled and synchronized. Evidence of temporally synchronized brain-to-brain coupling was especially marked in the medial prefrontal cortex, an area associated with "reward-based learning and memory, . . . empathy, and theory of mind," and the precuneus, an area on the superior parietal lobe that has been linked to "a wide spectrum of highly integrated tasks, including episodic memory retrieval, first-person perspective taking, and the experience of agency" (e4692–93). These are brain areas that one would expect to be coupled during experiences of collaboration and joint attention, and that is what this experiment showed— temporally correlated synchronization across a network of cortical regions associated with understanding and identifying with others and coordinating attention and memory. If stories exert social power by setting in motion and synchronizing neuronally based cognitive activity across the boundaries between self and other, the temporal coupling of responses in areas having to do with memory, perspective taking, empathy, and agency would be evidence of just the sort of brain-based interactions that the doubling of worlds in narrative understanding would produce.

   As is almost always the case, however, this experiment raises as many questions as it answers. Although the synchronization of cortical activity that it documents is powerful evidence of the intersubjective sharing of a story's intentionality, it isn't exactly clear how we should understand the different roles of the speakers and listeners in the experiment or how these compare to the various subject positions that can be coupled in the process of telling and following stories. The three speakers in the experiment are not identical to the author of a story, for example, because they recited a prescripted narrative that they did not create. But they are also not quite equivalent to a story's narrator, because that is a position within the narrative that the recitation actualizes along with other roles (a story's different characters, for example, or the explicit or implicit narratee). Like the oral recitation of a poem that can be regarded as a way of interpreting the work, a speaker enunciating a preestablished story belongs to its comprehenders as much as to its producers. The experiment nevertheless does indeed register the shared intentionality entailed in an exchange of narrative figuration inasmuch as all fourteen participants (three speakers, eleven listeners) responded in their different but correlated, synchronized ways to the configurative patterns of meaning in the narrative. But the point remains that the speaker-listener relationship in the experiment does not line up exactly with the relation of teller, tale, and audience. And this imprecision means that the experiment's claim to have recorded the brain-to-brain coupling entailed in telling and following stories is not entirely accurate.

Similarly, the questions narrative theorists endlessly debate about the relation between the various subject positions that can be configured in narrative exchanges—for example, the author, the implied author, the narrator, the narratee, the authorial audience, and the actual audience—are left ambiguous by this experiment.[16] These distinctions matter to the experience of a listener or reader because they indicate different modes of narrative intentionality that the subjectivity of the recipient may engage and double with—for example, coupling my consciousness with the intentionality of the narrator or the narratee, or projecting an implied author that my consciousness assumes it is in relation with, or aligning my individual response to the story with the perspectives of other respondents that I either know or imagine are (or have been or will be) coparticipants in its reception (fellow readers, listeners, critics, and interlocutors through whose responses a story lives on, the actual audience no author can ever fully anticipate). Interactions, couplings, and synchronizations of different kinds would occur in all of these doubled relations, but the instruments of neuroscience are not able to register what these experiences are like.

An important issue left open by this experiment is the relationship between its measurements of brain-to-brain coupling and the kinds of synchronization that occur across broader expanses of time and space in the social life of stories. Audiences from different social worlds and historical periods that respond to the same story are no doubt synchronizing their brains as they reactivate the intentionality of the narrative and thereby participate in the transmission of its we-intentionality across its history of reception, but this kind of cross-cultural, transgenerational collaboration is impossible to measure through a hyperscanning EEG experiment or an intersubject correlation analysis of fMRI images. The patterns registered in this experiment's recording of coupled brain activity provide material evidence of how different brains can synchronize in response to a story, and if this can happen across fourteen subjects who separately entered and left an fMRI machine at different moments as they recited or listened to a narrative, then the correlations across space and time measured in this particular case could plausibly be extended to imply similar synchronizations across even greater temporal and spatial divides. The scanning technologies may not be able to provide precise measurements of these widely dispersed interactions, but the experimental evidence nevertheless warrants the inference that similar brain-based synchronizations and processes of doubling are at work (or, better, in play) in the interactions across history and culture through which stories exercise their social power. When I hear a story from long ago or far away, I do often feel that my world is resonating with another world, and perhaps the brain-to-brain couplings registered in this fMRI experiment are the material, biological basis of that mysterious, ephemeral experience.

Stories as a Cognitive Archive: What Is It Like to Be Conscious?

Cognitive literary critics have recently argued that neuroscience has much to learn from literature because of its understanding of phenomena that defy objective measurement or physical analysis. The central issue here is the problem of qualia, the dilemma of how to explain the first-person, lived experience of a sensation like seeing red (see Humphrey 2006). This problem is the topic of Thomas Nagel's memorably titled essay "What Is It Like to Be a Bat?" (1974) in which he argues that conscious experience—for example, a first-person, lived sensation like seeing red—cannot be adequately explained in the objective terms of science. Nagel's critique is aimed at the program of neuroscientists like Francis Crick (1994, 3, 9) who, defiantly proclaiming "you're nothing but a pack of neurons," contends that "the neural correlate of 'seeing red'" is objectively definable. "The scientific belief is that our minds—the behavior of our brains—can be explained by the interactions of nerve cells (and other cells) and the molecules associated with them," Crick argues, and so "we may be able to say that you perceive red if and only if certain neurons (and/or molecules) in your head behave in a certain way" (7, 9). This assumption informs much work in "neuroaesthetics," the field pioneered by British neuroscientist Semir Zeki, who purports to explain artistic beauty as a response of the "reward system" in the frontal cortex (see Zeki and Ishizu 2011). His much-watched TED talk (which has thousands of views on YouTube) shows him pointing to a patch of color on an fMRI image where experiences of beautiful art and music intersect and pronouncing that this is the location of beauty in the brain.

There are a number of problems with this claim, among them that aesthetic experiences set in motion far-reaching to-and-fro interactions across the cortex and between the brain and the body that are not localizable to any region of neural anatomy (see Conway and Rehding 2013). Equally important, however, is the question of what fMRI images can and cannot show about consciousness. These striking color images look like snapshots of the brain in action—neurons firing in response to beauty—but this appearance is deceiving. For one thing, fMRI technology offers only an indirect measurement of cortical activity, tracking differences in blood flow to parts of the brain with a considerable temporal lag. Even more, however, Zeki's images are nothing more (or less) than visualizations—pictorial representations of statistical measurements of differential blood flow averaged across a group of twenty-one subjects—and are therefore more like graphs or charts than photos. Crick may be right that we only can have an experience of beauty or anything else if neurons fire, but these images are at most vivid statistical displays; they are not what it is like to be conscious of music or visual art.

A closer approximation of neuronal activity may be provided by single-cell measurements of the electrical activity of individual neurons, a more direct and specific technology of measurement than fMRI, but ordinarily not possible in human subjects due to ethical restrictions. Occasionally, however, as with epilepsy patients prior to surgery, it is necessary and permissible to insert probes into the brains of live human subjects and record electrical activity, and interesting experimental findings sometimes result—as in one notorious case in the neuroscience literature where a single neuron was discovered in the face recognition area of an epilepsy patient that responded exclusively to images of actress Jennifer Aniston and not to pictures of her and her ex-husband Brad Pitt or to other faces or objects (see Quiroga et al. 2005). This is what Crick is looking for—the neuronal activity underlying an experience—but it is not what it is like to be conscious of Jennifer Aniston.

Hence Nagel's skepticism that first-person experience can be captured by the terms and concepts of the physical sciences. As he argues, "Every subjective phenomenon is essentially connected with a single point of view, and it seems inevitable that an objective, physical theory will abandon that point of view" (1974, 437). Further, he claims, "even to form a conception of what it is like to be a bat (and a fortiori to know what it is like to be a bat) one must take up the bat's point of view" (442n). Whether humans without sonar echolation can ever do this is debatable, but what strikes a literary critic (and what Nagel does not seem to recognize) is that "point of view" is also a literary term with a long, sometimes controversial history in the theory of the novel. Whether and how a point of view (of a human, if not a bat) can be rendered in a work of fiction so that the reader can imaginatively recreate its lived immediacy is a nontrivial question that has been much debated in narrative theory.

When David Lodge (2002, 16) claims that "literature constitutes a kind of knowledge about consciousness which is complementary to scientific knowledge," it is no accident that the example he chooses is a novel by Henry James, a writer famously associated with point of view in fiction. After the cognitive scientist in Lodge's novel *Thinks . . .* (2001, 42–43) explains "the problem of consciousness" (that is, "how to give an objective, third-person account of a subjective, first-person phenomenon"), the other lead character who not coincidentally happens to be a creative writer replies: "Oh, but novelists have been doing that for the last two hundred years," and as proof she recites from memory the opening lines of *The Wings of the Dove*. As Lodge observes, "We read novels like *The Wings of the Dove* because they give us a convincing sense of what the consciousness of people other than ourselves is like" (2002, 30). This accomplishment is not unique to James (the other example Lodge's writer cites is a poem by Andrew Marvell), but James's experiments with point of view are of special cognitive interest because they seek to represent not primarily the what of the world but the how of its perception by consciousness. This thematization of perception lays bare processes, problems, and paradoxes that are involved whenever literature and other arts attempt to render subjective experience.

James's experiments with perspective and focalization are instructive because the access literature provides to qualia is not as straightforward as Lodge suggests. The artistic representation of experience is not, after all, a matter of simply offering up consciousness for direct inspection or of immersing us fully and immediately in another world. The like in what it is like can only be rendered by the as-if of aesthetic staging (see Iser 1993). When literary works from whatever genre or period attempt to re-create what it is like to be someone other than ourselves, they can only do so by using styles, conventions, and techniques that are not identical to the subjective experience they seek to represent. Cave (2016, 14) is correct when he argues that "literature offers a virtually limitless archive of the ways in which human beings think, how they imagine themselves and their world." To mine this archive, however, requires an appreciation of the aesthetic variability of the as-if in rendering the cognitive experience of what it is like to be conscious.

The curious thing about Lodge's example, consequently, is that James renders the consciousness of Kate Croy not immediately and directly but through a recognizable, finely wrought, and notoriously controversial literary style:

> She waited, Kate Croy, for her father to come in, but he kept her unconscionably, and there were moments at which she showed herself, in the glass over the mantel, a face positively pale with the irritation that had brought her to the point of going away without sight of him. It was at this point, however, that she remained; changing her place, moving from the shabby sofa to the armchair upholstered in a glazed cloth that gave at once—she had tried it—the sense of the slippery and of the sticky. (2003 [1902], 21)

Even in these two sentences one can recognize James's distinctive manner. Following his well-known method of representing a scene indirectly through the point of view of a "central intelligence" (which is why Lodge chooses this example), James's novel opens by depicting Kate's perceptions and reflections (her sight of herself in the mirror, for example, and her annoyance at her father's delay) and even her tactile sensations (the feel of the tacky upholstery). James is sometimes criticized for portraying characters with huge heads and nonexistent bodies, but here Kate Croy's consciousness is haptically embodied. Just as visible in this passage as what Kate is thinking and feeling, however, is James's writing (even how he renders the materiality of touch by the rhetorical trick of turning adjectives into nouns ["the slippery and the sticky"]).

This is not stream of consciousness (whatever that hopelessly vague term signifies) but rather a finely balanced structure of phrases and clauses that calls attention to its verbal play. The style itself implies a presence and a perspective other than the character's—giving us a doubled sense of observing Kate from an implied narrator's viewpoint while also inhabiting her interiority. We are there, watching with her, even as we also watch her—and also as we watch James and marvel at his style (or despair, because how can we do all three things at once—an understandable frustration that prompted his brother William to complain and to admonish Henry just to get on with it and tell us what's happening in the story). What it is like to be Kate Croy at this moment in time, as James portrays it in this passage, is a complex product of aesthetic staging.

Lodge credits the invention of free indirect style with giving novels extraordinary power to open up inside views into other lives (see 2002, 37–57). This technique is indeed a manifestation of the paradox of the alter ego, as I have argued, but it is not simply natural, immediate, and transparent. A biocultural hybrid, its doubling of self and other is both an enactment of basic, embodied cognitive processes and a contingent historical construct—a stylistic convention that only emerged through a long history of literary experimentation and that can be deployed in a variety of ways for different purposes. There is an enormous difference, for example, between the biting ironies of Flaubert's free indirect style in *Madame Bovary* and the generous sympathy informing James's depiction of Isabel Archer's consciousness as she sits up all night reflecting on the disappointments of her marriage in the famous chapter 42 of *The Portrait of a Lady* or the notoriously ambiguous, undecidable detachment of Joyce's rendering of Stephen Dedalus's sensibility in *A Portrait of the Artist as a Young Man*. Literature may have powers to render what it is like to be conscious that the objective measures of science lack, but the as of the as-if still leaves a gap between the re-creation of another point of view in art and the immediacy of first-person consciousness.

This gap is both disabling and empowering. It prevents literature from ever completely transcending the divide between one consciousness and another, but it also makes it possible for art to stage versions of other lives and to experiment with different ways of doing so. If the as of representation prevents a work of fiction from presenting qualia immediately and directly, it also allows writers to display and explore various aspects of perceptual experience through cognitively distinctive styles. One of the ways neuroscience can assist literary theory is by identifying and describing the cognitive processes that a particular narrative technique seeks to represent and re-create. It is not enough to specify the formal features or grammatical markers associated with techniques like point of view, stream of consciousness, or interior monologue. As Alan Palmer (2004, 64) points out, "There are vast areas of the mind that are not addressed within the speech category approach" that governs narratological analyses of fictional minds. Because different narrative methods for representing consciousness foreground different aspects of human understanding, a particular strategy for depicting the life of the mind will not be fully elucidated until its cognitive implications have been analyzed and explained, and for this work the ideas and theories of neuroscience can be immensely useful. Scientific concepts alone are not enough to explain the epistemological implications of a particular technique because the as of its staging of what it is like to be conscious in one way or another requires careful explication that is attuned to the aesthetics of style, but attempting to interpret the way a cognitive process is staged in a narrative without consulting the sciences of the mind is to deprive oneself of valuable analytical tools.

The need to analyze the cognitive assumptions and aims of a representational style is especially evident in the notorious difficulty of defining the aesthetic of impressionism in literature and painting. Impressionism is a fascinating example of the way in which literature, painting, and other arts provide a cognitive archive that can be mined for evidence of how the question of what it is like to be conscious has been explored by artists in different genres, periods, and cultures. As evidence of the biocultural diversity of our species' cognitive life, this archive is historically varied, inasmuch as the like in what it is like and the as of the as-if can be staged in a variety of different ways, even as it is also characterized by universal epistemological structures and processes that have been constant over recent evolutionary time.

Historically, the impressionist project began with a desire to radicalize the aesthetic of realism by exposing and thematizing its epistemological conditions of possibility. Both visual and literary impressionists had become impatient with the conventions of representation because they were inconsistent with the workings of consciousness and consequently seemed artificial. The paradox of impressionism, however, is that the attempt to render faithfully the perceptual processes through which consciousness knows the world thwarts mimetic illusion building. The result is art that can seem strange, baffling, and unrealistic and that calls attention to itself as art (the formal qualities of the picture plane or the textuality of narrative discourse). This paradox points the way to the abstraction and antimimetic textual play that characterize the aesthetic of modernism. The reasons for these changes have to do with the elusiveness of consciousness as a target of representation. Impressionism gives rise to modernism because of the instabilities of an aesthetic of qualia.

The term "impressionism" is so heterogeneous that it might seem to defy definition, covering artists ranging from the painters in Monet's school to the literary impressionists who led the novel's transition from realism to modernism (especially Henry James, Joseph Conrad, and Ford Madox Ford, but the term has sometimes been extended to include almost any writer who attempts to render subjective experience, from Walter Pater and Stephen Crane to Joyce, Proust, and Virginia Woolf). What "impressionism" generally designates, however, is an interest in developing representational techniques that would do justice to first-person perceptual experience.[17] How to render the subjective experience of a sensation or a perception with paint or words is the distinctive challenge of impressionist art, and the difficulties (perhaps impossibility) of attaining this goal are responsible not only for the heterogeneity of impressionism but also for its many paradoxes and contradictions.

Impressionism exposes the gap between the as of the as-if re-creation of another point of view in art and the immediacy of first-person consciousness by attempting to overcome it, and this is why it is such a paradoxical phenomenon. Consider, for example, the contradictory aims and effects of Monet's painting "Impression: Sunrise" (1872), often cited as emblematic of the impressionist aesthetic. An attempt to render a visual sensation at a particular moment, under specific conditions of light and atmosphere, this painting exemplifies Zola's description of impressionism as "a corner of nature seen through a temperament" (quoted in Rubin 1999, 48). Aiming to capture accurately and precisely the experiential effects of a moment, it is both objective and subjective. Hence the paradox that impressionism has been regarded as not only more scientific but also more personal and phenomenal in its approach to representation than the conventions of realism it challenges (see Lewis 2007). The claim to the greater realism of Monet's painting of the sunrise is both its truth to the atmospheric conditions of the moment and its truth to the perceiver's visual sensations. In a further important complication, however, it can only represent this perceptual experience in an arrangement of colored brush strokes, and so another contradiction of this painting—one that looks forward to modernism's focus on the picture plane—is that its atmospheric, sensational effects depend on relations between color contrasts (red versus blue), shapes (the intense, off-center circle of sun and the sketchily indicated ships), and brush strokes (vigorously and roughly applied in the sky and the water) that emphasize its tangibility as a made object (even signed and dated by its maker in the lower left corner).

The effects of these contradictions on the viewer are paradoxical and double, simultaneously immediate and reflective. Monet's painting is both an incitement to vicarious immersion in a momentary sensation and a call to reflect on the cognitive conditions it simulates as well as on the artistic techniques whereby it criticizes the unnaturalness of realism. As the art historian James Rubin (1999, 115) perceptively notes, "Monet's techniques concentrate on purely visual phenomena to create a fascinating interplay between presence and absence—an interplay that calls attention to representation and illusion." Oscillating between presence and absence, this painting seeks to render a first-person experience that it is not and cannot be, and its effort to create a simulacrum of experience foregrounds the material, technical means through which it seeks to do so. This contradiction has the paradoxical effect of promoting aesthetic reflection about the formal features of the work (the abstract play of colors on the picture plane that is a harbinger of modernist abstraction) even as it incites the viewer to re-create an as-if doubling of the original moment of sensation—a simulacrum of the moment that both is and is not what Monet experienced. The qualia of the sensation of the sunrise is both there and not there in Monet's painting, and this duality sets in motion an oscillation between sensuous immersion and cognitive, aesthetic reflection.

These oppositions are evident in the conflict between two famous beholders, John Ruskin and E. H. Gombrich, who disagree about impressionism because they emphasize contrary poles of its defining paradoxes. According to Ruskin's well-known formulation, "The whole technical power of painting depends on our recovery of what may be called the *innocence of the eye*; that is to say, of a sort of childish perception of these flat stains of colour, merely as such, without consciousness of what they signify, as a blind man would see them if suddenly gifted with sight" (1857, 6n; original emphasis). Ironically and inevitably, this account of primordial perception prior to the imposition of conventional categories relies on metaphors—fanciful comparisons to how a child or a blind person would see that are not strictly accurate. As the neuroscience of vision has discovered, the rear visual cortex will atrophy if it fails to receive stimuli during critical periods of early life that allow it to organize itself. This was one of the central findings of the now-classic experiments that won Thorstein Wiesel and David Hubel (see 1965) their Nobel Prize. Without establishing patterns of response to orientation, movement, and color, the visual brain loses its ability to make neuronal connections, and so a blind person who was suddenly granted vision literally could not see. Monet's painting is *not* how either a child or a sightless person would perceive the scene, then, but this "not" is evocative rather than merely erroneous because it makes possible a comparison that uses the as-if of figurative language to suggest in memorable terms what it is like to have an original sensation (an experience of qualia which, of course, is not strictly speaking reproducible). Ruskin may be scientifically wrong, but there is something figuratively right about the phrase "the innocent eye" as a metaphor for qualia that explains why it has endured.

Famously objecting that "the innocent eye is a myth," Gombrich (1960, 298) insists on the role of "the beholder's share" in perception and painting: "Seeing is never just registering. It is the reaction of the whole organism to the patterns of light that stimulate the back of our eyes." This is indeed a central doctrine of contemporary neuroscience, which understands vision as a to-and-fro process of assembling inputs back and forth across the visual cortex in interactions between the brain, the body, and the world (see Livingstone 2002). In ways Gombrich insufficiently credits, however, impressionism also entails purposive play with pattern. Monet's painting relies on gestalts and constructs for its effects, not only in the formal alignment and juxtaposition of shapes and colors on the picture plane but also in the viewer's ability to recognize features of the scene (the ships and the harbor, the rising sun, its reflection on the water) that both are and are not there. The oscillations between presence and absence characteristic of the viewing experience are not evidence of formlessness but are the product of an interplay of figures and patterns. Ruskin and Gombrich are both wrong as well as right about what Monet is up to. Ruskin correctly understands that impressionism is an attempt to render qualia, but Gombrich is right that to do so it must deploy the aesthetic and cognitive resources of the as-if to suggest what it is like.

Similar paradoxes characterize literary impressionism, as is evident in the notoriously contradictory pronouncements of its most prominent advocate, the novelist and critic Ford Madox Ford. According to Ford (1964 [1914], 41), "Any piece of Impressionism, whether it be prose, or verse, or painting, or sculpture, is the record of the impression of a moment." The goal is to produce "the sort of odd vibration that scenes in real life really have; you would give your reader the impression . . . that he was passing through an experience" (1964 [1914], 42) with "the complexity, the tantalisation, the shimmering, the haze, that life is" (1924, 204). As Ford and his sometime collaborator Joseph Conrad recognized, "Life did not narrate, but made impressions on our brains. We in turn, if we wished to produce on you an effect of life, must not narrate but render impressions" (1924, 194–95). Following this advice, impressionist narratives like *The Good Soldier* or *Lord Jim* disrupt temporal continuity, jumping back and forth across time to offer disconnected perspectives on events and characters that can be bewildering because they resist our attempt to build patterns. Ford claims that "the object of the novelist is to keep the reader entirely oblivious of the fact that the author exists—even of the fact that he is reading a book" (1924, 199). But these disorienting techniques would seem to have the opposite effect. Rather than promoting discursive invisibility, they call attention to the constructedness of the text and to the cognitive processes its disjunctions dramatize.

As with the oscillations between presence and absence set in motion by "Impression: Sunrise," this contradiction foregrounds the fact that qualia cannot be given directly and immediately in painting or literature but can only be re-created, simulated, and staged through manipulations of the as-if. Hence Ford's claim that "the Impressionist must always exaggerate" (1964 [1914], 36), advice that would seem to fly in the face of his doctrine that the author and the text must disappear. Distortion is inevitable in painting or literature, however, because representation necessarily renders something *as* something other than itself. Rather than seeking to disguise this dilemma through mimetic illusion making, the disruptions of impressionism expose it.

Impressionism consequently has much in common with Viktor Shklovsky's well-known aesthetic of defamiliarization. The purpose of art, according to Shklovsky (1965 [1917], 12), is "to make objects 'unfamiliar,' to make forms difficult, to increase the difficulty and length of perception" and thereby to "recover the sensation of life, . . . to make one feel things, to make the stone *stony*." The effects of such defamiliarizing techniques can be paradoxical, not only revivifying perception but also promoting reflection about how habit blunts sensation and calling attention to artistic forms that resist naturalization. This doubleness is akin to the effects of distraction and bewilderment that Ford describes as characteristically impressionist:

> Indeed, I suppose that Impressionism exists to render those queer effects of real life that are like so many views seen through bright glass—through glass so bright that whilst you perceive through it a landscape or a backyard, you are aware that, on its surface, it reflects the face of a person behind you. For the whole of life is really like that; we are almost always in one place with our minds somewhere quite other. (1964 [1914], 41)

This is an experience of doubling, an oscillation between presence and absence—simultaneously a heightening of perception and an interruption of automatic processing that prompts the viewer to reflect about an odd optical effect, a peculiarity that is aesthetically interesting even as it foregrounds otherwise unnoticed aspects of consciousness. This duality both renders qualia—what it is like to have a visual sensation—and calls attention to the way in which the staging of what it is like requires a manipulation of the as (here figured as an experience of decentered consciousness as if we were in two places at once).

If the as of representation prevents the impressionists from presenting qualia immediately and directly, it also allows them to foreground and explore various aspects of perceptual experience, and the differences in how they do this are reflected in the multifariousness of the impressionist aesthetic. For example, James makes point of view a central principle of novelistic composition because of his fascination with the constructive powers of consciousness—how we know the world by "guess[ing] the unseen from the seen" (1970c [1884], 389) and composing patterns from a limited perspective that leaves some things hidden and indeterminate. Readers of *What Maisie Knew* or *The Ambassadors* are given a simulacrum of what this composing power is like—an as-if experience of seeing the world as Maisie or Strether do—but also are able to note ironically what these characters probably fail to observe or too imaginatively fill out (so that we share the child's bewilderment even as we understand the narcissistic machinations of adults that baffle her, and we are not as surprised as Strether is when he learns that the "virtuous attachment" between Chad and Madame de Vionnet is not purely chaste). By thematizing a character's perspective on the world and dramatizing how it is constructed according to certain assumptions, habits, and expectations, James allows us to immerse ourselves in another consciousness (experiencing what it is like to share their point of view) even as we also observe its characteristic limitations and blind spots and notice the disjunctions between its hold on the world and other points of view that would construe things differently (the adults who cruelly laugh at Maisie's naive questions or Woollett's worries that Strether has been carried away by the Parisian Babylon). This doubleness calls attention to the constructive powers of cognitive pattern making that we ordinarily do not notice in everyday perception and that traditionally realistic fiction tacitly employs to portray objects and characters by unfolding a series of aspects that display them.

Conrad's and Ford's ambiguous, fragmentary narratives deploy different techniques for similar cognitive purposes. In *Lord Jim*, the inconsistencies between the different perspectives Marlow receives on the titular character resist synthesis into a coherent point of view and consequently leave him frustrated and bewildered: "They fed one's curiosity without satisfying it; they were no good for purposes of orientation" (1996 [1900], 49). Marlow's glimpses of Jim remain fragmentary and disconnected, and their refusal to synthesize foregrounds the drive to build consistency among elements in a pattern that is necessary for lucid comprehension. In Ford's impressionistic masterpiece *The Good Soldier*, the similar inability of the narrator Dowell to reconcile different versions of events as he revisits and revises his many mistaken assumptions and beliefs also leaves him baffled. "I don't know. I leave it to you," he repeatedly tells the reader even as his narrative draws to its inconclusive close (1990 [1915], 282). The notorious ambiguities of both of these novels challenge and defy the reader to do a better job of fitting evidence into consistent patterns. In wondering whether to trust or doubt their narrators' explanations and interpretations, we replay their uncertainties in our own experience, and the refusal of fragments to cohere calls attention to the ordinarily invisible work of cognitive pattern construction.

One of the curiosities of impressionist experimentation in both painting and literature is that it must resort to such complicated technical innovation in order to render the seemingly simple, self-evident presence of consciousness to itself. But this contradiction is also a defining characteristic of modernism. For example, after denouncing the "tyranny" of plot and the "ill-fitting vestments" of conventional representation that fail to capture life's "luminous halo," Virginia Woolf memorably demands in her classic manifesto "Modern Fiction" (1984 [1921], 149–50): "Let us record the atoms as they fall upon the mind in the order in which they fall." She recognizes as well, however, that rendering first-person experience in all of its immediacy requires techniques and conventions, and so she worries that her generation will be condemned to "a season of failures and fragments," "smashing" and "crashing" and "writing against the grain," because "the Edwardian tools are the wrong ones for us to use" and more adequate techniques have yet to be invented ("Mr. Bennett and Mrs. Brown," 1950 [1924], 117, 116, 114, 112). Hence the seeming paradox that the effort to render what it is like to be conscious produces a panoply of stylistic innovations, from Woolf and Joyce to Faulkner and beyond, a technical variety that the over-used umbrella term "stream of consciousness" drastically oversimplifies. The issue is not which of these modernists' distinctive modes of stylistic experimentation gets the "luminous halo" of qualia right. Is "Time Passes" in *To the Lighthouse* a more accurate representation of the "atoms" than "Sirens" or "Oxen of the Sun" in *Ulysses*? Is Benjy's narration in *The Sound and the Fury* a more faithful rendering of consciousness than his brother Quentin's or Jason's—or Mrs. Ramsay's, or Leopold Bloom's, or Molly's? The absurdity of these questions suggests that this is not the right way to frame the problem. What the experiments of the modernists and the impressionists reveal, rather, is that the quest to render the what it is like of qualia requires the deployment of the as-if of representation and that this is open to endless variation. That is why modernism, like impressionism, is a heterogeneous assembly of styles for rendering consciousness rather than a unified epistemology or a homogeneous aesthetic.

The point is not that James, Conrad, and Ford or any of the great modernists are more or less right about consciousness but rather that their different technical experiments with figuring what it is like to be conscious use the as-if to stage in the reading experience various dimensions of cognitive life that neuroscience explores from its different perspective. The variability of the as in the as-if and the like in what it is like is what gives rise to the variety of stylistic experimentation through which impressionism and modernism stage and explore consciousness, never getting "it" quite right because they are always staging what it is like, a process of experimentation, innovation, and variation that makes representation historical.[18] Literature can never completely, fully capture what it is like to be conscious any more than science can, but the experiments of impressionism and modernism can help us to understand why this is so, even as they attempt to transcend the limits of the as-if and convey an experience that is beyond their grasp.

Impressionism and modernism are especially clear and compelling examples of how the arts provide a cognitive archive that can offer perspectives on the embodied life of consciousness that complement what neuroscience can disclose. The focus of these aesthetic movements on what it is like to be conscious thematizes cognitive processes at work in the configuration of experience in any rendering of the as-relations through which we know each other and our worlds. The as-if of aesthetic staging in whatever historical, generic, or cultural mode manipulates and makes visible the ordinarily invisible patterns of seeing-as through which we construe the world and, in the process, may potentially transfigure and transform them.[19] Music, the visual arts, and literature stage the as-if in different ways, but they all have cognitive value because their manipulations of the as-structure of their particular aesthetic domains can affect the as-relations through which cognition operates.

In the case of narrative, as I have tried to show in this book, by taking up the figurations through which we experience the world and configuring them into the patterns of discourse and story (the telling and the told), the stories we exchange may then reconfigure the as-relations that animate and define our everyday cognitive lives. This circuit of the three types of mimesis has generated an archive of figuration—the record of the social and historical life of stories—that testifies to the playful plasticity of our embodied cognitive powers. This archive is an intersubjective reservoir of shared intentionality that is not only a witness to what it has been like to be conscious in different periods and cultures; it is also an invitation to us to synchronize with other brains through the traces of their cognitive lives that await us in the stories they have left behind. The cognitive archive of the world's stories is an invaluable record of the social powers of narrative in other times and places. Those powers are not merely locked in the past, however, but can reach across historical and cultural distance as we couple our brains with the patterns of concord and discord that other members of our species have configured into stories.

Epilogue

NEUROSCIENCE AND NARRATIVE theory have much to learn from each other. There is an explanatory gap between the neural correlates of consciousness and the lived experience of telling and following stories, but as I have tried to show, this gap can be a resource rather than an obstacle. The challenge, no doubt easier said than done, is to understand and take advantage of how the differences that divide these two fields provide complementary perspectives that are irreducible but (at least potentially) mutually illuminating. The problem is not how to reconcile the sciences and the humanities in a grand epistemological synthesis (E. O. Wilson's [1998] dream of consilience) or how to resolve the conflict between the so-called two cultures. What is required, rather, is to figure out how to conduct productive exchanges across this divide from positions of disciplinary strength, where each side recognizes what the other can do that its theories and methods cannot. Identifying places where such exchanges might occur and suggesting what they might look like has been one of this book's primary aims.

What might narrative theory learn from such an exchange? For one thing, as I have argued, the findings of contemporary neuroscience about cognition, language, and emotion make some literary and narratological theories less plausible than others (especially those still haunted by the legacy of structuralist narratology). I have also tried to show that some neuroscientific research (on the disjunctive temporality of brain functioning, for example, or on the action-perception circuit) can shed light on much-discussed topics in narrative theory (how stories organize time and how plots imitate actions).

The benefits are not all one way, however. As I have argued, neuroscientific investigations of simulation in cognition, metaphor, and social interactions need to be informed by literary and narrative theories that have analyzed with great precision and detail the paradoxical workings of as-relations and the as-if in fictional stagings of experience. These theories, drawn from the works of Nietzsche, Iser, and Ricoeur (among others), show why the as-structure of simulation is more variable and open ended than causal or mechanical models imply, which explains in turn why the grounding of metaphors in embodied experience is differentially graded on a spectrum from the concrete to the abstract. Hence the biocultural variability of embodied metaphors for experiences like anger or pain that are both universal across our species and culturally and historically differentiated. Similarly, as phenomenological theories of reading suggest, the doubling of self and other in our experience of the intentionality embedded in a text casts doubt on the unidirectional assumptions of simulation models that underlie simplistic claims about the ability of literary works to improve theory of mind and empathy. Understanding the relation between stories and the brain requires competence in narrative theory as well as in neuroscience. Neither can do this work alone.

If one of the long-standing goals of narratology has been to explain the triangular relationship between stories, language, and the mind—to understand how our ability to tell and follow stories correlates with basic linguistic and cognitive processes characteristic of our species—then it is incumbent on narrative theory to keep up with the science. It may have once been the case that so called first-generation cognitive science, based on an artificial intelligence model of the brain, lined up well with the assumptions of structuralist narratology. The logical, algorithmic relations between anatomically based modules of a computer-like brain might then correspond to the rules of operation of universal grammar or to the orderly structures of language (*langue*) underlying speech (*parole*), and it would have made sense for narratology to propose cognitive schemes, frames, or scripts analogous to these modules and preference rules defining the formulas governing their operation.

As I explain in chapter 1, however, this model of the brain has fallen out of favor as the science has evolved. Extensive and ever-growing evidence provided by new scanning technologies has revealed that a modular, computer-like conception of the brain is too rigid and orderly to account for the dynamic, recursive interactions across the cortex and between brain, body, and the world through which cognitive patterns form, dissolve, and re-form. Language is a whole-brain phenomenon (Huth et al. 2016), and different parts of the cortex can be repurposed to support various and variable cognitive functions (Anderson 2010), as when the brain learns to read by recycling parts of the visual cortex that had evolved for invariant object recognition (Dehaene 2009). Our capacity for language is based on recurring, interactive experiences, not innate grammar-like structures (Nadeau 2012), and emotions are similarly an anatomically variable function of personal and cultural experiences, not universal structures with defined "neural signatures" (Lindquist et al. 2012, Barrett 2017). A bushy conception of the brain as a dynamic assembly of interacting, mutually constituting elements has displaced the logical, orderly modular theory, and cognitive narratology needs to revise its research program accordingly.

Science is a historical enterprise, not simply a collection of facts, and its theories change as new evidence casts doubt on previously accepted models. Fields in the humanities like narratology that make assumptions about cognition and the body need to continually review and evaluate those assumptions in light of developments in the scientific research. Neuroscience will not settle all of our controversies, however. There is no danger that the scourge of scientific positivism will close off inquiry and debate. To begin with, falsification is asymmetrical. Science can invalidate some views that are inconsistent with well-documented findings, but it can't necessarily tell us what is right. Some theories turn out to be wrong, but much room remains for productive disagreement about how to proceed. Although theories of language and emotion based on a modular theory of the brain don't stand up well against growing bodies of evidence, many questions remain about how best to understand these aspects of our cognitive lives, and conflicting interpretive approaches are still viable. Just as there are multiple ways in which our evolutionarily developed cognitive equipment can be used to create different narrative and cultural worlds, so different hermeneutic programs for making sense of this pattern-forming activity can be productively pursued—but there are constraints on what works and what doesn't (see Armstrong 1990).

A dynamic, recursive model of the bushy brain is consistent with a variety of different ways of analyzing the interaction of brain, body, and world in the exchange of stories. Drawing on the work of Ricoeur and Iser, I have preferred a phenomenological model of the circuit of figuration that crosses back and forth between different aspects of experience as we exchange stories—how the configuration of action in narration and emplotment (mimesis$_2$) draws on prefigurative personal and cultural experience (mimesis$_1$) and can in turn transform the figurative cognitive processes of recipients (mimesis$_3$) (see chapter 1). But as I have also suggested, other pragmatically-oriented approaches in second-generation cognitive narratology offer promising insights, consistent with contemporary neuroscience, into the dynamic interactions through which stories are constructed and exchanged. For example, Terence Cave (2016) combines the theories of implication from relevance theory with Gibson's concept of affordances to propose a cognitive model of thinking with literature that emphasizes the improvisatory possibilities made available by narrative forms. Elaine Auyoung (2018) applies the concept of fluency from communication theory to clarify how mimetic fiction can come to seem real. Karin Kukkonen (2016) uses Bayesian models of predictive processing to explain how the probability design in a narrative plays with the expectations that guide our cognitive activity in reading and in life. James Phelan's (2017) rhetorical theory has much to say about the ways in which authors seek to influence their audiences by manipulating various aspects of narrative communication. This is not an exhaustive list but, I think, an indication of some of the many lines of inquiry that make this new period in the history of narrative theory exciting and promising.[1]

Some terms and concepts from classical structural narratology still provide useful tools for analyzing the circuit of figuration through which stories are produced and exchanged. For example, I have repeatedly invoked the foundational narratological distinction between story and discourse (Chatman 1978) in order to explore the interaction between the different temporal processes and modes of action that characterize the telling (the act of narration), the told (the organization of events), and their reception (the activities of narrative comprehension). Similarly, Gérard Genette's (1980) magisterial explanation of narrative anachronies lays bare disjunctions in the temporal organization of stories that are interestingly correlated to the peculiarities of our temporally decentered brains. These terms and concepts often need correction or supplementation, however, because a grammatically-oriented model lacks the ability to clarify and explain the epistemological and cognitive workings of narrative—for example, as I show in chapter 4, a linguistic model is inadequate to explain how the much-discussed ambiguities of free indirect discourse play with the experiential paradoxes of intersubjectivity or how stories from different historical periods configure the as-structures of cognition to stage what it is like to be conscious through different versions of the as-if. The lexicon of classical narratology, although sometimes dauntingly complex and obscure, can provide invaluable instruments for making sense of the processes through which narratives build and break patterns. What is wrong is to reify or ossify these terms by ontologizing them or freezing them into a taxonomy.

The drive to classify and taxonomize, a pervasive characteristic of narratology that goes back to Aristotle, is both a good and bad thing. Categorization is a basic cognitive activity at work across the different sensory processes of seeing-as through which our embodied brains play with patterns to configure our worlds. From opponency in vision to the exploratory activity of different sensory and perceptual processes, our responsiveness to differences is basic equipment for living. The error is to reify these categorizing and differentiating processes into cognitive modules or formal structures that provide more logic and order than is evident in the bushy brain's ever-shifting balancing act between building and breaking patterns. Modes of categorization do crucial cognitive work, and the terms and concepts of classical narratology can provide tools for understanding these processes, but a classificatory scheme cannot do justice to the to-and-fro between the competing imperatives of order and flexibility to which narratives contribute by playing with concord and discord.

Stories offer a potentially productive resource for exploring many of the issues that have recently emerged as central to the neuroscience of the bushy brain—for example, the processes of neuronal assembly, oscillatory binding, and brain-to-brain coupling that neuroscientists have come to recognize as crucial to the workings of the dynamic system of intracortical and brain-body-world interactions that constitute the so-called connectome (see Raichle 2011, Dehaene 2014). Because of its reliance on an outmoded conception of brain structure and cortical modularity, formalist cognitive narratology is not well equipped to provide the theoretical guidance this research needs, but one of my hopes is that neuroscientists might find useful suggestions about possible research questions and areas to explore in the correlations I lay out between narrative theories of time, action, and intersubjectivity and the corresponding cognitive science. The instruments available to neuroscience are not always adequate to these challenges. For example, as I have explained, the temporality and sociality of narrative interactions are especially recalcitrant to measurement by current scanning technologies. But often these limitations point to vital areas of brain functioning that neuroscientists increasingly recognize the need to account for—how timing is crucial to the oscillatory processes of neuronal synchronization, for example, and how coupled brains in collaborative interactions behave differently from brains in isolation. What stories do that neuroscience has a hard time measuring is often exactly what neuroscience needs to understand.

It is also important to keep in mind what literature can reveal about cognition that necessarily eludes the measuring instruments of science—the qualia of what it is like to be conscious, for example, that fictional narratives can stage in different ways beyond what the quantifications of empirical methods can register. It is essential as well that cognitive scientists not ignore or run roughshod over these limitations by oversimplifying matters whose complexities narrative theory can and should instruct them about—for example, how fictional stagings of other worlds double self and other in ways that are not reducible to unilinear simulations and that consequently may not necessarily produce prosocial effects. (For the same reasons, predictions about the necessarily antisocial effects of violent films or video games are also overly simplistic and deterministic.) One of the hallmarks of science is its inventiveness in designing experiments that circumvent the limitations of its measuring instruments, but narrative theory can help differentiate between illuminating creativity and blunt-edged obfuscation (as in experiments that invoke vague notions of literary fiction to test equally vague responses to theory of mind measures, neither of which do justice to the stylistic complications of narratives or to the variability of the reading process).

Some practitioners of cognitive literary studies have recently called for an empirical turn to test theoretical claims about reading and narrative against experimental evidence (for the best work of this kind, see *Scientific Study of Literature*, founded in 2011 as the journal of the International Society for the Empirical Study of Literature). This is in many respects a welcome development. Ascertaining what the facts are is not a simple and straightforward matter, however. The empirical turn sometimes seems motivated by an aversion to theoretical speculation, but experimental work can't do without theory. Experiments test hypotheses, and these hypotheses need to be based on good science and also on good theories about narrative and reading. Rather than regarding experimental work as an alternative to literary and phenomenological models of the reading process, empirical studies should look to narrative theory and phenomenology as a source of hypotheses to test and as frameworks for making sense of their findings. I have cited some important work in this field, by researchers like Richard Gerrig (2010, 2012) and David Miall (2011), because their experiments shed interesting light on important scientific and theoretical questions about memory-based processing and the role of emotions in guiding expectations. Empirical work is a process not of collecting facts but of designing informative experiments, and good experimental design requires an understanding of the issues deserving exploration, based on the best-regarded science and the relevant literary and narrative theory, and an appreciation of the limits as well as the powers of various methods for gathering evidence. Testing hypotheses is a theoretical enterprise, not an alternative to theory.

Experimental work on narrative and reading also needs to keep in mind how readers can make sense of stories differently not only because of their different levels of competence but also because of their different interpretive frameworks. Skepticism about a so-called WEIRD subject pool (Henrich, Heine, and Norenzayan 2010)—whether undergraduate students from Western, educated, industrial, rich, and developed countries are a neutral, unbiased source of evidence about cognitive processes—is also relevant to neuroscientific and psychological experiments about stories and reading. As biocultural hybrids, members of any subject pool will have some universal and some contingent, historically and culturally variable characteristics. In one sense the ability to tell and follow stories is natural to our species—even small children can do it! But it is also a cultural acquisition, something we learn to do, and something we can learn to do better (or so I as a teacher of literature believe).

Any description of how we tell and follow stories is likely to have a prescriptive dimension. For example, Iser's phenomenological description of the reading process also offers guidance about how to better understand stories (by attending more thoughtfully to how we fill gaps and indeterminacies, how we build and break illusions, how we project expectations that are in turn surprised, or how we double our consciousness with the consciousness held ready by the text). One of the ways in which we learn to read stories is by following the guidance of others who we think have something to teach us, and narrative theories at their best may help us become better readers of narrative. What counts as better is not measurable on a linear and univocal scale, however, that leads teleologically from bad to better to best. There are degrees of competence in reading, but at some point equally competent readers may begin to differentiate themselves by adopting opposing, sometimes mutually exclusive, hermeneutic allegiances and acquiring different reading practices, which in turn may reflect the contingencies of their cultural, historical situations.

One of the paradoxes of our biocultural hybridity as readers is that our universally shared cognitive equipment can be deployed in a variety of not always reconcilable ways, guided by different presuppositions and interests, so that equally valid interpretations of a text can disagree fundamentally about its meaning (see Armstrong 1990). Empirical studies of literature must remember that opposed reading practices may divide even the most competent readers because they belong to different interpretive communities, with different values and aims. These differences are not something that an empirical approach can or should hope to overcome by digging down to the simple facts of the matter. They are, rather, fundamental aspects of reading and interpretation that a scientific study of literature needs to understand—and that theoretical accounts of hermeneutic pluralism and its epistemological limits can help to explain.

Empirically tested scientific theory will not by itself tell you how to read, although knowing something about the cognitive processes that narratives draw on and set in motion may heighten our appreciation of the ways in which stories play with pattern. This is one of the limits to what science can tell the humanities and a reason not to fear its determinism. Interpretation is a circular process of projecting hypotheses about how parts fit together into wholes and adjusting these hypotheses as anomalies and inconsistencies emerge (see Armstrong 2013, 54–90). These guesses and the revisions we must make to them as we read and interpret are an open-ended, to-and-fro, interactive process that cannot be reduced to deterministic procedures or mechanical formulas. Our hermeneutic guesswork can be guided, however, by various models that offer suggestions about hypotheses to test, and that is a reason why narrative theories of whatever stripe (classical or postclassical, cognitive or linguistic, guided by formal interests or informed by concerns about gender, sexuality, or politics) can be sources of productive, interesting interpretations and, by inspiring creative guesses, can make us more insightful readers. For example, Genette's elaborate categorization of narrative temporality, voice, and focalization by itself won't make us more competent interpreters of stories, but his terms and concepts have unquestionably been a rich source of suggestions for how to understand narratives of all kinds.

Genette's work is also a good example of another question that scientific approaches to narrative need to deal with: what should be the database? Can an adequately comprehensive theory of narrative be constructed on the basis of a single work, even one as complex and ambitious as Proust's *In Search of Lost Time*? No theorist of narrative knows all of the world's literatures, from all periods and cultures. There have been, of course, many admirable, courageous attempts at encyclopedic coverage (for a recent example see Pettersson 2018), and one reason why Scholes and Kellogg's *Nature of Narrative* (2006 [1966]) continues to illuminate is the rare and productive partnership of this modernist and medievalist with complementary expertise. The examples I have offered in this book reflect my own limitations from a lifetime of work teaching and writing about a particular body of narratives (including a studies in fiction course, with examples from Balzac to Pynchon, that Bob Kellogg first suggested I teach when he was my chair at the University of Virginia, and that evolved into a seminar on realism and modernism when I was Bob Scholes' colleague at Brown). The narratives I know best— especially the works of literary impressionists James, Conrad, and Ford and modernists Joyce, Woolf, and Faulkner—are by no means representative of all stories, but as I have tried to show, their self-consciousness about the epistemological processes set in motion by representation and narration makes them particularly useful cases for foregrounding the cognitive workings of narrative figuration of interest to me. Any examples offered by a narrative theory will reflect the cultural, historical contingencies of their time and place—their situation in the cognitive archive—and this is a necessary consequence of our biocultural hybridity. But this hybridity should also make it possible to extrapolate from the particular to the general and to identify species-wide processes and properties deployed by any given example from this archive. That is my hope, in any case, and it is a wager that all students of narrative must make—and that an empirical, scientific approach cannot avoid.

Science also cannot dictate or determine the moral and pedagogical implications of narrative. The play of doubling in the exchange of stories and the variability of the as and the as-if in narrative figurations of experience resist reduction to mechanical, univocal formulations of the social powers of narrative, whether Steven Pinker's overly optimistic claims for the moral education of epistolary novels or Mark Bracher's well-intentioned but authoritarian, monolithic pedagogy of reverse engineering through habitual reinforcement of preferred cognitive categories. Stories can have noxious as well as beneficial moral consequences, fueling conflict and violence or promoting empathy and compassion. Narratives can reinforce boundaries between us and them, or they can challenge prevailing conceptions of justice and injustice and encourage democratic conversation about reconfiguring our sense of responsibility toward others. This book tries to explain this contradictory state of affairs in scientific as well as humanistic terms. The three-fold exchange of figurative patterns (the pre-, con-, and refiguration cycle) as we tell and follow stories is grounded in various neurobiological processes and the interactions they enable and constrain between our brains, bodies, and worlds. This cycle of figuration is open ended and unpredictable, however, which is a good thing for many reasons having to do not only with our neurobiological health (preventing cognitive patterns from getting locked into rigid habits) but also with the creative potentialities of our existential and cultural lives. Neuroscientifically informed analyses of the figurative processes involved in narrative can help explain why this is so, but they do not let us off the hook from making difficult moral and social choices.

Neither neuroscience nor narrative theory can claim to have the last word about stories. Narratives are crucial to the life of our species, and it is unlikely that such a complex phenomenon would yield its secrets to any one approach. Active conversation between neuroscience and narrative theory across the explanatory gap about how we tell and follow stories is yet another chapter in a long history of reflection and debate about this aspect of our cognitive lives. Turning to science for answers to questions long debated in narrative theory will not end these arguments. Plenty will remain to disagree about, but those disputes are likely to be more rigorous and productive if neuroscience is part of the conversation.

NOTES

Chapter 1: Neuroscience and Narrative Theory

1. For classic statements of the structuralist theory of narrative, see Barthes 1975, Todorov 1969, and Lotman 1990. Also see Phelan 2006, 286–91, for a lucid summary of the assumptions and history of models of narrative as a formal system.

2. As I show in this chapter, formalist models and modes of analysis still pervade Herman's 2013 book *Storytelling and the Sciences of Mind*, even though he claims to have embraced enactivism and to have abandoned the structuralist assumptions of his earlier narratological work. This may reflect his attempt at "rapprochement," but my critique of his project is meant to suggest that this compromise is inadequate and incoherent.

3. This opposition is a reprise of the debates between structuralism and its phenomenological and pragmatic opponents. See, for example, Ricoeur's critique of the *langue-parole* distinction as static and not historical and interactive enough to account for the sentence-level construction of new meaning in his classic essay "Structure, Word, Event" (1968) as well as Merleau-Ponty's anti-Saussurean insistence on bodily gesture as the source of our "natural power of expression" and his analysis of conventions as "the depository and the sedimentation of acts of speech" (2012 [1945], 187, 202) rather than transcendental structures.

4. Nadeau's fascinating book provides a thorough and rigorous (although technically difficult) explanation of the neuroscientific case against universal grammar. See Changeaux 2012, 206–8, for a more concise and accessible explanation of why contemporary neuroscience has rejected the Chomksyan model of "mental organs" as "innate," "determined genetically," and "suited to a given species." For comprehensive reviews of the neuroscientific findings that cast doubt on the claim that language is based on inborn, universal cognitive structures, see Evans and Levinson 2009 and Christiansen and Chater 2008. Nancy Easterlin (2012, 163–79) provides an insightful critique of structural linguistics and its literary applications from a cognitive and evolutionary perspective. Berwick and Chomsky (2016) have recently attempted to reconcile the assumption of an innate "language faculty" with contemporary neurobiology and evolutionary theory. The scientific community generally remains skeptical, however, for reasons outlined in reviews by cognitive linguist Vyvyan Evans (2016, 46), who politely notes that their "position seems less reasonable today than it once did," and by neuroscientist Elliot

Murphy (2016, 8), who more pointedly criticizes their reliance "on outdated assumptions" about "how the brain actually operates (via oscillations and their various coupling operations)" and shows in detail that their assertions about the localization of linguistic operations do not fit the experimental evidence. Also see the highly critical review by the language columnist for the *Economist* (Greene 2016). For a favorable review, see Tattersall 2016.

5. See Ingarden 1973 (1931), 1973 (1937), Iser 1974, 1978, and Jauss 1982. For a brief survey of phenomenological theories of literature and their relation to the epistemological concepts that define this philosophical movement, see my article "Phenomenology" (2012, 378–82) in *Contemporary Literary and Cultural Theory* (2012).

6. Ricoeur took up the problems of metaphor and narrative as he became convinced that phenomenology needed to take a "hermeneutic turn" in order to engage arguments about sexual desire, politics, and language that had contested the status of consciousness as the controlling center of meaning. Many theorists saw this dislocation of the cogito as a refutation of phenomenology, but Ricoeur regarded it as a productive, even necessary, challenge to reconsider and revise phenomenology's theories of meaning creation (see Valdés 1991, Armstrong 2012). His analyses of metaphor, narrative, and the conflict of interpretations sought to extend and complicate the phenomenological account of being-in-the-world as paradoxically bound and free, located in a body, historical circumstances, and linguistic structures that simultaneously constrain meaning and enable semantic innovation. These existential paradoxes of embodied, situated meaning creation informed Ricoeur's (1966) earliest reflections on "the voluntary and the involuntary," and he returned to them in his late book *Oneself as Another* (1992). These concerns were, however, always implicit in his explorations of metaphor and narrative.

7. On the confusion between plot and story, see Chatman 1978, 19–20, and Brooks 1984, 12–13.

8. See Genette 1980, which devotes separate chapters to mood (161–211) and voice (212–62). As Jakob Lothe (2000, 41) observes, however, "in much narrative theory perspective has come to indicate both narrator and vision," although, he argues, these are "two narrative agencies" that "actually supplement rather than duplicate each other." My point is that the role of seeing-as in both agencies explains why each tends to shade into the other.

9. These are the opposing interpretations offered by Ian Watt (1979) and Albert Guerard (1958), two of the most famous interpreters of the novel. On ambiguity in Conrad, also see my *Challenge of Bewilderment* (1987).

10. See chapter 3 for a further analysis of the configurative processes of seeing-as that characterize metaphor. Also see the chapter "The Cognitive Powers of Metaphor" in my *Conflicting Readings* (1990, 67–88) and my critique of blending theory in *How Literature Plays with the Brain* (2013, 87–88). Easterlin (2012, 163–79) also provides a thorough and illuminating critique of blending along lines similar to mine.

11. See also Ricoeur's classic essay "Structure, Word, Event" (1968) in which he argues for the importance of attending to the eventfulness of language—the enunciation of words in potentially ever-new combinations as unpredictable sentences deploy preexisting linguistic structures in innovative ways that in turn may transform those structures (as innovative metaphors and narratives can do). Ricoeur's essays on language and metaphor exposed the problems of reification and reductionism in mid-twentieth-century structuralism, and his theory of narrative can similarly be used to correct these mistakes now as they manifest themselves in the formalist project of twenty-first-century postclassical narratology.

12. Other important second-generation theories that I analyze below include Karin Kukkonen's (2014a, 2014b, 2016) Bayesian model of narrative as predictive processing and Elaine Auyoung's (2013, 2018) analysis of representational immersion.

13. Monika Fludernik addresses the compatibility of her model with Ricoeur's theory of narrative in *Towards a "Natural" Narratology* (1996, 22–24). Except for a brief dismissive comment on Iser's theory of the imaginary (42–43; see Iser 1993), however, she otherwise seems unaware of the phenomenological tradition and the resources it offers for analyzing experientiality and narrativity. This is an unfortunate missed opportunity and an odd blindness given the historical connections between Freiburg, where she is based, and the careers of Husserl and Heidegger as well as the geographical proximity of this town in the Black Forest to Konstanz just seventy-five miles south on the Bodensee, where Iser and Jauss developed their theories of readerly reception.

14. Fludernik (1996, 31–35) credits Jonathan Culler (1975) as the source of her argument about the power of narratives to produce naturalization, which Culler in turn bases on the arguments of the Russian formalists about how conventions routinize and dull perception. On the relation between the neuroscience of habituation and Viktor Shklovsky's (1965 [1917]) well-known aesthetic of defamiliarization, see Armstrong 2013, 48–53, 111–16.

15. For instructive analyses of Joyce's word play in the *Wake*, see especially Attridge 1992, Norris 2004, and Derrida 1984.

16. Two of the foundational texts for the theory that cognition is embodied, enactive, and extended are Varela, Thompson, and Rosch 1991 and Clark 2011. Also see Noë 2009. Reflecting on the tension between these perspectives, Andy Clark (2008, 57) argues that "the true cognitive role of the body . . . is to act as a bridge enabling biological intelligence and the wider world to intermingle in the service of adaptive success." Clark's recent work on predictive processing (see 2016) acknowledges the importance of brain-based biological intelligence that his earlier work on the extended mind (see 2011) may seem to have relegated to the sidelines. See chapters 3 and 4 in this book for analyses of the intracortical, brain-based cognitive processes involved in the extended mind's use of affordances.

Chapter 2: The Temporality of Narrative and the Decentered Brain

1. In a vacuum, electrical energy and light travel at the same velocity, but the speed of electricity carried by a wire will of course be less than this theoretical maximum. In ordinary electronic devices, this speed can be anywhere from 50 to 90 percent of the speed of light (70–90 percent in a copper wire). These rates are many times faster than the rates at which electro-chemical signals are propagated through axons in the brain (at most 150 meters per second in a well-myelinated axon).

2. See Lothe 2000, 54–62, for a lucid explanation of Genette's temporal categories. On snares, equivocations, and other strategies for setting the reader's curiosity in motion and postponing its satisfaction, see Roland Barthes's (1974, 76) classic analysis in *S/Z* of what he calls the "hermeneutic code" and "the considerable labor the discourse must accomplish if it hopes to *arrest* the enigma, to keep it open" in defiance of the expectation that the truth will be revealed.

3. On music and time, see Koelsch 2012, Drake and Bertrand 2003, and Samson and Ehrlé 2003. On dance, see Hagendoorn 2004 and Sheets-Johnstone 1966, 2011. Theater, cinema, and even video games can also manipulate, organize, and reconfigure our sense of time because they are fundamentally narrative arts (see Bushnell 2016).

4. See Husserl 1964 [1928] and Merleau-Ponty 2012 [1945], 432–57. For lucid explanations of Husserl's theory of temporal horizons, see Thompson 2007, 312–59, and Gallagher and Zahavi 2012, 77–97. On the implications of these theories for reading, literature, and art, see Armstrong 2013, 91–130.

5. The phrase "We live forward, but we understand backward" originates with the Danish philosopher Søren Kierkegaard (1938, 127) and is quoted by William James in *Pragmatism* (1978 [1908], 107). Also see Armstrong 2013, 91–130.

6. On the prism spectacle experiment, see Stratton 1897 and Snyder and Pronko 1952. This is, of course, a double reversal because the images on the retina are upside-down to begin with, and the spectacles reverse the brain's habit of reading them as rightside up, a habit that then gets reestablished once the wearer becomes accustomed to this new distortion.

7. The phi phenomenon (so named after the angle phi that separates the dots in the experiment) was first studied by Max Wertheimer (1912) and refers to the apparent motion that we perceive between two static points that flash at particular intervals. Nelson Goodman then asked what would happen if the dots were different colors, and Paul Kolers and Michael von Grünau (1976) did the experiment on what became known as the "color phi" phenomenon (see Goodman 1978, 82–83, on his proposal and their experiment). Daniel Dennett (1991, 114–28) uses this phenomenon to support his multiple drafts model of consciousness, which describes consciousness not as a theater viewed by an observer but as an assemblage of "parallel, multitrack processes of interpretation and elaboration of sensory inputs" that undergo "continuous 'editorial revision'" (111). This ongoing

process of interpretation and revision is characterized by the temporal recursivity that I analyze in this section.

8. See Leys 2011, 452–63, for an insightful critique of the ways in which Massumi here and elsewhere misrepresents scientific experiments and then on the basis of those misrepresentations goes on to make extravagant, unwarranted metaphysical claims.

9. As the editors explain, Dickens's source for this anecdote is a story in *Tales of the Genii* (1764) by James Ridley that "relates how the Sultan's vizier builds a palace that is designed to cave in and crush a pair of evil enchanters who have seized the Sultan's throne" (476).

10. Given his lifelong interest in freedom, limitation, and temporality, it is no accident that Ricoeur felt compelled to undertake a major study of narrative and time. Ricoeur began his career with an ambitious study of *Freedom and Nature: The Voluntary and the Involuntary* (1966), and he returned to these existential questions in his late book *Oneself as Another* (1992). On the relation between narrative, freedom, and fate, see especially Morson 1994.

11. Shaun Gallagher (2005, 238–43) questions, however, whether motor control and free will are identical problems. "There is a distinction between fast, automatic reflex actions and slower, voluntary action," he argues. "Free will cannot be squeezed into time-frames of 150–350 msecs" because it requires "conscious deliberation" over "an extended duration equivalent to a specious present" (238–39). Not all phenomenological thinkers equate freedom with conscious deliberation, however. For example, see Merleau-Ponty (2012 [1945], 458–83), who argues that often "deliberation follows the decision" (460) that I find I have already made prereflectively when I look back and ask why I acted as I did, and my reflections then disclose an implicit choice in the original prereflective action that I only come to recognize after the fact. At precisely what temporal moment freedom begins is a question that defies definitive answer. But no matter what the answer might be, the fact that neurobiological time is asynchronous and not homogeneous is what makes possible not only the prospective and retrospective deliberations of voluntary action but also the steering of motor acts that we experience as agency.

12. For example, see the exchange that unfolded in *Critical Inquiry* after Frank attempted to answer the criticisms of spatial form Kermode makes in *The Sense of an Ending* (1967): Frank 1977, Kermode 1978, and Frank 1978. See Mitchell 1980 for an analysis of the aesthetic issues involved in this dispute. As Mitchell notes, however, the criticisms of spatial form were often political rather aesthetic: "The most polemical attacks [against Frank's theory] have come from those who regard spatial form as an actual, but highly regrettable, characteristic of modern literature and who have linked it with anti-historical and even fascist ideologies" (541), especially the views of Wyndham Lewis and Ezra Pound, a connection Kermode also makes in his 1978 essay. Frank replies that "it is really no longer permissible to identify the revolt against linear time in modern literature as a whole . . .

with the repulsive social-political ideas of a few (or one [i.e., Ezra Pound]) of the Anglo-American writers of the post-World War I generation" (96), and he quotes in his defense the theorist of the avant-garde Renato Poggioli: "We must deny the hypothesis that the relation between avant-garde art (or art generally) and politics can be established a priori. Such a connection can only be determined a posterori, from the viewpoint of the avant-garde's own political opinions and convictions" (quoted in Frank 1977, 101). The disruption and foregrounding of the temporal processes of meaning making brought about by spatial form can serve a variety of epistemological, aesthetic, and social purposes. To lay bare how time is working in the construction of meaning leaves open how this knowledge will be used, and its political consequences are not predetermined. See chapter 4 for a further analysis of what neuroscience can (and cannot) tell us about the social powers of literature.

13. This process of temporal framing should not be confused with the frames of first-generation cognitive narratology. The temporal parsing of phenomena into ever-shifting windows of integration is not the same as the fixed, static "mental models" or "cognitive schemata" of structuralist narratology. Unlike cognitive frames that encode rules for interpreting typical situations, the perceptual framing that Varela describes refers to configurative processes of seeing-as that organize cognition in a reciprocal, recursive manner through shifting, mutually formative part-whole relationships. Temporal windows of integration are aspects of the activity of cognitive configuration—of how binding occurs at different temporal levels—and not reified, rule-governed cognitive structures.

14. The best-known instance of such selective memory loss is the case of a patient referred to in the neuroscience literature as H. M. (later identified as Henry Molaison), whose hippocampus was surgically removed in an attempt to relieve his epileptic seizures. After the surgery, as Eric Kandel (2006, 127–33) explains, "H. M. remained the same intelligent, kind, and amusing man he had always been, but he was unable to convert any new memories into permanent memory. . . . [H]e had perfectly good short-term memory, lasting for minutes," and he retained "implicit (or procedural) memory" for various habitual, embodied abilities. For example, he could learn new skills, like "tracing the outline of a star," and he "retained what he had learned through practice—even though he had no recollection of the task." What he had lost was the ability to form new explicit memories of people, events, or experiences, a process of consolidation that passes through the hippocampus. For a riveting account of this case, see Dittrich 2016.

15. An interesting attempt to overcome this limitation is Uri Hasson's method of intersubject correlation analysis (ISC) that compares the time course of fMRI images of specific brain regions of different subjects in response to the same stimulus. See Hasson et al. 2004 for an explanation of the method and Hasson et al. 2008 for an ISC analysis of how viewers respond to different films. See Armstrong 2013, 5, for an evaluation of these findings. For a detailed survey of the various technologies for studying the brain and their limitations, see "The Tools: Imaging

the Living Brain" in Baars and Gage 2010, 95–125. Also see chapter 4 in this book on other recent efforts to develop methods and technologies for analyzing the neurobiological processes underlying collaborative interactions.

Chapter 3: Action, Embodied Cognition, and the As-If of Narrative Figuration

1. See the analysis in chapter 1 of the dispute between first- and second-generation cognitive literary theorists. Giving primacy to embodied action over the schemes, frames, and preference rules of traditional cognitive narratology, proponents of enactive narratology eschew the taxonomies of structuralist theory and instead explore the various ways in which stories draw on and set in motion embodied processes of cognition. Important examples include Bolens 2012, Caracciolo 2014, and Kukkonen 2017. Also see the analysis below of work by Kuzmičová 2012, Cave 2016, and Auyoung 2018.

2. As Jakob Lothe (2000, 77) observes, the relation between action and character in Aristotle's *Poetics* is more complex and contradictory than this oft-quoted pronouncement suggests: "Is it right to make characters subordinate to those fictional events which precisely *they* have initiated and constituted? . . . The problem is already apparent in Aristotle, for although he ranks the action above the characters, several of the key terms in his *Poetics* (such as 'reversal and recognition' . . .) are closely related to the concept of character." E. M. Forster (1927, 126) also famously disputes the claim that action trumps character: "We know better. We believe that happiness and misery exist in the secret life, which each of us leads privately and to which (in his characters) the novelist has access." Robert Scholes and Robert Kellogg (2006 [1966], 236) note that Forster's claim "is very much the assertion of a modern, mimetically oriented novelist." How fictional character is produced and perceived is a complicated question that I take up in the next chapter's analysis of narrative and the problem of other minds.

3. On the neuroscience of habituation, see Eric Kandel's (2006, 198–220) discussion of his well-known experiments on the sea slug (also see Noë 2009, 99–128). On the implications of these experiments for aesthetic experience, see Armstrong 2013, 111–16.

4. Whether intentions are intrinsic to actions is one of the main objections to mirror neuron theory raised by Hickok (2009, 2014) and other skeptics like Patricia Churchland (2011), who offers the example of the ambiguity of raising one's hand. I have more to say about this controversy in my analysis of grounded versus ungrounded cognition. See also my evaluation of the mirror neuron evidence in *How Literature Plays with the Brain* (2013, 139–42).

5. This is not, however, the linear and mechanical process that the notion of preference rules implies (in set of conditions C, prefer to see A as B). See Jahn 1997, 2005, and my critique of structuralist cognitive narratology in chapter 1. As Heidegger explains, the fore-structure of understanding is a recursive, to-and-fro process, manifested in how we perpetually shift back and forth between our

expectations and our explications of possibilities they project; see the chapter titled "Understanding and Interpretation" [*Verstehen und Auslegung*] in *Being and Time* (1962 [1927], 188–95).

6. Fictionality may take various historical shapes, but it is wrong to claim that it was invented by any particular genre or cultural form, as Catherine Gallagher (2006, 337) notoriously does in asserting that the eighteenth-century novel "discovered fiction." Some of the characteristics of eighteenth-century life that, in her view, gave rise to "the kind of cognitive provisionality one practices in reading fiction"—the "affective speculation," for example, of women envisioning potential marriage partners or the economic imaginings of entrepreneurs "calculating risks" in the marketplace (346–47)—go back to fundamental characteristics of our species as exploratory, hypothesis-generating animals that have a long evolutionary history (see Clark 2016). In contrast to Gallagher, Iser finds in the pastoral poetry of much earlier periods a "paradigm of literary fictionality" (1993, 22–86) in its characteristic doubling of worlds that exemplifies the generative capacity of the as if (his primary examples are Theocritus, Virgil, and Spenser). Provisionality is an inherent characteristic of action and perception, and it lends itself to the playful transformations of what Iser calls "the fictive and the imaginary," which in turn can give rise to various historical forms of fictionality, but none of these versions of the as if deserves to be privileged over any other.

7. On the role of Broca's area in organizing events and comprehending sequences in action-perception circuits, also see Saygin et al. 2004, Fadiga et al. 2009, Berthoz and Petit 2008, 53, and Jeannerod 2006, 163–64.

8. See Terence Cave's similar analysis of inference in cognition and reading based on the relevance theory of Deirdre Wilson and Dan Sperber (2012) in his important book *Thinking with Literature* (2016). See my analysis below of Cave's theory of literary affordances. Also see Clark (2016) for the Bayesian model of cognition as probabilistic prediction on which Kukkonen 2016 draws. On the role of hypotheses and presuppositions in literary interpretation, also see my *Conflicting Readings* (1990).

9. See the analysis in chapter 2 of the futurity of emotions in what Jenefer Robinson calls "affective appraisals."

10. The mirror neuron literature is vast. For a summary of the foundational experiments and the controversy surrounding them, see Armstrong 2013, 137–42. Recent accounts of the state of research are provided by Ferrari and Rizzolati 2014 and Rizzolati and Fogassi 2014. Thorough explanations of the Parma group's findings are provided by Rizzolati and Sinigaglia 2008 and Iacoboni 2008. For skeptical analyses see Hickok (2008, 2014), Churchland (2011), and Caramazza et al. (2014).

11. Roel Willems and Daniel Casasanto likewise note that "it remains an open question whether people can understand words referring to actions they have never performed as completely as they understand words for actions they have performed themselves"; "the way people act in the world influences their semantic

representations," but "people can also understand language about actions they have never performed." As they observe, "This creates a potential tension between embodiment and abstraction" (2011, 3).

12. Localization dies hard, however. For example, see Semir Zeki's attempt (2011, 2012) to identify the region of the brain that is responsible for beauty in music and the visual arts. See Armstrong 2013, 1–25, and chapter 4 for a critique of this approach.

13. As Clare Pettit (2016, 143) notes, this "awkward pagoda" is "the most famous of all of James's late metaphors." She interestingly characterizes Jamesian metaphor as "a sophisticated model of embodied knowledge" that "suggests that the roots of our abstract world lie deep in physical practice" (142). The classic criticism of this figure comes from F. R. Leavis (1948). Ruth Bernard Yeazell's chapter titled "The Imagination of Metaphor" (1976, 37–63) offers a still unsurpassed analysis of the cognitive play of Jamesian figuration. Also see my more detailed interpretation of this passage in *The Challenge of Bewilderment* (1987, 59–60).

14. For an explanation of Joyce's use of siglas, see Finn Fordham's (2012) informative introduction to *Finnegans Wake*. The 1929 recording of Joyce reading the opening lines of the Anna Livia Plurabelle chapter is available in the Internet Archive (https://archive.org/details/JamesJoyceReadsannaLiviaPlurabelleFromFinnegansWake1929) and on YouTube (https://www.youtube.com/watch?v=M8kFqiv8Vww).

15. Caroline Levine (2015, 9) gets this definition slightly but importantly wrong in her influential argument about the politics of form: "With affordances, then, we can begin to grasp the constraints on form that are imposed by materiality itself." This reified, objectivist conception of materiality is precisely what Gibson opposes. As I explain in more detail in what follows, the constraints characterizing an affordance are a matter of the reciprocal relations between the user's dispositions and the potentialities opened up by the interaction of these with the environment (Gibson's is an *ecological* theory of perception). They are not determined in advance or "imposed by materiality itself." Levine's impersonal, materialist conception of form ignores how (as a Gibsonian analysis would emphasize) the affordances of a social or literary form depend on the uses to which we put them. As Lambros Malafouris (2013, 18) explains, "In the human engagement with the material world there are no fixed attributes of agent entities and patient entities and no clean ontological separations between them; rather, there is a constitutive intertwining between intentionality and affordance." Affordances are as much immaterial as they are material because they are potentialities that are undefined until they are engaged by a particular organism, an agent whose perception of the possible actions available in an environment depends as much on its cognitive equipment as on what is "there" in the world. Affordances are thus futural and horizonal, depending for their potentialities on reciprocal interactions with users that are unpredictable, and this openness to variation and innovation cannot be accounted for by an impersonal notion of form as materiality. Their immateriality also allows affordances to have an aesthetic dimension, a playful as-if

quality that a purely materialist theory is bound to overlook (as is the case with the peculiar neglect of the aesthetic in Levine's theory of form). Malafouris's favorite example is the unpredictable play of the potter's wheel, where "the being of the potter is co-dependent and interweaved with the becoming of the clay" (20).

16. James Phelan provides an especially insightful analysis of this complex issue in his fascinating chapter "Somebody Telling Somebody Else: Audiences and Probable Impossibilities" (2017, 30–59). As he explains, "Probable deviations are not one-off or anomalous phenomena but rather instructive examples that indicate how tellers frequently rely on the unfolding of readerly dynamics in their construction of textual dynamics" (43). His account of how readerly and textual dynamics interact in instances of "plausible violations of probability" (59) is consistent with the analysis I offer here of how the various modalities of action that intertwine in a narrative play with the reader's probability predictions.

17. Here is the entire passage Kukkonen cites. The protagonist Ferdinand "has just had a brush with death," Kukkonen explains, "and escapes with a potentially treacherous landlady as his guide to the next town and safety": "Common fear was a comfortable sensation to what he felt in this excursion. The first steps he had taken for his preservation, were the effects of mere instinct, while his faculties were extinguished or suppressed by despair; but, now as his reflection began to recur, he was haunted by the most intolerable apprehensions. Every whisper of the wind through the thickets, was swelled into the hoarse menaces of murder, the shaking of the boughs was construed into the brandishing of poignards, and every shadow of a tree, became the apparition of a ruffian eager for blood. In short, at each of these occurrences, he felt what was infinitely more tormenting than the stab of a real dagger; and at every fresh filip of his fear, he acted as remembrancer to his conductress, in a new volley of imprecations, importing that her life was absolutely connected with his opinion of his own safety" (quoted in 2014b, 368).

Chapter 4: Neuroscience and the Social Powers of Narrative

1. This doubling is characteristic of all stories, not only those that portray psychological interiority. Regardless of their subject matter, stories double my world with another world as the patterns of intentionality that characterize my habits of understanding interact with the different configurative patterns of the narrative. In some realistic fictions that represent the psychological lives of characters, this doubling may connect the reader to another's inner thoughts and feelings, although this of course is not something all stories try to do.

2. Frith cites Pronin, Berger, and Molouki 2007 to support his claim that we more easily identify causes of behavior in others than ourselves. This study of the so-called introspection illusion documented a perhaps unsurprising asymmetry in conformity assessments—that is, a tendency to judge others as more conformist than we are.

3. Cohn calls free indirect discourse "narrated monologue," an oxymoronic term whose contradiction (a first-person monologue voiced in third-person narra-

tion) reflects this ambiguity. She distinguishes this form in turn from "quoted monologue" (defined as "a character's mental discourse") and "psycho-narration" ("the narrator's discourse about a character's consciousness") (see 1978, 14). The narratological literature on free indirect discourse is immense. Central to its many debates is Gérard Genette's problematic distinction (1980, 161–262) between voice and focalization (or "mood," in his vocabulary)—"who says" versus "who sees"—two seemingly different states of affairs from a narratological standpoint that are blended indistinguishably in free indirect discourse. See Walsh 2010 for an insightful summary and analysis of this controversy.

4. See the analysis of the mirror neuron controversy in chapter 3 and also in Armstrong 2013, 136–42. See Iacoboni 2008 and Rizzolatti and Sinigaglia 2008 on the evidence in favor of the theory and Hickok 2014 on the reasons for skepticism. For recent reports of the state of the research by proponents of the theory, see Ferrari and Rizzolatti 2014 and Rizzolatti and Fogassi 2014.

5. The work of popular fiction referred to here is the Harry Potter series, which has been shown to enhance performance on some measures of theory of mind and empathy (see Vezzali et al. 2015). On the effects of romance novels versus domestic fiction and science fiction/fantasy, see Fong, Mullin, and Mar 2013. This study correlated performance on an interpersonal sensitivity task with respondents' familiarity with various literary genres as indicated by their answers to an author recognition test, but the article reporting their results unfortunately does not specify which authors were included in each category. The distinction between romance and science fiction/fantasy seems relatively straightforward but the boundary between romance and domestic fiction much less so.

6. See James Phelan's thoughtful struggle with the ethical dilemmas posed by this novel (2005, 98–131). "Nabokov is doing something extraordinary, however distasteful," he argues: "Occupying the perspective of a pedophile, asking us to take that perspective seriously, and, indeed, . . . asking us, at least to some extent, to sympathize with him" (130). Phelan attempts to give Nabokov every benefit of the doubt (more than I find myself able to do), but he finally concludes that "because the attention Nabokov and the authorial audience give to Humbert's perspective comes at the expense of Dolores's, Nabokov's very construction of the novel mirrors Humbert's dominance at the level of action" (130–31). Phelan is torn about how to evaluate the novel because he believes that priority should be granted to "the authorial audience," which he regards as a perspective inscribed in the text, yet he confesses that "as flesh-and-blood reader, I find that perspective to have significant strengths and problems" (130). The "authorial audience" is not an independent, objective state of affairs, however, but a doubled, intersubjective structure that is produced over the history of reception by the different engagements of "flesh and blood readers" with Nabokov's text, and the disturbing dissonances between me and not me generated across this history are part of this work's heteronomous existence (see chapter 2). No author can understand in advance how she will be understood in the future. As Gadamer (1993 [1960], 296–97) points

out, "Not just occasionally, but always, the meaning of a text goes beyond its author. . . . It is enough to say that we understand in a different way, if we understand at all" (see Armstrong 2011). There is no reason to privilege either pole in the author-audience relationship—no reason to defer to the "authorial audience"—because their interaction is how a text lives and is passed on. The ethical dilemmas posed by the acts of identification Humbert's narration invites are integral to this interaction, and the risk Nabokov runs is that readers (like me) may not be willing to play along with him (as Phelan generously tries to do) because the cruelty and disregard with which Dolores is treated interfere irreparably with the text's call for our participation. As Phelan rightly concludes, "The author who created this book is someone to be admired but also someone to be wary of" (131). Different readers will come to different conclusions about whether admiration or wariness is more in order, but in either case these dilemmas are vivid proof that simulation is an inadequate model for the mismatches that may occur between the reader's appraisals and those dramatized in a text.

7. See the chart on page 101 of this fascinating study for a detailed breakdown of Alderson-Day, Bernini, and Fernyhough's results. For example, when asked "Do you ever hear characters' voices when you are reading?" the responses were "Never 166 (11%), Very occasionally 157 (10%), Some of the time 446 (28%), Most of the time 468 (30%), All of the time 329 (21%)." The question "How vivid are characters' voices when you read?" elicited these responses: "No voices present 125 (8.0%), Vaguely present 307 (19.6%), Voices with some vivid qualities 555 (35.4%), Voices with lots of vivid qualities 363 (23.2%), As vivid as hearing an actual person 216 (13.8%)."

8. On the *Pamela* controversy, see Keymer 2001, and on Fielding's critique of Richardson, see Battestin 1961.

9. See Martin Hoffman's authoritative *Empathy and Moral Development* (2000) for a nuanced analysis of the contingencies and complications that characterize the path from fellow feeling to compassion and moral altruism.

10. Hoffman (2000, 297) cautions, however, against exaggerating the dangers of in-group bias: "There is nothing inherently wrong with bias in favor of family and friends. . . . In-group empathic bias is normal and acceptable as long as it allows people to help strangers as well." He cites research demonstrating that "at least in America, bystanders are prone to help strangers"—although, he notes, "to a lesser degree than family and friends."

11. See Konvalinka and Roepstorff 2012 for a useful analysis of the technical difficulties of performing EEG and fMRI studies of multiple-brain interactions and a review of the innovative procedures neuroscientists have employed to attempt to overcome them. Advances in portable EEG technology have facilitated such so-called hyperscanning studies, as has the recent development of NIRS (near-infrared spectroscopy), which measures changes in blood flow through detectors on the scalp. The hyperscanning movement's ultimate goal, still a long way off (if

attainable at all), is something approximating what Nobel laureate David Hubel once described when he was asked about the brain-scanning technology he would like to have available in an ideal world (2011), which he said was a cap fitted onto the skull of a mobile subject that could measure single-cell neuronal activity at all levels of the brain. Hubel had in mind only a single brain. For hyperscanning studies of collaboration, a group of subjects would need to be fitted out with such caps and the measurements taken from them would then have to be calibrated.

12. Whether this kind of reciprocity challenges Tomasello's claims for the uniqueness of the human ability to collaborate is an interesting question. For explorations of animal-animal and animal-human cooperative activity, see Prum 2013 and Weil 2012. See Tomasello 2014 for an analysis of the differences between human collaboration and the sorts of cooperative behavior observable in apes. Given how much we share with other species because of our evolutionary histories, it would be strange if there were no continuities across the animal-human divide, but Tomasello also makes a compelling case that differences in the capacity for collaboration ("we intentionality") have made possible kinds of cultural learning and sharing among humans that are less in evidence, if at all, among other species.

13. See, for example, Clark's 2016 research on "predictive processing" and the top-down hypothesis-generating capacities of the brain, which recognizes the importance of brain-based cognitive processes inside the head.

14. See chapter 1 on the error of referring to our processes of configurative seeing-as by using the terminology of "schemas, scripts, and preference rules" that Bracher employs.

15. An example of how this boundary can shift is Hurricane Maria that struck Puerto Rico on 16 September 2017, which at first was a misfortune that caused great suffering to the island's residents but could not be blamed on any particular individual's or government agency's malfeasance. This misfortune then resulted in injustice when the federal government's relief efforts lagged behind the response to similar natural disasters in Florida and Texas. The first days without electrical power on Puerto Rico were unfortunate but not necessarily unfair; the fact that residents months later were still without electricity, however, could rightly be considered an injustice.

16. For a lucid explanation of these concepts see Phelan 2018. The lively discussion that this target essay provoked provides an excellent overview of the current state of the debate about these much-discussed distinctions (see especially the responses by Alber, Lothe, and Prince).

17. As one recent study (Parkes 2011, ix) observes, "Literary impressionism is usually described as a set of stylistic and formal strategies designed to heighten our sense of individual perceptual experience," and the term "impression," although variously defined, "signifies the mark of sensory experience on human consciousness." On the variety of novelists who have been characterized as impressionist, see

Kronegger (1973) and Matz (2001). For more on the epistemological implications of the narrative experiments of James, Conrad, and Ford that I analyze here, see my *Challenge of Bewilderment* (1987).

18. This is the key point that David Herman misunderstands when he claims that modernist writers all share a commitment to an "ecologically valid," anti-Cartesian model of embodied, enactive cognition (see 2011, 243–72). In his eagerness to defend Woolf, Joyce, Lawrence, and other modern novelists against the charge that they are guilty of the cognitive fallacy of splitting mind and body by turning the novel inward, Herman homogenizes their epistemologies—they do not all agree, after all, on what it is like to be conscious—even as he overlooks the historical specificity of any representation of consciousness. The different versions of conscious life displayed in the cognitive archive should not be evaluated according to their epistemological validity but rather should be appreciated for their distinctive deployment of the as of the as if in disclosing particular aspects of cognitive life (and in the process concealing, disguising, and possibly distorting others). Even if the modernists were all Cartesianist, that would not be a bad thing but instead a sign of their cultural and historical particularity (it would perhaps be more accurate to say that different modern writers vary in their distance from and proximity to this outlook, with Pater, Proust, and Beckett closest and Lawrence and Joyce farthest away). The representational styles in the archive are not teleological stages in a movement toward the "truth" of twenty-first-century cognitive science but evidence of our biocultural diversity, which is characterized by shifting and variable combinations of cognitive universals and historical, cultural differences.

19. Alva Noë makes a similar argument (2015) that works of art are "strange tools" that lay bare the patterns of organization through which we experience the world in order to make possible their reorganization.

Epilogue

1. Among others, see Bernini 2018, Bolens 2012, Caracciolo 2014, Gosetti-Ferencei 2018, Kuzmičová 2012, Park 2012, 2018, and Troscianko 2014.

WORKS CITED

Abbott, H. Porter. 2002. *The Cambridge Introduction to Narrative*. Cambridge: Cambridge University Press.

Alber, Jan. 2009. "Impossible Storyworlds—And What to Do with Them." *StoryWorlds* 1 (1): 79–96.

———. 2018 "Rhetorical Ways of Covering Up Speculations and Hypotheses, or Why Empirical Investigations of Real Readers Matter." *Style* 52 (1–2): 34–39.

Alber, Jan, and Monika Fludernik, eds. 2010a. *Postclassical Narratology: Approaches and Analyses*. Columbus: Ohio State University Press.

———. 2010b. Introduction. In Alber and Fludernik 2010a, 1–34.

Alber, Jan, Henrik Skov Nielsen, and Brian Richardson. 2013. Introduction to *A Poetics of Unnatural Narrative*, ed. Jan Alber, Henrik Skov Nielsen, and Brian Richardson, 1–15. Columbus: Ohio State University Press.

Alderson-Day, Ben, Marco Bernini, and Charles Fernyhough. 2017. "Uncharted Features and Dynamics of Reading: Voices, Characters, and Crossing of Experiences." *Consciousness and Cognition* 49:98–109.

Alexandrov, Vladimir E. 1982. "Relative Time in *Anna Karenina*." *Russian Review* 41 (2): 159–68.

Anderson, Michael L. 2010. "Neural Reuse: A Fundamental Organizational Principle of the Brain." *Behavioral and Brain Sciences* 33 (4): 245–66.

Aristotle 1990 [355 BCE]. *Aristotle's Poetics*. Trans. Hippocrates Apostle, Elizabeth A. Dobbs, and Morris A. Parslow. Grinnell, IA: Peripatetic Press.

Armstrong, Paul B. 1987. *The Challenge of Bewilderment: Understanding and Representation in James, Conrad, and Ford*. Ithaca, NY: Cornell University Press.

———. 1990. *Conflicting Readings: Variety and Validity in Interpretation*. Chapel Hill: University of North Carolina Press.

———. 2005. *Play and the Politics of Reading: The Social Uses of Modernist Form*. Ithaca, NY: Cornell University Press.

———. 2011. "In Defense of Reading: Or, Why Reading Still Matters in a Contextualist Age." *New Literary History* 42 (1): 87–113.

———. 2012. "Phenomenology." In *Contemporary Literary and Cultural Theory: The Johns Hopkins Guide*, ed. Michael Groden, Martin Kreiswirth, and Imre Szeman, 378–82. Baltimore, MD: Johns Hopkins University Press.

———. 2013. *How Literature Plays with the Brain: The Neuroscience of Reading and Art*. Baltimore, MD: Johns Hopkins University Press.

———. 2015. "How Historical is Reading? What Literary Studies Can Learn from Neuroscience (and Vice Versa)." *REAL: Yearbook of Research in English and American Literature* 31:201–18.

———. 2018. "Henry James and Neuroscience: Cognitive Universals and Cultural Differences." *Henry James Review* 39 (2): 133–51.

Arstila, Valtteri, and Dan Lloyd. 2014a. Introduction to part 4, "Fragments of Time," in Arstila and Lloyd 2014b, 199–200.

———, eds. 2014b. *Subjective Time: The Philosophy, Psychology, and Neuroscience of Temporality*. Cambridge, MA: MIT Press.

Attridge, Derek. 1992. "The Peculiar Language of *Finnegans Wake*." In *Critical Essays on James Joyce's "Finnegans Wake,"* ed. Patrick A. McCarthy, 73–84. New York: G. K. Hall.

Auerbach, Erich. 2003 [1953]. *Mimesis: The Representation of Reality in Western Literature*. Princeton, NJ: Princeton University Press.

Augustine, Saint. 1961 [397–400]. *Confessions*. Trans R. S. Pine-Coffin. London: Penguin.

Auyoung, Elaine. 2013. "Partial Cues and Narrative Understanding in *Anna Karenina*." In Bernaerts et al. 2013b, 59–78.

———. 2018. *When Fiction Feels Real: Representation and the Reading Mind*. Oxford: Oxford University Press.

Aziz-Zadeh, Lisa, Stephen M. Wilson, Giacomo Rizzolatti, and Marco Iacoboni. 2006. "Congruent Embodied Representations for Visually Presented Actions and Linguistic Phrases Describing Actions." *Current Biology* 16 (18): 1818–23.

Baars, Bernard J., and Nicole M. Gage. 2010. *Cognition, Brain, and Consciousness: Introduction to Cognitive Neuroscience*. Amsterdam: Elsevier.

Bagdasaryan, Juliana, and Michel Le Van Quyen. 2013. "Experiencing Your Brain: Neurofeedback as a New Bridge Between Neuroscience and Phenomenology." *Frontiers in Human Neuroscience* 7:680.

Bak, Thomas H., Dominic G. O'Donovan, John H. Xuereb, Simon Boniface, and John R. Hodges. 2001. "Selective Impairment of Verb Processing Associated with Pathological Changes in Brodmann Areas 44 and 45 in the Motor Neurone Disease-Dementia-Aphasia Syndrome." *Brain* 124 (1): 103–20.

Bal, P. Matthijs, and Martijn Veltkamp. 2013. "How Does Fiction Reading Influence Empathy? An Experimental Investigation on the Role of Emotional Transportation." *PloS One* 8 (1): e55341.

Balzac, Honoré. 2004 [1834]. *Père Goriot*. Trans. Henry Reed. New York: Signet.

Banfield, Ann. 1982. *Unspeakable Sentences: Narration and Representation in the Language of Fiction*. Boston: Routledge & Kegan Paul.

Bang, Dan, and Chris D. Frith. 2017. "Making Better Decisions in Groups." *Royal Society Open Science* 4 (8): 170–93.

Barrett, Lisa Feldman. 2007. "The Experience of Emotion." *Annual Review of Psychology* 58:373–403.

———. 2017. *How Emotions Are Made: The Secret Life of the Brain*. New York: Houghton Mifflin Harcourt.

Barsalou, Lawrence W. 1999. "Perceptual Symbols Systems." *Behavioral and Brain Sciences* 22:577–660.

———. 2008. "Grounded Cognition." *Annual Review of Psychology* 59:617–45.

Barthes, Roland. 1974. *S/Z*. Trans. Richard Miller. New York: Hill and Wang.

———. 1975. "An Introduction to the Structural Analysis of Narrative." *New Literary History* 6 (2): 237–72.

Battestin, Martin C. 1961. Introduction in Fielding 1961 [1741], v–xl.

Bear, Mark, Barry W. Connors, and Michael A. Paradiso. 2007. *Neuroscience: Exploring the Brain*. 3rd ed. Baltimore, MD: Lippincott Williams & Wilkins.

Belluck, Pam. 2013. "For Better Social Skills, Scientists Recommend a Little Chekhov." *New York Times*, 4 October, A1.

Bernaerts, Lars, Dirk De Geest, Luc Herman, and Bart Vavaeck. 2013a. Introduction in Bernaerts et al. 2013b, 1–22.

———, eds. 2013b. *Stories and Minds: Cognitive Approaches to Literary Narrative*. Lincoln: University of Nebraska Press.

Bernini, Marco. 2018. "Affording Innerscapes: Dreams, Introspective Imagery and the Narrative Exploration of Personal Geographies." *Frontiers of Narrative Studies* 4 (2): 291–311.

Berthoz, Alain, and Jean-Luc Petit. 2008. *The Physiology and Phenomenology of Action*. Trans. Christopher Macann. Oxford: Oxford University Press.

Berwick, Robert C., and Noam Chomsky. 2016. *Why Only Us: Language and Evolution*. Cambridge, MA: MIT Press.

Bhattacharya, Joydeep. 2017. "Cognitive Neuroscience: Synchronizing Brains in the Classroom." *Current Biology* 27 (9): R346–R348.

Blamires, Harry. 1996. *The New Bloomsday Book: A Guide through "Ulysses."* London: Routledge.

Bloom, Paul. 2010. *How Pleasure Works*. New York: Norton.

Bolens, Guillemette. 2012. *The Style of Gestures: Embodiment and Cognition in Literary Narrative*. Baltimore, MD: Johns Hopkins University Press.

Boulenger, Véronique, Alice C. Roy, Yves Paulignan, Viviane Deprez, Marc Jeannerod, and Tatjana A. Nazir. 2006. "Cross-Talk between Language Processes and Overt Motor Behavior in the First 200 msec of Processing." *Journal of Cognitive Neuroscience* 18 (10): 1607–15.

Bourke, Joanna. 2014. "Pain: Metaphor, Body, and Culture in Anglo-American Societies between the Eighteenth and Nineteenth Centuries." *Rethinking History* 18 (4): 475–98.

Boyd, Brian. 2009. *On the Origin of Stories: Evolution, Cognition, and Fiction*. Cambridge, MA: Harvard University Press.

Bracher, Mark. 2013. *Literature and Social Justice: Protest Novels, Cognitive Politics, and Schema Criticism*. Austin: University of Texas Press.

Brooks, Peter. 1984. *Reading for the Plot: Design and Intention in Narrative*. New York: Knopf.

Brown, Donald E. 1991. *Human Universals*. Philadelphia: Temple University Press.

Bruner, Jerome S. 1986. *Actual Minds, Possible Worlds*. Cambridge, MA: Harvard University Press.

Buckner, Randy L., and Daniel C. Carroll. 2007. "Self-Projection and the Brain." *Trends in Cognitive Science* 11 (2): 49–57.

Buonomano, Dean V. 2014. "The Neural Mechanisms of Timing of Short Timescales." In Arstila and Lloyd 2014b, 329–42.

Burke, Kenneth. 1966. *Language as Symbolic Action*. Berkeley: University of California Press.

Busch, Niko A., and Rufin VanRullen. 2014. "Is Visual Perception Like a Continuous Flow or a Series of Snapshots?" In Arstila and Lloyd 2014b, 161–78.

Bushnell, Rebecca. 2016. *Tragic Time in Drama, Film, and Videogames: The Future in the Instant*. London: Palgrave Macmillan.

Buzsáki, György. 2006. *Rhythms of the Brain*. Oxford: Oxford University Press.

Cacciari, Cristina, Nadia Bolognini, Irene Senna, Maria Concetta Pellicciari, Carlo Miniussi, and Costanza Papagno. 2011. "Literal, Fictive and Metaphorical Motion Sentences Preserve the Motion Component of the Verb: A TMS Study." *Brain and Language* 119 (3): 149–57.

Calvo-Merino, Beatriz, Daniel E. Glaser, Julie Grèzes, Richard E. Passingham, and Patrick Haggard. 2004. "Action Observation and Acquired Motor Skills: An FMRI Study with Expert Dancers." *Cerebral Cortex* 15 (8): 1243–49.

Caracciolo, Marco. 2014. *Narratologia: The Experientiality of Narrative; An Enactivist Approach*. Berlin: De Gruyter.

Caramazza, Alfonso, Stefano Anzellotti, Lukas Strnad, and Angelika Lingnau. 2014. "Embodied Cognition and Mirror Neurons: A Critical Assessment." *Annual Review of Neuroscience* 37:1–15.

Cave, Terence. 2016. *Thinking with Literature: Towards a Cognitive Criticism*. Oxford: Oxford University Press.

Chalmers, David J. 1995. "Facing up to the Problem of Consciousness." *Journal of Consciousness Studies* 2 (3): 200–219.

Changeux, Jean-Pierre. 2012. *The Good, the True, and the Beautiful: A Neuronal Approach*. Trans. Laurence Garey. New Haven, CT: Yale University Press.

Chatman, Seymour. 1978. *Story and Discourse: Narrative Structure in Fiction and Film*. Ithaca, NY: Cornell University Press.

Chatterjee, Anjan. 2010. "Disembodying Cognition." *Language and Cognition* 2 (1): 79–116.

Chen, Joyce L., Virginia B. Penhune, and Robert J. Zatorre. 2008. "Listening to Musical Rhythms Recruits Motor Regions of the Brain." *Cerebral Cortex* 18 (12): 2844–54.

Cheng, Yawei, Chenyi Chen, Ching-Po Lin, Kun-Hsien Chou, and Jean Decety. 2010. "Love Hurts: An fMRI Study." *Neuroimage* 51 (2): 923–29.

Christiansen, Morten H., and Nick Chater. 2008. "Language as Shaped by the Brain." *Behavioral and Brain Sciences* 31 (5): 489–509.

Churchland, Patricia. 2011. *Braintrust: What Neuroscience Tells Us about Morality*. Princeton, NJ: Princeton University Press.

Cikara, Mina, and Jay J. Van Bavel. 2014. "The Neuroscience of Intergroup Relations: An Integrative Review." *Perspectives on Psychological Science* 9 (3): 245–74.

Clark, Andy. 2008. "Pressing the Flesh: A Tension in the Study of the Embodied, Embedded Mind?" *Philosophy and Phenomenological Research* 76 (1): 37–59.

———. 2011. *Supersizing the Mind: Embodiment, Action, and Cognitive Extension*. Oxford: Oxford University Press.

———. 2016. *Surfing Uncertainty: Prediction, Action, and the Embodied Mind*. Oxford: Oxford University Press.

Cohn, Dorrit. 1978. *Transparent Minds: Narrative Modes for Presenting Consciousness in Fiction*. Princeton, NJ: Princeton University Press.

Colombetti, Giovanni. 2014. *The Feeling Body: Affective Science Meets the Enactive Mind*. Cambridge, MA: MIT Press.

Conrad, Joseph. 1996 [1900]. *Lord Jim*, ed. Thomas C. Moser. New York: Norton.

Conway, Bevil R., and Alexander Rehding. 2013. "Neuroaesthetics and the Trouble with Beauty." *PLoS Biology* 11 (3): e1001504.

Cook, Amy. 2018. "4E Cognition and the Humanities." In *The Oxford Handbook of 4E Cognition*, ed. Albert Newen, Leon De Bruin, and Shaun Gallagher, 875–90. Oxford: Oxford University Press.

Crick, Francis. 1994. *The Astonishing Hypothesis: The Scientific Search for the Soul*. New York: Simon & Schuster.

Cross, Ian. 2003. "Music, Cognition, Culture, and Evolution." In Peretz and Zatorre 2003, 42–56.

Culler, Jonathan. 1975. *Structuralist Poetics: Structuralism, Linguistics, and the Study of Literature*. Ithaca, NY: Cornell University Press.

D'Aloia, Adriano. 2012. "Cinematic Empathy: Spectator Involvement in the Film Experience." In Reynolds and Reason 2012, 91–107.

Damasio, Antonio R. 1994. *Descartes' Error: Emotion, Reason, and the Human Brain*. New York: Putnam.

———. 1999. *The Feeling of What Happens: Body and Emotion in the Making of Consciousness*. New York: Houghton Mifflin Harcourt.

Deacon, Terrence W. 2012. *Incomplete Nature: How Mind Emerged from Matter*. New York: Norton.

Decety, Jean, and Jason M. Cowell. 2015. "The Equivocal Relationship between Morality and Empathy." In Decety and Wheatley 2015, 279–302.

Decety, Jean, and Claus Lamm. 2009. "Empathy versus Personal Distress: Recent Evidence from Social Neuroscience." In Jean Decety and William Ickes, eds., *The Social Neuroscience of Empathy*, 199–213. Cambridge, MA: MIT Press.

Decety, Jean, and Thalia Wheatley, eds. 2015. *The Moral Brain: A Multidisciplinary Perspective*. Cambridge, MA: MIT Press.

Dehaene, Stanislas. 2009. *Reading in the Brain: The New Science of How We Read*. New York: Penguin.

———. 2014. *Consciousness and the Brain: Deciphering How the Brain Codes Our Thoughts*. New York: Penguin.

De Jaegher, Hanne, Ezequiel Di Paolo, and Ralph Adolphs. 2016. "What Does the Interactive Brain Hypothesis Mean for Social Neuroscience? A Dialogue." *Philosophical Transactions of the Royal Society B* 371:20150379.

De Jaegher, Hanne, Ezequiel Di Paolo, and Shaun Gallagher. 2010. "Can Social Interaction Constitute Social Cognition?" *Trends in Cognitive Sciences* 14 (10): 441–47.

Delton, Andrew W., and Max M. Krasnow. 2015. "Adaptationist Approaches to Moral Psychology." In Decety and Wheatley 2015, 19–34.

Dennett, Daniel C. 1991. *Consciousness Explained*. New York: Little, Brown.

Derrida, Jacques. 1984. "Two Words for Joyce." In *Post-Structuralist Joyce: Essays from the French*, ed. Derek Attridge and Daniel Ferrer, 145–59. Cambridge: Cambridge University Press.

Desai, Rutvik H., Lisa L. Conant, Jeffrey R. Binder, Haeil Park, and Mark S. Seidenberg. 2013. "A Piece of the Action: Modulation of Sensory-Motor Regions by Action Idioms and Metaphors." *NeuroImage* 83:862–69.

Dickens, Charles. 2008 [1861]. *Great Expectations*, ed. Margaret Cardwell and Robert Douglas-Fairhurst. Oxford: Oxford University Press.

Dikker, Suzanne, Lu Wan, Ido Davidesco, Lisa Kaggen, Matthias Oostrik, James McClintock, Jess Rowland, Mingzhou Ding, David Poeppel, and Dana Bevilacqua. 2017. "Brain-to-Brain Synchrony Tracks Real-World Dynamic Group Interactions in the Classroom." *Current Biology* 27 (9): 1375–80.

Dittrich, Luke. 2016. *Patient H. M.: A Story of Memory, Madness, and Family Secrets*. New York: Random House.

Donald, Merlin. 2012. "The Slow Process: A Hypothetical Cognitive Adaptation for Distributed Cognitive Networks." In Schulkin 2012, 25–42.

Dove, Guy. 2011 "On the Need for Embodied and Dis-embodied Cognition." *Frontiers in Psychology* 1:242.

Drake, Carolyn, and Daisy Bertrand. 2003. "The Quest for Universals in Temporal Processing in Music." In Peretz and Zatorre 2003, 21–31.

Dreyfus, Hubert L. 1992. *What Computers Still Can't Do: A Critique of Artificial Reason*. Cambridge, MA: MIT Press.

Droit-Volet, Sylvie. 2014. "What Emotions Tell Us About Time." In Arstila and Lloyd 2014b, 477–506.

Dudai, Yadin. 2011. "The Engram Revisited: On the Elusive Permanence of Memory." In Nalbantian, Matthews, and McClelland 2011, 29–40.

Easterlin, Nancy. 2012. *A Biocultural Approach to Literary Theory and Interpretation*. Baltimore, MD: Johns Hopkins University Press.

———. 2015. "Thick Context: Novelty in Cognition and Literature." In Zunshine 2015, 613–32.

Eco, Umberto. 1976. *A Theory of Semiotics*. Bloomington: Indianapolis University Press.

Edelman, Gerald M. 1987. *Neural Darwinism: The Theory of Neuronal Group Selection*. New York: Basic Books.

Edelman, Gerald M., and Giulio Tononi. 2000. *A Universe of Consciousness: How Matter Becomes Imagination*. New York: Basic Books.

Ekman, Paul. 1999 "Basic Emotions." In *Handbook of Cognition and Emotion*, ed. Tim Dagliesh and Mick Power, 45–60. New York: John Wiley & Sons.

Evans, Nicholas, and Stephen C. Levinson. 2009. "The Myth of Language Universals: Language Diversity and Its Importance for Cognitive Science." *Behavioral and Brain Sciences* 32 (5): 429–92.

Evans, Vyvyan. 2016. "Why Only Us: The Language Paradox." *New Scientist*, 27 February.

Fadiga, Luciano, Laila Craighero, and Alessandro D'Ausilio. 2009. "Broca's Area in Language, Action, and Music." *Annals of the New York Academy of Sciences* 1169 (1): 448–58.

Fauconnier, Giles, and Mark Turner. 2002. *The Way We Think: Conceptual Blending and the Mind's Hidden Complexities*. New York: Basic Books.

Faulkner, William. 1994 [1929]. *The Sound and the Fury*, ed. David Minter. New York: Norton.

Fazio, Patrik, Anna Cantagallo, Laila Craighero, Alessandro D'Ausilio, Alice C. Roy, Thierry Pozzo, Ferdinando Calzolari, Enrico Granieri, and Luciano Fadiga. 2009. "Encoding of Human Action in Broca's Area." *Brain* 132 (7): 1980–88.

Fernyhough, Charles. 2016. *The Voices Within: The History and Science of How We Talk to Ourselves*. New York: Basic Books.

Ferrari, Pier Francesco, and Giacomo Rizzolatti. 2014. "Mirror Neuron Research: The Past and the Future." *Philosophical Transactions of the Royal Society B* 369:20130169.

Fielding, Henry. 1961 [1741]. *Joseph Andrews; Shamela*, ed. Martin Battestin. Boston: Houghton Mifflin.

Flaubert, Gustave. 2003 [1857]. *Madame Bovary*. Trans. Geoffrey Wall. New York: Penguin.

Flesch, William. 2007. *Comeuppance: Costly Signaling, Altruistic Punishment, and Other Biological Components of Fiction*. Cambridge, MA: Harvard University Press.

Fludernik, Monika. 1996. *Towards a "Natural" Narratology*. London: Routledge.
———. 2014. Afterword, *Style* 48 (3): 404–8.
Fodor, Jerry A. 1983. *The Modularity of Mind*. Cambridge, MA: MIT Press.
Fong, Katrina, Justin B. Mullin, and Raymond A. Mar. 2013. "What You Read Matters: The Role of Fiction Genre in Predicting Interpersonal Sensitivity." *Psychology of Aesthetics, Creativity, and the Arts* 7 (4): 370–76.
Ford, Ford Madox. 1924. *Joseph Conrad: A Personal Remembrance*. Boston: Little, Brown.
———. 1964 [1914]. "On Impressionism" in *Critical Writings of Ford Madox Ford*, ed. Frank MacShane, 33–55. Lincoln: University of Nebraska Press.
———. 1990 [1915]. *The Good Soldier*, ed. Thomas C. Moser. Oxford: Oxford University Press.
Fordham, Finn. 2012. Introduction. In Joyce 2012 [1939], vii–xxxiv.
Forster, E. M. 1927. *Aspects of the Novel*. London: Edward Arnold.
Frank, Joseph. 1945. "Spatial Form in Modern Literature." In Frank 1991, 5–66.
———. 1977. "Spatial Form: An Answer to Critics." In Frank 1991, 67–106.
———. 1978. "Spatial Form: Some Further Reflections." In Frank 1991, 107–32.
———. 1991. *The Idea of Spatial Form*. New Brunswick, NJ: Rutgers University Press.
Fraps, Thomas. 2014. "Time and Magic—Manipulating Subjective Temporality." In Arstila and Lloyd 2014b, 263–85.
Freud, Sigmund. 1958 [1908]. "The Relation of the Poet to Day-Dreaming." In *On Creativity and the Unconscious: Papers on the Psychology of Art, Literature, Love, Religion*, ed. Benjamin Nelson, 44–54. New York: Harper & Row.
Friston, Karl, and Christopher Frith. 2015. "A Duet for One." *Consciousness and Cognition* 36:390–405.
Frith, Chris D. 2012. "The Role of Metacognition in Human Social Interactions." *Philosophical Transactions Royal Society B* 367: 2213–23.
Frith, Uta, and Chris D. Frith. 2010. "The Social Brain: Allowing Humans to Boldly Go Where No Other Species Has Been." *Philosophical Transactions Royal Society B* 365: 165–75.
Gadamer, Hans-Georg. 1993 [1960]. *Truth and Method*. 2nd rev. ed. Trans. Joel Weinsheimer and Donald G. Marshall. New York: Continuum.
Gallagher, Catherine. 2006. "The Rise of Fictionality." In *The Novel*, 2 vols., ed. Franco Moretti, 1:336–63. Princeton, NJ: Princeton University Press.
Gallagher, Shaun. 2005. *How the Body Shapes the Mind*. Oxford, UK: Clarendon Press.
———. 2012. *Phenomenology*. New York: Palgrave Macmillan.
Gallagher, Shaun, and Dan Zahavi. 2008. *The Phenomenological Mind: An Introduction to Philosophy of Mind and Cognitive Science*. New York: Routledge.
———. 2012. *The Phenomenological Mind*. 2nd ed. New York: Routledge.

Gallese, Vittorio, and George Lakoff. 2005. "The Brain's Concepts: The Role of the Sensory-Motor System in Conceptual Knowledge." *Cognitive Neuropsychology* 22 (3–4): 455–79.

Garrels, Scott R., ed. 2011. *Mimesis and Science: Empirical Research on Imitation and the Mimetic Theory of Culture and Religion.* East Lansing: Michigan State University Press.

Genette, Gérard. 1980. *Narrative Discourse: An Essay in Method.* Ithaca, NY: Cornell University Press.

Gerrig, Richard J. 2010. "Readers' Experiences of Narrative Gaps." *StoryWorlds* 2 (1): 19–37.

———. 2012. "Why Literature is Necessary, and Not Just Nice." In *Cognitive Literary Studies: Current Themes and New Directions,* ed. Isabel Jaén and Jacques Simon, 35–52. Austin: University of Texas Press.

Gerrig, Richard J., and Philip G. Zimbardo. 2005. *Psychology and Life.* 17th ed. Boston: Pearson.

Gibbs, Raymond W. Jr., and Tweenie Matlock. 2008. "Metaphor, Imagination, and Simulation: Psycholinguistic Evidence." In *The Cambridge Handbook of Metaphor and Thought,* ed. Raymond W. Gibbs, 161–76. New York: Cambridge University Press.

Gibson, James J. 1979. *The Ecological Approach to Visual Perception.* Boston: Houghton Mifflin.

Glenberg, Arthur M., and Michael P. Kaschak. 2002. "Grounding Language in Action." *Psychonomic Bulletin & Review* 9 (3): 558–65.

Gombrich, E. H. 1960. *Art and Illusion.* Princeton, NJ: Princeton University Press.

Gomes, Gilberto. 1998. "The Timing of Conscious Experience: A Critical Review and Reinterpretation of Libet's Research." *Consciousness and Cognition* 7 (4): 559–95.

Goodman, Nelson. 1978. *Ways of Worldmaking.* Indianapolis, IN: Hackett.

Gosetti-Ferencei, Jennifer Anna. 2018. *The Life of Imagination: Revealing and Making the World.* New York: Columbia University Press.

Greene, Joshua D. 2015. "The Cognitive Neuroscience of Moral Judgment and Decision Making." In Decety and Wheatley 2015, 197–220.

Greene, Robert Lane. 2016. "The Theories of the World's Best-Known Linguist Have Become Rather Weird." *Economist,* 26 March, 96.

Gross, Daniel M. 2010. "Defending the Humanities with Charles Darwin's *The Expression of the Emotions in Man and Animals* (1872)." *Critical Inquiry* 37 (1): 34–59.

Guerard, Albert J. 1958. *Conrad the Novelist.* Cambridge, MA: Harvard University Press.

Hagendoorn, Ivar. 2004. "Some Speculative Hypotheses about the Nature and Perception of Dance and Choreography." *Journal of Consciousness Studies* 11 (3–4): 79–110.

Haggard, Patrick, Sam Clark, and Jeri Kalogeras. 2002. "Voluntary Action and Conscious Awareness." *Nature Neuroscience* 5 (4): 382–85.

Haggard, Patrick, Yves Rossetti, and Mitsuo Kawato, eds. 2008. *Sensorimotor Foundations of Higher Cognition: Attention and Performance*. Vol. 22. Oxford: Oxford University Press.

Hakemulder, Jèmeljan. 2000. *The Moral Laboratory: Experiments Examining the Effects of Reading Literature on Social Perception and Moral Self-Concept*. Amsterdam: John Benjamins.

Hasson, Uri, Asif A. Ghazanfar, Bruno Galantucci, Simon Garrod, and Christian Keysers. 2012. "Brain-to-Brain Coupling: A Mechanism for Creating and Sharing a Social World." *Trends in Cognitive Sciences* 16 (2): 114–21.

Hasson, Uri, Ohad Landesman, Barbara Knappmeyer, Ignacio Vallines, Nava Rubin, and David J. Heeger. 2008. "Neurocinematics: The Neuroscience of Film." *Projections* 2 (1): 1–26.

Hasson, Uri, Yuval Nir, Ifat Levy, Galit Fuhrmann, and Rafael Malach. 2004. "Intersubject Synchronization of Cortical Activity during Natural Vision." *Science* 303 (5664): 1634–40.

Hauk, Olaf, and Friedemann Pulvermüller. 2004. "Neurophysiological Distinction of Action Words in the Fronto-Central Cortex." *Human Brain Mapping* 21:191–201.

Hebb, Donald O. 2002 [1949]. *The Organization of Behavior: A Neurophysiological Theory*. Mahwah, NJ: Erlbaum.

Heidegger, Martin. 1962 [1927]. *Being and Time*. Trans. John Macquarrie and Edward Robinson. New York: Harper & Row.

Hein, Grit, and Tania Singer. 2008. "I Feel How You Feel but Not Always: The Empathic Brain and Its Modulation." *Current Opinion in Neurobiology* 18 (2): 153–58.

Henrich, Joseph, Steven J. Heine, and Ara Norenzayan. 2010. "The Weirdest People in the World?" *Behavioral and Brain Sciences* 33 (2–3): 61–83.

Herman, David. 2002. *Story Logic: Problems and Possibilities of Narrative*. Lincoln: University of Nebraska Press.

———. 2010. "Narrative Theory after the Second Cognitive Revolution." In Zunshine 2010, 155–75.

———. 2011. "1880–1945: Re-Minding Modernism." In *The Emergence of Mind: Representations of Consciousness in Narrative Discourse in English*, ed. David Herman, 243–72. Lincoln: University of Nebraska Press.

———. 2013. *Storytelling and the Sciences of Mind*. Cambridge, MA: MIT Press.

Hickok, Gregory. 2009. "Eight Problems for the Mirror Neuron Theory of Action Understanding in Monkeys and Humans." *Journal of Cognitive Neuroscience* 21 (7): 1229–43.

———. 2014. *The Myth of Mirror Neurons: The Real Science of Communication and Cognition*. New York: Norton.

Hoffman, Martin. 2000. *Empathy and Moral Development: Implications for Caring and Justice*. Cambridge: Cambridge University Press.

Hogan, Patrick Colm. 2003. *The Mind and Its Stories: Narrative Universals and Human Emotion*. Cambridge: Cambridge University Press.

———. 2010. "Literary Universals." In Zunshine 2010, 37–60.

———. 2011a. *Affective Narratology: The Emotional Structure of Stories*. Lincoln: University of Nebraska Press.

———. 2011b. *What Literature Teaches Us about Emotion*. Cambridge: Cambridge University Press.

Hubel, David. 2011. "Thinking in the Brain." Cognitive Literary Studies Seminar, Mahindra Humanities Center, Harvard University, 8 December.

Humphrey, Nicholas. 2006. *Seeing Red: A Study in Consciousness*. Cambridge, MA: Harvard University Press.

Hunt, Lynn Avery. 2007. *Inventing Human Rights: A History*. New York: Norton.

Husserl, Edmund. 1964 [1928]. *The Phenomenology of Internal Time Consciousness*. Trans. James S. Churchill. Bloomington: Indiana University Press.

———. 1970 [1954]. *The Crisis of European Sciences and Transcendental Phenomenology*. Trans. David Carr. Evanston, IL: Northwestern University Press.

Hutchison, William D., Karen D. Davis, Andres M. Lozano, Ronald R. Tasker, and Jonathan O. Dostrovsky. 1999. "Pain-Related Neurons in the Human Cingulate Cortex." *Nature Neuroscience* 2 (5): 403–5.

Huth, Alexander G., Wendy A. de Heer, Thomas L. Griffiths, Frédéric E. Theunissen, and Jack L. Gallant. 2016. "Natural Speech Reveals the Semantic Maps that Tile Human Cerebral Cortex." *Nature* 532 (7600): 453–58.

Hutto, Daniel D. 2007. "The Narrative Practice Hypothesis: Origins and Applications of Folk Psychology." *Royal Institute of Philosophy Supplements* 60: 43–68.

Hyman, John. 2010 "Art and Neuroscience." In *Beyond Mimesis: Representation in Art and Science*, ed. Roman Frigg and Mathew J. Hunter, 245–54. Heidelberg: Springer.

Iacoboni, Marco. 2008. *Mirroring People: The Science of Empathy and How We Connect with Others*. New York: Farrar, Straus & Giroux.

Ingarden, Roman. 1973 [1931]. *The Literary Work of Art*. Trans. George G. Grabowicz. Evanston, IL: Northwestern University Press.

———. 1973 [1937]. *The Cognition of the Literary Work of Art*. Trans. Ruth Ann Crowley and Kenneth R. Olson. Evanston, IL: Northwestern University Press.

Iser, Wolfgang. 1974. *The Implied Reader: Patterns of Communication in Prose Fiction from Bunyan to Beckett*. Baltimore, MD: Johns Hopkins University Press.

———. 1978. *The Act of Reading: A Theory of Aesthetic Response*. Baltimore, MD: Johns Hopkins University Press.

———. 1993. *The Fictive and the Imaginary: Charting Literary Anthropology*. Baltimore, MD: Johns Hopkins University Press.

Jacobs, Arthur M. 2015. "Neurocognitive Poetics: Methods and Models for Investigating the Neuronal and Cognitive-Affective Bases of Literature Reception." *Frontiers in Human Neuroscience* 9:1–22.

Jahn, Manfred. 1997. "Frames, Preferences, and the Reading of Third-Person Narratives: Towards a Cognitive Narratology." *Poetics Today* 18 (4): 441–68.

———. 2005. "Cognitive Narratology." In *Routledge Encyclopedia of Narrative Theory*, ed. David Herman, Manfred Jahn, and Marie-Laure Ryan, 67–71. London: Routledge.

James, Henry. 1970a [1888]. *Partial Portraits*. Ann Arbor: University of Michigan Press.

———. 1970b [1883]. "Alphonse Daudet." In James 1970a [1883], 193–239.

———.1970c [1884]. "The Art of Fiction." In James 1970a [1884], 375–408.

———. 1987. *The Complete Notebooks of Henry James*, ed. Leon Edel and Lyall H. Powers. Oxford: Oxford University Press.

———. 2003 [1902]. *The Wings of a Dove*, ed. J. Donald Crowley and Richard A. Hocks. New York: Norton.

———. 2009 [1904]. *The Golden Bowl*, ed. Ruth Bernard Yeazell. New York: Penguin.

James, William. 1950 [1890]. *Principles of Psychology*. 2 vols. New York: Dover.

Jauss, Hans Robert. 1982. *Toward an Aesthetic of Reception*. Trans. Timothy Bahti. Minneapolis: University of Minnesota Press.

Jeannerod, Marc. 2006. *Motor Cognition: What Actions Tell the Self*. Oxford: Oxford University Press.

Johns, Louise C., and Jim Van Os. 2001. "The Continuity of Psychotic Experiences in the General Population." *Clinical Psychology Review* 21 (8): 1125–1141.

Joyce, James. 2007 [1916]. *A Portrait of the Artist as a Young Man*, ed. John Paul Riquelme. New York: Norton.

———. 2012 [1939]. *Finnegans Wake*, ed. Robbert-Jan Henkes, Erik Bindervoet, and Finn Fordham. Oxford: Oxford University Press.

Kandel, Eric. 2006. *In Search of Memory: The Emergence of a New Science of Mind*. New York: Norton.

Kearney, Richard. 2015. "The Wager of Carnal Hermeneutics." In *Carnal Hermeneutics*, ed. Richard Kearney and Brian Treanor, 15–56. New York: Fordham University Press.

Keen, Suzanne. 2007. *Empathy and the Novel*. Oxford: Oxford University Press.

———. 2011. "Introduction: Narrative and Emotions." *Poetics Today* 32 (1): 1–53.

———. 2015. "Intersectional Narratology in the Study of Narrative Empathy." In *Narrative Theory Unbound: Queer and Feminist Interventions*, ed. Robyn Warhol and Susan S. Lanser, 123–46. Columbus: Ohio State University Press.

Keller, Peter E. 2008. "Joint Action in Music Performance." In *Enacting Intersubjectivity: A Cognitive and Social Perspective on the Study of Interactions*, ed. Francesca Morganti, Antonella Carassa, and Giuseppe Riva, 205–21. Amsterdam: IOS Press.

Kelso, J. A. S. 1995. *Dynamic Patterns: The Self-Organization of Brain and Behavior.* Cambridge, MA: MIT Press.

———. 2000. "Fluctuations in the Coordination Dynamics of Brain and Behavior." In *Disorder versus Order in Brain Function: Essays in Theoretical Neurobiology,* ed. Peter Århem, Clas Blomberg, and Hans Liljenström, 185–203. Singapore: World Scientific Publishing.

Kermode, Frank. 1967. *The Sense of an Ending.* New York: Oxford University Press.

———. 1978. "Spatial Form: Some Further Reflections." *Critical Inquiry* 5 (2): 275–90.

Keymer, Thomas. 2001. Introduction to Samuel Richardson, *Pamela; or, Virtue Rewarded,* vii–xxxvi. Oxford: Oxford University Press.

Kidd, David Comer, and Emanuele Castano. 2013. "Reading Literary Fiction Improves Theory of Mind." *Science* 342 (6156): 377–80.

———. 2017. "Panero et al. (2016): Failure to Replicate Methods Caused the Failure to Replicate Results." *Journal of Personality and Social Psychology* 112 (3): e1–e4.

Kierkegaard, Søren. 1938. *The Journals of Søren Kierkegaard.* Trans. Alexander Dru. London: Oxford University Press.

Koelsch, Stefan. 2012. *Brain and Music.* Oxford: Wiley-Blackwell.

Kolers, Paul, and Michael von Grünau. 1976. "Shape and Color in Apparent Motion." *Vision Research* 16 (4): 329–35.

Konvalinka, Ivana, and Andreas Roepstorff. 2012. "The Two-Brain Approach: How Can Mutually Interacting Brains Teach Us Something About Social Interaction?" *Frontiers in Human Neuroscience* 6:215.

Kronegger, Maria Elisabeth. 1973. *Literary Impressionism.* New Haven, CT: College and University Press.

Kukkonen, Karin. 2014a. "Bayesian Narrative: Probability, Plot and the Shape of the Fictional World." *Anglia* 132 (4): 720–39.

———. 2014b. "Presence and Prediction: The Embodied Reader's Cascades of Cognition." *Style* 48 (3): 367–84.

———. 2016. "Bayesian Bodies: The Predictive Dimension of Embodied Cognition and Culture." In *The Cognitive Humanities: Embodied Mind in Literature and Culture,* ed. Peter Garratt, 153–67. London: Palgrave Macmillan.

———. 2017. *A Prehistory of Cognitive Poetics: Neoclassicism and the Novel.* Oxford: Oxford University Press.

Kukkonen, Karin, and Marco Caracciolo. 2014. "Introduction: What is the 'Second Generation'?" *Style* 48 (3): 261–74.

Kuzmičová, Anežka. 2012. "Presence in the Reading of Literary Narrative: A Case for Motor Enactment." *Semiotica* 189:23–48.

Lacey, Simon, Randall Stilla, and Krish Sathian. 2012. "Metaphorically Feeling: Comprehending Textural Metaphors Activates Somatosensory Cortex." *Brain and Language* 120 (3): 416–21.

Lakoff, George, and Mark Johnson. 1980. *Metaphors We Live By*. Chicago: University of Chicago Press.

———. 1999. *Philosophy in the Flesh: The Embodied Mind and Its Challenge to Western Thought*. New York: Basic Books.

Lawrence, Karen. 1981. *The Odyssey of Style in "Ulysses."* Princeton, NJ : Princeton University Press.

Lawtoo, Nidesh. 2013. *The Phantom of the Ego: Modernism and the Mimetic Unconscious*. East Lansing: Michigan State University Press.

Leavis, F. R. 1948. *The Great Tradition*. London: Chatto & Windus.

LeDoux, Joseph. 1996. *The Emotional Brain: The Mysterious Underpinnings of Emotional Life*. New York: Simon & Schuster.

Lessing, Gotthold Ephraim. 1962 [1766]. *Laocoön: An Essay on the Limits of Painting and Poetry*. Trans. Edward Allen McCormick. Baltimore, MD: Johns Hopkins University Press.

Levine, Caroline. 2015. *Forms: Whole, Rhythm, Hierarchy, Network*. Princeton, NJ: Princeton University Press.

Lewis, Mary Tompkins. 2007. "The Critical History of Impressionism." In *Critical Readings in Impressionism and Post-Impressionism*, ed. Mary Tompkins Lewis, 1–19. Berkeley: University of California Press.

Leys, Ruth. 2011. "The Turn to Affect: A Critique." *Critical Inquiry* 37 (3): 434–72.

Libet, Benjamin. 1993. "The Experimental Evidence for Subjective Referral of a Sensory Experience Backwards in Time: Reply to P. S. Churchland." In *Neurophysiology of Consciousness*, 205–20. Boston: Birkhäuser.

———. 2002. "The Timing of Mental Events: Libet's Experimental Findings and Their Implications." *Consciousness and Cognition* 11:291–99.

———. 2003. "Timing of Conscious Experience: Reply to the 2002 Commentaries on Libet's Findings." *Consciousness and Cognition* 12:321–31.

———. 2004. *Mind Time: The Temporal Factor in Consciousness*. Cambridge, MA: Harvard University Press.

Libet, Benjamin, Elwood W. Wright Jr., Bertram Feinstein, and Denies K. Pearl. 1979. "Subjective Referral of the Timing for a Conscious Sensory Experience: A Functional Role for the Somatosensory Specific Projection System in Man." *Brain* 102:193–224.

Lindenberger, Ulman, Shu-Chen Li, Walter Gruber, and Viktor Müller. 2009. "Brains Swinging in Concert: Cortical Phase Synchronization while Playing Guitar." *BMC Neuroscience* 10 (1): 22.

Lindquist, Kristen A., Tor D. Wager, Hedy Kober, Eliza Bliss-Moreau, and Lisa Feldman Barrett. 2012. "The Brain Basis of Emotion: A Meta-Analytic Review." *Behavioral and Brain Sciences* 35 (3): 121–43.

Lipps, Theodor. 1903. "Einfühlung, innere Nachahmung und Organempfindungen." In *Archiv für die Gesamte Psychologie*, vol. 1, pt. 2:185–204. Leipzig: Engelmann.

Livingstone, Margaret. 2002. *Vision and Art*. New York: Abrams.

Lloyd, Dan. 2016. "Inside Daniel Dennett: The Temporal Connectome." Paper presented at the conference of the Association for the Scientific Study of Consciousness, Buenos Aires, 15–18 June.

Lodge, David. 2001. *Thinks . . .* New York: Penguin.

———. 2002. *Consciousness and the Novel*. Cambridge, MA: Harvard University Press.

Lothe, Jakob. 2000. *Narrative in Fiction and Film*. Oxford: Oxford University Press.

———. 2018. "Characters and Narrators in Narrative Communication: James Phelan's Rhetorical Poetics of Narrative." *Style* 52 (1–2): 83–87.

Lotman, Yuri M. 1990. *Universe of the Mind: A Semiotic Theory of Culture*. Trans. Ann Shukman. Bloomington: Indiana University Press.

Maess, Burkhard, Stefan Koelsch, Thomas C. Gunter, and Angela D. Friederici. 2001. "Musical Syntax is Processed in Broca's Area: An MEG Study." *Nature Neuroscience* 4 (5): 540–45.

Malabou, Catherine. 2008. *What Should We Do with Our Brain?* Trans. Sebastian Rand. New York: Fordham University Press.

Malafouris, Lambros. 2013. *How Things Shape the Mind: A Theory of Material Engagement*. Cambridge, MA: MIT Press.

Mar, Raymond A., Keith Oatley, Jacob Hirsh, Jennifer dela Paz, and Jordan B. Peterson. 2006. "Bookworms versus Nerds: Exposure to Fiction versus Non-Fiction, Divergent Associations with Social Ability, and the Simulation of Fictional Social Worlds." *Journal of Research in Personality* 40 (5): 694–712.

Massumi, Brian. 1995. "The Autonomy of Affect." *Cultural Critique* 31:83–109.

———. 2002. *Parables for the Virtual: Movement, Affect, Sensation*. Durham, NC: Duke University Press.

Matz, Jesse. 2001. *Literary Impressionism and Modernist Aesthetics*. Cambridge: Cambridge University Press.

McCloud, Scott. 1993. *Understanding Comics: The Invisible Art*. New York: William Morrow.

McHugh, Roland. 1991. *Annotations to "Finnegans Wake."* Rev. ed. Baltimore, MD: Johns Hopkins University Press.

Merleau-Ponty, Maurice. 1963 [1942]. *The Structure of Behavior*. Trans. Alden L. Fisher. Boston: Beacon.

———. 1968 [1964]. *The Visible and the Invisible*, ed. Claude Lefort. Trans. Alphonso Lingis. Evanston, IL: Northwestern University Press.

———. 2012 [1945]. *Phenomenology of Perception*. Trans. Donald A. Landes. New York: Routledge.

Metz, Christian. 1974. *Film Language: A Semiotics of the Cinema*. Trans. Michael Taylor. Chicago: University of Chicago Press.

Miall, David S. 2011. "Emotions and the Structuring of Narrative Response." *Poetics Today* 32 (2): 323–48.

Mitchell, W. J. T. 1980. "Spatial Form in Literature: Toward a General Theory." *Critical Inquiry* 6 (3): 539–67.

Mölder, Bruno. 2014. "Constructing Time: Dennett and Grush on Temporal Representation." In Arstila and Lloyd 2014b, 217–38.

Morson, Gary Saul. 1994. *Narrative and Freedom: The Shadows of Time*. New Haven, CT: Yale University Press.

Mumper, Micah L. and Richard J. Gerrig. 2019. "How Does Leisure Reading Affect Social Cognitive Abilities?" *Poetics Today* 40 (3): 454–73.

Murphy, Elliot. 2016. "The Human Oscillome and Its Explanatory Potential." *Biolinguistics* 10:6–20.

Nadeau, Stephen E. 2012. *The Neural Architecture of Grammar*. Cambridge, MA: MIT Press.

Nagel, Thomas. 1974. "What Is It Like to Be a Bat?" *Philosophical Review* 83: 435–50.

———. 2012. *Mind and Cosmos*. Oxford: Oxford University Press.

Nalbantian, Suzanne, Paul M. Matthews, and James L. McClelland, eds. 2011. *The Memory Process: Neuroscientific and Humanistic Perspectives*. Cambridge, MA: MIT Press.

Niedenthal, Paula M. 2007. "Embodying Emotion." *Science* 316 (5827): 1002–5.

Nietzsche, Friedrich. 1994 [1872]. *The Birth of Tragedy Out of the Spirit of Music*. Trans. Shaun Whiteside. New York: Penguin.

———. 2015 [1873]. *Über Wahrheit und Lüge im außermoralischen Sinne [On Truth and Lie in an Extramoral Sense]*. Stuttgart: Reclam.

Nodjimbadem, Kim. 2015. "What Happens to Your Body When You Walk on a Tightrope?" *Smithsonian.com*, 13 October. www.smithsonianmag.com/science - nature/what-happens-your-body-when-you-walk-tightrope-180956897.

Noë, Alva. 2004. *Action in Perception*. Cambridge, MA: MIT Press.

———. 2009. *Out of Our Heads: Why You are Not Your Brain, and Other Lessons from the Biology of Consciousness*. New York: Hill and Wang.

———. 2015. *Strange Tools: Art and Human Nature*. New York: Hill and Wang.

Norris, Margot. 2004. "*Finnegans Wake.*" In *The Cambridge Companion to James Joyce*, ed. Derek Attridge, 149–70. Cambridge: Cambridge University Press.

Nussbaum, Martha C. 1997. *Cultivating Humanity: A Classical Defense of Reform in Liberal Education*. Cambridge, MA: Harvard University Press.

Oatley, Keith. 2016. "Fiction: Simulation of Social Worlds." *Trends in Cognitive Sciences* 20 (8): 618–28.

Palmer, Alan. 2004. *Fictional Minds*. Lincoln: University of Nebraska Press.

Pan, Yafeng, Xiaojun Cheng, Zhenxin Zhang, Xianchun Li, and Yi Hu. 2017. "Cooperation in Lovers: An fNIRS-Based Hyperscanning Study." *Human Brain Mapping* 38 (2): 831–41.

Panero, Maria Eugenia, Deena Skolnick Weisberg, Jessica Black, Thalia R. Goldstein, Jennifer L. Barnes, Hiram Brownell, and Ellen Winner. 2016. "Does

Reading a Single Passage of Literary Fiction Really Improve Theory of Mind? An Attempt at Replication." *Journal of Personality and Social Psychology* 111 (5): e46–e54.

Park, Sowon. 2012. "The Feeling of Knowing in *Mrs. Dalloway*: Neuroscience and Woolf." In *Contradictory Woolf*, ed. Derek Ryan and Stella Bolaki, 108–14. Liverpool, UK: Liverpool University Press.

———. 2018. "The Unconscious Memory Network," 22 May. https://unconsciousmemory.english.ucsb.edu.

Parkes, Adam. 2011. *A Sense of Shock: The Impact of Impressionism on Modern British and Irish Writing*. Oxford: Oxford University Press.

Patel, Aniruddh. 2008. *Music, Language, and the Brain*. New York: Oxford University Press.

Peretz, Isabelle, and Robert Zatorre, eds. 2003. *The Cognitive Neuroscience of Music*. Oxford: Oxford University Press.

Petitot, Jean, Francisco J. Varela, Bernard Pachoud, and Jean-Michel Roy, eds. 1999. *Naturalizing Phenomenology: Issues in Contemporary Phenomenology and Cognitive Science*. Stanford, CA: Stanford University Press.

Pettersson, Bo. 2018. *How Literary Worlds Are Shaped: A Comparative Poetics of Literary Imagination*. Berlin: De Gruyter.

Pettitt, Clare. 2016. "Henry James Tethered and Stretched: The Materiality of Metaphor." *Henry James Review* 37:139–53.

Phelan, James. 2002. "Narrative Progression." In Richardson 2002, 211–16.

———. 2005. *Living to Tell about It: A Rhetoric and Ethics of Character Narration*. Ithaca, NY: Cornell University Press.

———. 2006. "Narrative Theory, 1966–2006: A Narrative." In Scholes and Kellogg 2006 [1966], 283–336.

———. 2015. "Rhetorical Theory, Cognitive Theory, and Morrison's 'Recitatif': From Parallel Play to Productive Collaboration." In Zunshine 2015, 120–35.

———. 2017. *Somebody Telling Somebody Else: A Rhetorical Poetics of Narrative*. Columbus: Ohio State University Press.

———. 2018. "Authors, Resources, Audiences: Toward a Rhetorical Poetics of Narrative." *Style* 52 (1–2): 1–34.

Phillips, David P. 1974. "The Influence of Suggestion on Suicide: Substantive and Theoretical Implications of the Werther Effect." *American Sociological Review* 39 (3): 340–54.

Pinker, Steven. 1994. *The Language Instinct: How the Mind Creates Language*. New York: Harper.

———. 2011. *The Better Angels of Our Nature: Why Violence Has Declined*. New York: Viking.

Pöppel, Ernst, and Yan Bao. 2014. "Temporal Windows as a Bridge from Objective to Subjective Time." In Arstila and Lloyd 2014b, 241–62.

Prince, Gerald. 2018. "Response to James Phelan." *Style* 52 (1–2): 42–45.

Pronin, Emily, Jonah Berger, and Sarah Molouki. 2007. "Alone in a Crowd of Sheep: Asymmetric Perceptions of Conformity and Their Roots in an Introspection Illusion." *Journal of Personality and Social Psychology* 92:585–95.

Prum, Richard O. 2013. "Coevolutionary Aesthetics in Human and Biotic Artworlds." *Biology and Philosophy* 28:811–32.

Pulvermüller, Friedemann. 2018. "Neural Reuse of Action Perception Circuits for Language, Concepts and Communication." *Progress in Neurobiology* 160:1–44.

Pulvermüller, Friedemann, and Luciano Fadiga. 2010. "Active Perception: Sensorimotor Circuits as a Cortical Basis for Language." *Nature Reviews Neuroscience* 11 (5): 351–60.

Quiroga, R. Quian, Leila Reddy, Gabriel Kreiman, Christof Koch, and Itzhak Fried. 2005. "Invariant Visual Representation by Single Neurons in the Human Brain." *Nature*, 23 June, 1102–7.

Rabinowitch, Tal-Chen, Ian Cross and Pamela Burnard. 2012. "Musical Group Interaction, Intersubjectivity and Merged Subjectivity." In Reynolds and Reason 2012, 109–20.

Rabinowitz, Peter. 2002. "Reading Beginnings and Endings." In Richardson 2002, 300–313.

Raichle, Marcus E. 2011. "The Restless Brain." *Brain Connectivity* 1 (1): 3–12.

Raposo, Ana, Helen E. Moss, Emmanuel A. Stamatakis, and Lorraine K. Tyler. 2009. "Modulation of Motor and Premotor Cortices by Actions, Action Words and Action Sentences." *Neuropsychologia* 47 (2): 388–96.

Rapp, David N. 2008. "How Do Readers Handle Incorrect Information during Reading?" *Memory and Cognition* 36 (3): 688–701.

Rauscheker, Josef P. 2003. "Functional Organization and Plasticity of the Auditory Cortex." In Peretz and Zatorre 2003, 357–65.

Reynolds, Dee, and Matthew Reason, eds. 2012. *Kinesthetic Empathy in Creative and Cultural Practices*. Bristol, UK: Intellect Books.

Richardson, Alan. 2011. "Defaulting to Fiction: Neuroscience Rediscovers the Romantic Imagination." *Poetics Today* 32 (4): 663–92.

Richardson, Brian, ed. 2002. *Narrative Dynamics: Essays on Time, Plot, Closure, and Frames*. Columbus: Ohio State University Press.

———. 2015. *Unnatural Narrative: Theory, History, and Practice*. Columbus: Ohio State University Press.

Richardson, Michael J., Kerry L. Marsh, Robert W. Isenhower, Justin R. L. Goodman, and Richard C. Schmidt. 2007. "Rocking Together: Dynamics of Intentional and Unintentional Interpersonal Coordination." *Human Movement Science* 26:867–91.

Ricoeur, Paul. 1966. *Freedom and Nature: The Voluntary and the Involuntary*. Trans. Erazim V. Kohák. Evanston, IL: Northwestern University Press.

———. 1968. "Structure, Word, Event." In *The Philosophy of Paul Ricoeur*, ed. Charles E. Regan and David Stewart, 109–19. Boston: Beacon.

————. 1977. *The Rule of Metaphor: Multi-Disciplinary Studies of the Creation of Meaning in Language.* Trans. Robert Czerny, Kathleen McLaughlin, and John Costello. Toronto: University of Toronto Press.

————. 1980a. "Mimesis and Representation." In Ricoeur 1991, 137–55.

————. 1980b. "Narrative Time." *Critical Inquiry* 7 (1): 169–90.

————. 1984a. *Time and Narrative.* Vol. 1. Trans. Kathleen McLaughlin and David Pellauer. Chicago: University of Chicago Press.

————. 1984b. "Narrated Time." In Ricoeur 1991, 338–54.

————. 1987. "Life: A Story in Search of a Narrator." In Ricoeur 1991, 425–37.

————. 1991. *A Ricoeur Reader: Reflection and Imagination,* ed. Mario J. Valdés. Toronto: University of Toronto Press.

————. 1992. *Oneself as Another.* Trans. Kathleen Blamey. Chicago: University of Chicago Press.

Rizzolatti, Giacomo, and Laila Craighero. 2004. "The Mirror-Neuron System." *Annual Review of Neuroscience* 27:169–92.

Rizzolatti, Giacomo, and Leonardo Fogassi. 2014. "The Mirror Mechanism: Recent Findings and Perspectives." *Philosophical Transactions of the Royal Society B* 369:20130420.

Rizzolatti, Giacomo, and Corrado Sinigaglia. 2008. *Mirrors in the Brain: How Our Minds Share Actions and Emotions.* Oxford: Oxford University Press.

Robinson, Jenefer. 2005. *Deeper Than Reason: Emotion and Its Role in Literature, Music, and Art.* Oxford, UK: Clarendon Press.

Rubin, James H. 1999. *Impressionism.* New York: Phaidon.

Rüschemeyer, Shirley-Ann, Marcel Brass, and Angela D. Friederici. 2007. "Comprehending Prehending: Neural Correlates of Processing Verbs with Motor Stems." *Journal of Cognitive Neuroscience* 19 (5): 855–65.

Ruskin, John. 1857. *The Elements of Drawing.* London: Smith, Elder.

Ryan, Marie-Laure. 2001. *Narrative as Virtual Reality: Immersion and Interactivity in Literature and Electronic Media.* Baltimore, MD: Johns Hopkins University Press.

Ryan, Vanessa. 2012. *Thinking without Thinking in the Victorian Novel.* Baltimore, MD: Johns Hopkins University Press.

Ryle, Gilbert. 2009 [1949]. *The Concept of Mind.* New York: Routledge.

Sänger, Johanna, Ulman Lindenberger, and Viktor Müller. 2011. "Interactive Brains, Social Minds." *Communicative and Integrative Biology* 4 (6): 655–63.

Samson, Séverine, and Nathalie Ehrlé. 2003. "Cerebral Substrates for Musical Temporal Processes." In Peretz and Zatorre, 192–203.

Sartre, Jean-Paul. 1962 [1947]. *What Is Literature?* Trans. Bernard Frechtman. New York: Harper & Row.

Saygin, Ayse Pinar, Stephen M. Wilson, Nina F. Dronkers, and Elizabeth Bates. 2004. "Action Comprehension in Aphasia: Linguistic and Non-Linguistic Deficits and Their Lesion Correlates." *Neuropsychologia* 42 (13): 1788–1804.

Schacter, Daniel L. 2002. *The Seven Sins of Memory: How the Mind Forgets and Remembers.* Boston: Houghton Mifflin.

Schacter, Daniel L., and Donna Rose Addis. 2007. "The Cognitive Neuroscience of Constructive Memory: Remembering the Past and Imagining the Future." *Philosophical Transactions of the Royal Society B* 362:773–86.

Schilbach, Leonhard, Bert Timmermans, Vasudevi Reddy, Alan Costall, Gary Bente, Tobias Schlicht, and Kai Vogeley. 2013. "Toward a Second-Person Neuroscience." *Behavioral and Brain Sciences* 36 (4): 393–414.

Schlesinger, I. M. 1968. *Sentence Structure and the Reading Process.* The Hague, Paris: Mouton.

Scholes, Robert, and Robert Kellogg. 2006 [1966]. *The Nature of Narrative.* Oxford: Oxford University Press.

Schulkin, Jay, ed. 2012. *Action, Perception, and the Brain.* New York: Palgrave Macmillan.

Schulkin, Jay, and Patrick Heelan. 2012. "Action and Cephalic Expression: Hermeneutical Pragmatism." In Schulkin 2012, 218–57.

Schwan, Stephan, and Sermin Ildirar. 2010. "Watching Film for the First Time: How Adult Viewers Interpret Perceptual Discontinuities in Film." *Psychological Science* 21 (7): 970–76.

Sheets-Johnstone, Maxine. 1966. *The Phenomenology of Dance.* Madison: University of Wisconsin Press.

———. 2011. *The Primacy of Movement.* 2nd rev. ed. Amsterdam: John Benjamins.

Shimamura, Arthur P. 2013a. *Experiencing Art: In the Brain of the Beholder.* Oxford: Oxford University Press.

———. 2013b. "Psychocinematics: Issues and Directions." In *Psychocinematics: Exploring Cognition and the Movies,* ed. Arthur P. Shimamura, 1–26. Oxford: Oxford University Press.

Shklar, Judith. 1990. *The Faces of Injustice.* New Haven, CT: Yale University Press.

Shklovsky, Viktor. 1965 [1917]. "Art as Technique." In *Russian Formalist Criticism: Four Essays.* Trans. Lee T. Lemon and Marion J. Reis, 3–24. Lincoln: University of Nebraska Press.

Silbert, Lauren J., Christopher J. Honey, Erez Simony, David Poeppel, and Uri Hasson. 2014. "Coupled Neural Systems Underlie the Production and Comprehension of Naturalistic Narrative Speech." *Proceedings of the National Academy of Sciences* 111 (43): e4687–e4696.

Silva, Alcino J. 2011. "Molecular Genetic Approaches to Memory Consolidation." In Nalbantian, Matthews, and McClelland 2011, 41–54.

Singer, Tania, Ben Seymour, John O'Doherty, Holger Kaube, Raymond J. Dolan, and Chris D. Frith. 2004. "Empathy for Pain Involves the Affective but Not Sensory Components of Pain." *Science* 303 (5661): 1157–62.

Smith, Tim J., Daniel Levin, and James E. Cutting. 2012. "A Window on Reality: Perceiving Edited Moving Images." *Psychological Science* 21 (2): 107–13.

Snyder, Frederick W., and N. H. Pronko. 1952. *Vision with Spatial Inversion.* Wichita, KS: University of Wichita Press.

Speer, Nicole K., Jeremy R. Reynolds, Khena M. Swallow, and Jeffrey M. Zacks. 2009. "Reading Stories Activates Neural Representations of Visual and Motor Experiences." *Psychological Science* 20 (8): 989–99.

Sperber, Dan, and Deirdre Wilson. 1995 [1986]. *Relevance: Communication and Cognition.* 2nd ed. Oxford, UK: Blackwell.

Spolsky, Ellen. 2015. *The Contracts of Fiction: Cognition, Culture, Community.* Oxford: Oxford University Press.

Starr, G. Gabrielle. 2013. *Feeling Beauty: The Neuroscience of Aesthetic Experience.* Cambridge, MA: MIT Press.

Stein, Edith. 1964 [1917]. *On the Problem of Empathy.* Trans. W. Stein. The Hague: Nijhoff.

Sternberg, Meir. 1987. *The Poetics of Biblical Narrative: Ideological Literature and the Drama of Reading.* Bloomington: Indiana University Press.

Stevens, Catherine, and Shirley McKechnie. 2005. "Thinking in Action: Thought Made Visible in Contemporary Dance." *Cognitive Processing* 6 (4): 243–52.

Stickgold, Robert. 2011. "Memory in Sleep and Dreams: The Construction of Meaning." In Nalbantian, Matthews, and McClelland 2011, 73–95.

Stratton, George M. 1897. "Vision without Inversion of the Retinal Image." *Psychological Review* 4:341–40.

Suddendorf, Thomas, and Michael C. Corballis. 2007. "The Evolution of Foresight: What is Mental Time Travel, and Is It Unique to Humans?" *Behavioral and Brain Sciences* 30 (3): 299–351.

Tabibnia, Golnaz, and Matthew D. Lieberman. 2007. "Fairness and Cooperation Are Rewarding." *Annals of the New York Academy of Sciences* 1118 (1): 90–101.

Tattersall, Ian. 2016. "At the Birth of Language." *New York Review of Books* 63 (13): 27–28.

Thompson, Evan. 2007. *Mind in Life: Biology, Phenomenology, and the Sciences of Mind.* Cambridge, MA: Harvard University Press.

Thompson, Evan, Antoine Lutz, and Diego Cosmelli. 2005. "Neurophenomenology: An Introduction for Neurophilosophers." In *Cognition and the Brain: The Philosophy and Neuroscience Movement*, ed. Andrew Brook and Kathleen Akins, 40–97. Cambridge: Cambridge University Press.

Todorov, Tzvetan. 1969. "The Structural Analysis of Narrative." Trans. Arnold Weinstein. *Novel: A Forum on Fiction* 3 (1): 70–76.

Tomasello, Michael. 2003. *Constructing a Language: A Usage-Based Theory of Language Acquisition.* Cambridge, MA: Harvard University Press.

———. 2014. *A Natural History of Human Thinking.* Cambridge, MA: Harvard University Press.

Tomasello, Michael, Malinda Carpenter, Josep Call, Tanya Behne, and Henrike Moll. 2005. "Understanding and Sharing Intentions: The Origins of Cultural Cognition." *Behavioral and Brain Sciences* 28 (5): 675–91.

Torgovnick, Marianna. 1981. *Closure in the Novel*. Princeton, NJ: Princeton University Press.

Trehub, Sandra E. 2003. "Musical Predisposition in Infancy: An Update." In Peretz and Zatorre 2003, 3–20.

Troscianko, Emily T. 2014. *Kafka's Cognitive Realism*. London: Routledge.

Turner, Mark. 1996. *The Literary Mind: The Origins of Thought and Language*. Oxford: Oxford University Press.

Valdés, Mario J. 1991. "Introduction: Paul Ricoeur's Post-Structuralist Hermeneutics." In Ricoeur 1991, 3–40.

van Gelder, Tim. 1999. "Wooden Iron? Husserlian Phenomenology Meets Cognitive Science." In Petitot et al. 1999, 245–65.

Vannuscorps, Gilles, and Alfonso Caramazza. 2016. "Typical Action Perception and Interpretation Without Motor Simulation." *Proceedings of the National Academy of Sciences* 113 (1): 86–91.

Varela, Francisco J. 1999. "The Specious Present: A Neurophenomenology of Time Consciousness." In Petitot et al. 1999, 266–314.

Varela, Francisco J., Jean-Philippe Lachaux, Eugenio Rodriguez, and Jacques Martinerie. 2001. "The Brainweb: Phase Synchronization and Large-Scale Integration." *Nature Reviews Neuroscience* 2 (4): 229–39.

Varela, Francisco J., Evan Thompson, and Eleanor Rosch. 1991. *The Embodied Mind: Cognitive Science and Human Experience*. Cambridge, MA: MIT Press.

Vessel, Edward A., G. Gabrielle Starr, and Nava Rubin. 2012 "The Brain on Art: Intense Aesthetic Experience Activates the Default Mode Network." *Frontiers in Human Neuroscience* 6:66.

Vezzali, Loris, Sofia Stathi, Dino Giovannini, Dora Capozza, and Elena Trifiletti. 2015. "The Greatest Magic of Harry Potter: Reducing Prejudice." *Journal of Applied Social Psychology* 45 (2): 105–21.

Walsh, Richard. 2010. "Person, Level, Voice." In Alber and Fludernik, 2010a, 35–57.

Walton, Kendall L. 1990. *Mimesis as Make-Believe: On the Foundations of the Representational Arts*. Cambridge, MA: Harvard University Press.

Watt, Ian. 1979. *Conrad in the Nineteenth Century*. Berkeley: University of California Press.

Wehrs, Donald R. 2017. Introduction to *The Palgrave Handbook of Affect Studies and Textual Criticism*, ed. Donald R. Wehrs and Thomas Blake, 1–93. Cham, Switzerland: Palgrave Macmillan.

Weil, Kari. 2012. *Thinking Animals: Why Animal Studies Now?* New York: Columbia University Press.

Wertheimer, Max. 1912. "Experimentelle Studien über das Sehen von Bewegung." *Zeitschrift für Psychologie* 61:161–265.

West, M. J., and A. P. King. 1988. "Female Visual Displays Affect the Development of Male Song in the Cowbird." *Nature* 334: 244–46.

Westmacott, Robyn, Sandra E. Black, Morris Freedman, and Morris Moscovitch. 2004. "The Contribution of Autobiographical Significance to Semantic Memory: Evidence from Alzheimer's Disease, Semantic Dementia, and Amnesia." *Neuropsychologia* 42 (1): 25–48.

Wicker, Bruno, Christian Keysers, Jane Plailly, Jean-Pierre Royet, Vittorio Gallese, and Giacomo Rizzolatti. 2003. "Both of Us Disgusted in My Insula: The Common Neural Basis of Seeing and Feeling Disgust." *Neuron* 40 (3): 655–64.

Wiesel, Thorstein N. and David Hubel. 1965. "Extent of Recovery from the Effects of Visual Deprivation in Kittens." *Journal of Neurophysiology* 28:1060–72.

Wilkowski, Benjamin M., Brian P. Meier, Michael D. Robinson, Margaret S. Carter, and Roger Feltman. 2009. "'Hot-headed' Is More Than an Expression: The Embodied Representation of Anger in Terms of Heat." *Emotion* 9 (4): 464–77.

Willems, Roel M., and Daniel Casasanto. 2011. "Flexibility in Embodied Language Understanding." *Frontiers in Psychology* 2 (116): 1–11.

Willems, Roel M., Peter Hagoort, and Daniel Casasanto. 2010. "Body-Specific Representations of Action Verbs: Neural Evidence from Right-and Left-Handers." *Psychological Science* 21 (1): 67–74.

Wilson, Deirdre, and Dan Sperber. 2012. *Meaning and Relevance.* Cambridge: Cambridge University Press.

Wilson, Edmund O. 1998. *Consilience: The Unity of Knowledge.* New York: Vintage.

Wittgenstein, Ludwig. 1980. *Remarks on the Philosophy of Psychology.* Vol 2. Oxford, UK: Blackwell.

Wittman, Marc. 2014. "Embodied Time: The Experience of Time, the Body, and the Self." In Arstila and Lloyd 2014b, 507–23.

Woolf, Virginia. 1950 [1924]. "Mr. Bennett and Mrs. Brown." In *The Captain's Deathbed and Other Essays*, 94–119. New York: Harcourt Brace Jovanovich.

———. 1984 [1921]. "Modern Fiction." In *The Common Reader: First Series*, ed. Andrew McNeillie, 146–54. New York: Harcourt.

Yao, Bo, Pascal Belin, and Christoph Scheepers. 2011. "Silent Reading of Direct Versus Indirect Speech Activates Voice-Selective Areas in the Auditory Cortex." *Journal of Cognitive Neuroscience* 23 (10): 3146–52.

Yarrow, Kielan, and Sukhvinder Obhi. 2014. "Temporal Perception in the Context of Action." In Arstila and Lloyd 2014b, 455–75.

Yeazell, Ruth Bernard. 1976. *Language and Knowledge in the Late Novels of Henry James.* Chicago: University of Chicago Press.

Zeki, Semir. 2003. "The Disunity of Consciousness." *Trends in Cognitive Sciences* 7 (5): 214–18.

———. 2004. "The Neurology of Ambiguity." *Consciousness and Cognition* 13:173–96.

———. 2012. "The Neurobiology Behind Beauty: Semir Zeki @ TEDxUCL." 2 July. www.youtube.com/watch?v=NlzanAwoRP4.

Zeki, Semir, and Tomohiro Ishizu. 2011. "Toward A Brain-Based Theory of Beauty." *PloS One* 6 (7) e21852 (July): 1–10.

Zeman, Adam, Fraser Milton, Alicia Smith, and Rick Rylance. 2013 "By Heart: An fMRI Study of Brain Activation by Poetry and Prose." *Journal of Consciousness Studies* 20 (9–10): 132–58.

Zunshine, Lisa, ed. 2010. *Introduction to Cognitive Cultural Studies.* Baltimore, MD: Johns Hopkins University Press.

———, ed. 2015. *The Oxford Handbook of Cognitive Literary Studies.* Oxford: Oxford University Press.

INDEX

Abbott, H. Porter, 56
action, 105–49; embodied and disembodied metaphors and, 125–34; grounded cognition and, 117–21; interactions in narrative and narration, 134–44; narrative affordances and, 144–49; paradoxes of simulation and, 117–25; understanding, 6–7, 123, 126, 157. *See also* action-perception circuit; imitation; pattern-forming activity
action-perception circuit, 7, 11, 13, 106–17, 199, 216n7
Addis, Donna Rose, 85
Adolphs, Ralph, 102
aesthetic experiences, 85–86, 107, 161, 181, 186, 215n3
affective appraisals, 98–101
affect theory, 62–63, 96, 213n8. *See also* emotions
affordances, 42, 44, 144–49, 178, 201, 211n16, 217n15
agency, 102, 175–76, 184
aggression, 161, 163
Alber, Jan, 15, 50
Alderson-Day, Ben, 165–66, 220n7
ambiguity, 30, 35, 155–56, 158, 167, 196, 215n4
anachronies, 12, 35, 70, 202
Anderson, Michael L., 22, 118, 124
anger, 7, 21, 43, 94–97, 132–34, 159, 200. *See also* emotions
anticipation and retrospection, 36, 58–73, 85–86, 99–100, 147
anticipatory understanding, 94, 97, 121
anxiety, 141, 142, 158, 159
aphasia, 23
Aristotle: desire to classify narratives and, 202; on imitation of action, 105;

on memory, 83; *Poetics*, 215n2; temporality and, 27; theory of catharsis and, 159–60, 163; theory of plots and, 4, 11, 27, 32, 69
arithmetic problems, 83
Armstrong, Paul B.: *Challenge of Bewilderment*, 210n9, 217n13, 222n17; *Conflicting Readings*, 216n8; *How Literature Plays with the Brain*, 215n4
Arstila, Valtteri, 56
artificial intelligence theory, 18, 20, 47, 200
as-if relations, 8, 28, 110, 119–21, 124, 126, 130, 140–41, 179–82, 190, 200, 207, 222n18; body loop, 158, 160; challenging habits and patterns, 179–81, 198; identification and, 158–60; impressionism and, 193, 195, 197
Asperger's syndrome, 162
as-relations and as-structure, 17, 18, 29, 111–12, 121, 149, 207; aesthetic movements and, 197; doubling and, 161, 168, 222n18; intentionality and, 44; simulation and, 7, 128–29, 151, 163, 200
attention and awareness, 49, 64, 77, 83, 86, 124, 147; awareness of an intention, 68; children's attentional engagement with their parents, 169–70; conscious awareness, 54, 57, 59, 74, 98–99; emotions focusing, 101; initial awareness, 59–60, 62–63; joint attention, 170, 182–84
attunement, 93–94, 97, 100–101, 107, 171, 182
Auerbach, Erich, 129
Augustine, 4, 26, 27

Austen, Jane: *Pride and Prejudice*,
  51–52
authorial audience, 185, 219–20n6
autism, 162
Auyoung, Elaine, 44, 138–40, 146, 202,
  211n12
Aziz-Zadeh, Lisa, 127

Baars, Bernard, 55, 87
Bal, P. Matthijs, 168
Balzac, Honoré de: *Père Goriot*, 33,
  128–29, 130; "Sarrasine," 88
Banfield, Ann, 14, 83–84
Bang, Dan, 172
Barnes, Djuna: *Nightwood*, 83
Barrett, Lisa Feldman, 21, 95
Barsalou, Lawrence, 100, 113–14, 117,
  118–20
Barthes, Roland: *S/Z*, 88, 212n2
Bayesian models of predictive pro-
  cessing, 45, 147, 202, 211n12, 216n8
Bear, Mark, 107
Beckett, Samuel, 222n18
Berlin, Isaiah, 34
Bernaerts, Lars (ed.): *Stories and Minds:
  Cognitive Approaches to Literary
  Narrative*, 14
Bernini, Marco, 165–66, 220n7
Berthoz, Alain: *The Physiology and
  Phenomenology of Action* (with Petit),
  106, 134, 144–45
Berwick, Robert C., 209n4
bias, 72, 84, 170, 220n10
binding, 54, 61, 62, 74, 81, 89
biocultural hybrids, 23–24, 25, 47, 149,
  180, 189, 205, 206–7
blending, 40–41, 210n10
Bloom, Paul, 160–61, 163
Bolens, Guillemette, 43–44, 135,
  148–49, 152–53
Bourke, Joanna, 132–33
Bracher, Mark, 180–81, 207
bracketing, 143
brain, anatomy of, 20–23; amygdala, 21,
  68, 95; anterior cingulate cortex, 160;
  brain stem, 68; Broca's area, 23,
  114–15, 216n7; cerebrum, 23, 60;
  cortex, 4, 20–22, 54–55, 68, 98, 186,
  200; frontal cortex, 186; hippocam-

pus, 68, 87, 98, 214n14; insula, 160;
  motor cortex, 6, 22, 66, 87, 109,
  112–14, 122–27, 136–38, 157;
  premotor cortex, 112, 127, 138;
  thalamus, 68, 98; visual cortex, 20,
  22, 50, 54, 68, 95, 123–24, 193, 200;
  Wernicke's area, 23
brain, conceptions of: asynchronous
  temporal processes, 6, 54–65, 104,
  213n11; bushy, 9, 19, 46, 201, 203;
  chaos and rules in terms of network
  behavior, 19–20; computer model
  superseded, 18, 20, 54, 77, 200–201,
  210n4; default mode network
  (DMN), 85–86; imagined in a vat, 3;
  interactive brain hypothesis, 102;
  plasticity of, 20–21, 124; stability vs.
  instability, 78–79, 81, 84; synchronization and desynchronization
  processes, 5, 19, 54–59, 76, 103,
  171–72, 203; web, 68, 70, 124–25
brain-body interactions: as-if body loop,
  158, 160; language and, 23; participatory sense-making and, 103; seeing-as
  and, 17–19
brain-body-world interactions, 4, 5, 11,
  62, 89; asynchrony and, 58, 213n11;
  cortical functions and, 20–22, 203;
  measuring equipment and, 90
brain-to-brain coupling, 9, 171, 182,
  185–86, 203
Brontë, Charlotte: *Jane Eyre*, 48
Brooks, Peter, 30
Brown, Donald E., 24
Bruner, Jerome, 39, 177
Buckner, Randy L., 85
Buonomano, Dean V., 56, 74
Burke, Kenneth, 136
Busch, Niko, 74–75
Butler, Octavia: *Parable of the Sower*,
  162
Buzsáki, György, 56, 67, 77

Cacciari, Cristina, 127
Calvino, Italo: *If on a Winter's Night a
  Traveler*, 83
Caracciolo, Marco, 42–43, 148
Caramazza, Alfonso, 122
Carroll, David C., 85

Carroll, Lewis: *Alice's Adventures in Wonderland,* 145
Cartesian model, 5, 38, 53, 222n18
Casasanto, Daniel, 216–17n11
Castano, Emanuele, 151, 152, 161–63, 169
categorization process, 17–18, 202, 206, 221n14. *See also* frames and scripts
catharsis, 27, 160, 163
Cave, Terence, 42, 85, 138, 142, 145–46, 178, 188, 201, 216n8
Changeux, Jean-Pierre, 23, 209n4
characters, 88, 101, 141, 155–56, 165–66, 189, 215n2
Chatman, Seymour, 12, 30
Chatterjee, Anjan, 118
Chekhov, Anton, 162
Cheng, Yawei, 160
Chomsky, Noam, 14, 209n4
Churchland, Patricia, 215n4
Cikara, Mina, 170
circularity of literary interpretation, 18, 205–6
Clark, Andy, 42, 106, 147, 177–78, 211n16, 216n8, 221n13
classification. *See* taxonomic, rule-based approach
closure, 80, 81
cognition, 3, 60–61, 122, 199; distributed, 177–86; embodied cognition, 5, 9, 13, 15, 17, 26–29, 45–48, 53, 105, 116, 118, 211n16, 222n18; emotion interconnected with, 95; figuration in narrative and, 26–37; 4e cognition, 4, 5, 7, 15, 41; grounded cognition, 117–22; integration in, 55, 73–83; motor cognition, 13, 108; performance deficits and cognitive ability, 121–22; social cognition, 119, 120, 151–52, 162, 165, 169
cognitive archive of stories, 186–98, 206, 222n18
cognitive formalism, 6, 14–15, 20, 22, 209n1
cognitive narratology, 9, 14–18, 201
cognitive science: first-generation, 15, 16–17, 20, 42, 200, 215n1; narrative theory and, 26, 52, 168, 200; relation to literary theories of memory and

imagination, 85; second-generation, 15–17, 43, 105, 201, 211n12, 215n1
Cohn, Dorrit, 153, 155–56, 218–19n3
cointentionality, 13
collaboration, 169–73, 182, 221n12. *See also* synchronization
color, 3, 54, 112, 186, 192
color phi phenomenon, 61–62, 212n7
comic panels, 75
conceptual blending, 40–41
concordant discordance, 12, 29, 32, 41, 46–48, 52, 54, 69–70, 74, 100, 103, 105, 142, 203; affordances and, 145–46; benefit of, 46, 117
concretization, 141
configuration. *See* figuration/configuration/refiguration
conflict of interpretations, 14, 34, 192, 199, 201, 205, 210n6
connectome, 9, 203
Conrad, Joseph, 191, 194, 206; *Lord Jim,* 34–35, 79–80, 143–44, 194, 196
consciousness, 3; archive of world's stories and, 186–98, 222n18; doubling and, 70; electrochemical activity and, 52; evolution and, 84; 4e cognition and, 4; impressionism and, 190–97; intentional binding in, 61; lag in, 54, 59–60, 66–67, 69–70, 98, 99, 142; memory and problem solving requiring, 83; modernism and, 196–97; multiple drafts model of, 212n7; neural models of, 2, 55, 190; phenomenology and, 210n6; reading fiction and, 153–56, 164; social powers of narrative and, 153, 186–98. *See also* attention and awareness; point of view
consilience, 52, 199
consistency building, 12, 35, 93, 139, 144–45, 165, 196
consonance, 12, 36
conventions, 7, 42, 48–51, 120, 125–28, 145, 191–93, 211n14
Cowell, Jason, 170
Crane, Stephen, 191
Crick, Francis, 186–87
Cross, Ian, 102, 173–75
Culler, Jonathan, 211n14

empathy, 7, 13, 150, 152–69, 200;
doubling and, 150, 158, 160; effects
of literary fiction, 150–52, 162–63,
166–68; effects of nonfiction, 169;
in-group bias and, 220n10. *See also*
identification
empirical turn in cognitive literary
studies, 204–5
emplotment: correlated to temporality
of the brain, 54; as natural cognitive
capability, 49, 111, 115. *See also*
figuration/configuration/refiguration;
plot-formation; probability
enactivism, 5, 9, 15, 16, 42, 53, 105,
209n2, 211n16, 222n18
engrams, 86
epilepsy, 55, 187
episodic dimension, 74, 78, 83, 87–88
equilibrium and disequilibrium, 78–81,
83, 84
Erdrich, Louise, 162
essentialism, 180. *See also* biocultural
hybrids; universals
Evans, Vyvyan, 209n4
evolution: consciousness and, 84;
cooperative behavior and, 221n12;
cultural, 169, 190; emotions and, 96;
neural reuse and, 23
expectations, 1, 56, 59, 91; emotion and,
99–100; gap filling and, 44; patterns
and, 45, 70, 125, 139; predictions
about probability and, 147, 172, 202;
of reciprocation, 173. *See also*
anticipation and retrospection;
fore-structure; surprise
experientiality, 47
explanatory gap, 2–3, 8, 52–53, 199,
207
extended mind, 177–78
eye movements (saccades), 49–50, 107

fabula, 30
Fadiga, Luciano, 112, 114
familiarity, 48–49, 70, 109, 117, 148.
See also defamiliarization;
habituation
Faulkner, William, 48, 206; *The Sound
and the Fury*, 73, 92–93, 197
Fazio, Patrik, 115

fear, 27, 36, 94–95, 101, 158, 160, 163,
218n17. *See also* emotions
Fernyhough, Charles, 165–66, 220n7
fictionality, 216n6
Fielding, Henry: *Shamela*, 167; *Tom
Jones*, 51
figuration/configuration/refiguration 2,
7, 17–19, 26–38, 41, 47, 68, 77–78,
84, 111, 180, 207. *See also* action-
perception circuit; emplotment;
mimesis
film, 47–50, 212n3, 214n15
first-person experience, 186, 190, 191
Flaubert, Gustave: *Madame Bovary*,
155, 189
flexibility and openness to change, 1, 11,
19, 22, 78, 84, 116–17, 119, 180–81.
See also consistency building; habit
formation; pattern-forming activity;
surprise
Fludernik, Monika, 15, 16, 46–47, 49,
51, 211nn13–14
fluency, 138–40, 142, 144, 202
fMRI measurement, 8, 23, 85–86,
89–90, 109, 113, 124, 126–27, 161,
183, 185–87, 220n11
focalization, 37, 188, 206, 219n3.
See also free indirect discourse;
perspectives; point of view
folk psychology, 155
Ford, Ford Madox, 35, 191, 194–95,
197, 206; *The Good Soldier*, 35–36,
194, 196
Fordham, Finn, 217n14
fore-structure, 58, 94, 109–12, 121, 125,
215–16n5
forgetting, 83–90. *See also* memory
Forster, E. M., 29, 215n2
4e cognition, 4, 5, 7, 15
frames and scripts, 14–15, 18–19, 47,
75, 200, 214n13, 221n14
Frank, Joseph, 71–72, 213n12
Fraps, Thomas, 61
free indirect discourse, 155–56, 189,
218–19n3
free riders, 173
free will, 66, 68, 213n11
Freud, Sigmund, 86
Friston, Karl, 103, 172

illusions, 33, 35–36, 85, 92, 116, 138–44, 205.
imagination, 6, 80, 84–86, 89, 138
imitation, 7, 27, 105, 161, 167, 171, 199. *See also* mimesis
immersion, 33–36, 45–46, 48, 72, 92, 138, 140, 142, 144, 157, 166, 192
impressionism: literary, 194–97, 206, 221–22n17; visual arts, 190–94
improvisation, 44–45, 146
infants, 38, 102, 108, 169, 174
inferences, 60–61, 115, 119–21, 124, 165, 216n8
Ingarden, Roman, 26, 141, 146
injustice, 181, 207, 221n15
innate language faculty, 209n4
innocent eye, 192–93
instability, 78–79, 81, 84
integration, 54, 57, 73–83, 90
intentional binding, 61, 62
intentionality, 108, 121, 135, 200; of actions, 108–9; as-relations and, 44; of emotions, 95–98; operative or non-thetic intentionality, 38, 63, 98; shared (we-intentionality), 169–79, 181–84, 221n12; textual, 36, 200, 218n1
intergenerational transmission, 104, 149, 198, 206
International Society for the Empirical Study of Literature, 204
interruption in narrative continuity, 143–44, 194, 202
intersubject correlation analysis (ISC), 214n15
intersubjectivity, 11, 36, 90–104, 153–54, 198, 202–3. *See also* paradox of the alter ego
intuition, 62, 83, 129, 136
irony, 51–52, 82, 120
Iser, Wolfgang, 2, 200, 201; on anticipation and retrospection, 147; on consistency building, 145; on fictionality, 216n6; *The Fictive and the Imaginary,* 110–11; on illusion-building and breaking, 141; on paradoxical duplication of "real" and "alien me," 159; reading theory of, 26, 32, 81–82, 140, 146, 205, 211n13;

theory of the imaginary, 211n13; virtual dimension and, 141; world-making and, 39

Jahn, Manfred, 15, 17, 18–19
James, Henry, 36, 129, 145, 187–89, 191, 206, 217n13; *The Ambassadors,* 37, 40, 44, 195–96; *The Golden Bowl,* 129–30; *The Portrait of a Lady,* 80, 189; *The Turn of the Screw,* 79; *What Maisie Knew,* 195–96; *The Wings of the Dove,* 188–89
James, William, 5, 12, 15, 26–27, 93, 189, 212n5
Jauss, Hans Robert, 26, 211n13
Jeannerod, Marc, 60, 108, 113, 122, 136, 142
Johnson, Mark: *Metaphors We Live By* (with Lakoff), 125; *Philosophy in the Flesh* (with Lakoff), 125–26, 132
joint attention, 170, 182–84
Joyce, James, 48, 50–51, 71–72, 92, 191, 206, 222n18; *Finnegans Wake,* 50–51, 52, 130–31, 211n15, 217n14; *A Portrait of the Artist as a Young Man,* 107–8, 111–12, 189; *Ulysses,* 31, 52, 82, 92, 131, 197

Kandel, Eric, 214n14, 215n3
Kaschak, Michael P., 145
Kearney, Richard, 17
Keen, Suzanne, 97, 150–51, 168
Kellogg, Robert, 206; *The Nature of Narrative* (with Scholes), 51, 206, 215n2
Kermode, Frank, 12, 213n12
Kidd, David Comer, 151, 152, 161–63, 169
Kierkegaard, Søren, 212n5
kinematic theory of narrative, 44, 148–49, 152–53
kinesic intelligence, 152
kinesic style, 135, 148–49
kinesthetic empathy, 138–39, 152–53, 158–59
Kolers, Paul, 212n7
Konstanz School, 26, 211n13
Konvalinka, Ivana, 172–73, 220n11
Kuhn, Thomas, 52

mood, 31, 99, 210n8, 219n3. *See also* emotions

morality, 151–52, 166–67, 207. *See also* social powers of narrative

Morse code, 76

motion agnosia, 82–83

motor cognition, 6–7, 13, 22, 87, 108–9, 113–14, 122–23, 125, 127, 136–38, 157

movies, 47–49, 212n3

multiple-plot novels, 33–34

Mumper, Micah, 164–65, 168–69

Murphy, Elliott, 209–10n4

music, 8, 9, 56, 60, 77, 88, 102, 103, 111, 114, 173–76, 212n3. *See also* rhythm

musical group interaction (MGI), 174

Nabokov, Vladimir: *Lolita*, 165, 219–20n6

Nadeau, Stephen E., 19–20, 23, 209n4

Nagel, Thomas, 52, 187; "What Is It Like to Be a Bat?" 186

narrative: brain processes enabling, 11, 88; episodic dimension of, 74, 78; kinematic theory of, 44; natural vs. unnatural, 46–53; rhetorical definition of, 43; social work of, 91, 150–52, 166–69, 177–82, 207; temporality and, 6, 55, 73–83. *See also* discourse; figuration/configuration/refiguration; mimesis; telling and following stories; temporality

narrative theory, 2, 11–19, 24–37, 206; endings of stories and, 65–66, 80–81; figurative activity and, 26–37; as guide to reading, 205; learning from neuroscience, 5, 8–10, 13–25, 199, 200, 202; research questions for neuroscience, 9–10, 203–4; structuralism and, 209n1; universal grammar and, 14, 83–84; worldmaking and, 37–46. *See also* narratology

narrative universals, 24–25

narrativity, 47

narratology: classificatory schemes of, 6, 14, 46; closure in fiction and, 80–81; fabula and sjužet, 30; relation between language, cognition, and

narrative, 13–14, 200; natural narratology, 46–47, 50; post-classical, 15; relation to changes in science, 9, 14, 15, 201; second-generation, 15–16, 43, 201; structuralist cognitive narratology, 9, 14, 199, 203, 215n5. *See also* cognitive narratology; narrative theory

narrator's voice, 31, 33, 37, 160, 165–66, 184–85, 189, 210n8, 218n3. *See also* focalization

natural vs. unnatural narratives, 46–53, 130

network thinking and connectivity, 85–86, 124

neural correlates of consciousness (NCCs), 2, 5, 52, 55, 67, 186, 202

neural reuse, 22–23, 25, 124

neuroaesthetics, 8–9, 186

neurobiology, 2, 6, 9, 11, 13, 19, 21–22, 47; of brain-body interaction, 114, 117, 207; of collaborative meaning making, 103; of emotions, 95; of grounded cognition, 122; of morality, 151; temporality and, 56–58, 76, 213n11

neuronal activity, 5, 19, 52–53, 55–57, 68, 74, 89, 112, 138, 160, 187, 200. *See also* Hebb's law

neurophenomenology, 2, 3, 9

neuroscience: complementary to narrative theory, 5, 8–10, 13–25, 199, 200, 202; of emotions, 21, 43, 95, 199, 201; evolution of, 5–6, 9, 200–1, 209n4; learning from narrative theory, 8–10, 13–25; limitations of, 89–90, 185, 186–88, 203–5; of memory and forgetting, 56, 68, 83–90, 204; research questions to explore in relation to narrative theory, 203–4; second-person, 8, 171, 216–17n11

niche construction, 42

Nicolai, Friedrich: *The Joys of Young Werther*, 167

Niedenthal, Paula: "Embodying Emotion," 120–21

Nietzsche, Friedrich, 40, 118–19, 176, 200

Noë, Alva, 53, 106–7, 135, 177, 222n19

novelty, 70, 95, 116–17, 119
Nussbaum, Martha, 150–51

Oatley, Keith, 151, 163–64
Obhi, Sukhvinder, 61
observational learning, 161

pain, 7, 132–34, 157, 160–61, 200
Palmer, Alan, 154, 190
paradox of the alter ego, 8, 90–91,
    153–56, 159, 189
Parma mirror-neuron group, 122,
    126–27, 216n10
Pater, Walter, 191, 222n18
pattern-completion inference mecha-
    nism, 119, 124, 140
pattern-forming activity, 2, 7, 13, 46,
    49–51, 68, 201; Hebbian firing and
    wiring, 86–87; need for, 1, 11, 18;
    oscillation and, 35, 55–57, 103, 182,
    192–96; play between building and
    breaking in narrative, 1, 12, 143–44,
    202; recurring patterns in narratives,
    24, 49, 178, 179
Peirce, Charles Sanders, 5
perception: action, role of, 7, 11, 13,
    106–17, 122; conventions' effect on,
    211n14; ecological theory of, 144–45;
    horizonal absences in, 139–40, 147;
    integration in, 140; intersubjectivity
    and, 153; motor, 67; natural, 48–49;
    speech, 136; temporality of, 60–63,
    67–69, 75–76, 81, 98; visual, 192–93.
    See also action-perception circuit;
    defamiliarization; habituation
performance deficits and cognitive
    ability, 121–22
perspectives, 34–37, 53, 79, 81–85, 88,
    90–92, 110, 139–40, 167, 170,
    182–85, 194–97
Petit, Jean-Luc: The Physiology and
    Phenomenology of Action (with
    Berthoz), 106, 134, 144–45
Petit, Philippe, 158
Pettitt, Clare, 217n13
Phelan, James, 14, 26, 43, 78, 80–81,
    202, 218n16, 219–20n6, 221n16
phenomenology: definition of intention-
    ality in, 38, 108; hermeneutic, 5,

210n6; paradox of the alter ego and,
    8, 153; phenomenological model of
    literature, 2, 38, 201, 210n5;
    suspension of natural attitude and,
    143
Pinker, Steven, 14, 150–51, 166–68,
    207
pity, 27, 36, 101, 157, 163
plasticity, 20–21, 111, 124, 198
play. See games and play
plot-formation, 12, 32, 35, 70, 77–79,
    91–92, 196. See also action;
    emplotment
plot vs. story, 29, 210n7
Poggioli, Renato, 214n12
point of observation, 81–82, 106
point of view, 48, 187–90, 195. See also
    focalization; perception
Pöppel, Ernst, 75–76
postmodernism, 50–51, 82
Pound, Ezra, 213–14n12
pragmatism, 38
predictive processing, 45, 67, 147, 202,
    211n16, 221n13
preference rules, 6, 14, 15, 17–19,
    43–44, 68–69, 170, 200, 215n5
prefiguration. See figuration/
    configuration/refiguration
prism spectacle experiment, 60, 63,
    212n6
probability, 146–47, 202, 218n16
Proust, Marcel, 191, 222n18; In Search
    of Lost Time, 56, 206
psychology, 16, 21, 94, 118–20, 151,
    156–57, 163–65, 168
Pulvermüller, Friedemann, 112, 114,
    136

qualia, 186, 188, 190–95, 197, 203
quasi judgments, 141

rabbit-duck figure, 17, 35, 76, 143
Rabinowitz, Peter, 80
Raichle, Marcus, 67, 76
Raposo, Ana, 127
Rapp, David, 69
ratchet effect, 169
reading: cortical capacities and, 22, 200;
    differences among readers, 22–23,

204–5; not linear logical processing, 19; scanning left to right bias in visual art, 72; temporality of integration in, 73–83; word decoding, 81. *See also* immersion; pattern-forming activity

realism, 51, 128, 191, 192, 206

reciprocity, 68, 173, 179, 221n12

reductionism, 2–3, 5, 186–87, 199

reenactment, 7, 118–24, 134–44, 160

refiguration. *See* figuration / configuration / refiguration

relativism, 24

relevance theory, 42, 201, 216n8

reliable vs. unreliable narration, 56, 79, 196

rhythm, 67, 75–78, 102–3, 112, 114, 131, 174–76

Richardson, Alan, 85–86

Richardson, Samuel: *Clarissa,* 51; *Pamela,* 167, 220n8

Ricoeur, Paul, 2, 104, 200, 201; on configuration, 47, 78; on eventfulness of language, 211n11; Fludernik on, 211n13; on illusion of sequence, 73–74; on imitation of action, 105–6; *langue-parole* distinction critiqued by, 209n3; on metaphor, 40, 210n6; on narrative intelligence, 177; *Oneself as Another,* 210n6, 213n10; on recollection and reading, 63–64; on split reference, 110, 180; "Structure, Word, Event," 211n11; on temporality, 26, 27, 28–29, 30, 58, 213n10; theory of plots and, 4, 11, 12, 43; on world-making, 38–39

Ridley, James, 213n9

Rizzolatti, Giacomo, 122

Robinson, Jenefer, 98, 100–101, 141, 216n9

Routledge Encyclopedia of Narrative Theory, 15

Rubin, James, 192

Rüschemeyer, Shirley-Ann, 127

Ruskin, John, 192–93

Russian formalism, 30, 211n14

Ryan, Marie-Laure, 45–46; *Narrative as Virtual Reality,* 46

Ryan, Vanessa, 142

Ryle, Gilbert, 40

Sartre, Jean-Paul, 159

Sathian, Krish, 114

Saussure, Ferdinand de, 14, 125, 209n3

scaffolding, 41

scanning technologies. *See* EEG measurement; fMRI measurement

Schacter, Daniel, 84, 85

Schilbach, Leonhard, 171, 173

Schlesinger, I. M., 81

Scholes, Robert, 206; *The Nature of Narrative* (with Kellogg), 51, 206, 215n2

Schwan, Stephan, 48–49

seeing-as, 2, 17–19, 26–46, 47, 120, 180, 198, 202, 210n8, 214n13; circularity of literary interpretation and, 18, 205–6; emplotment and, 30; frames and scripts and, 47, 221n14

segmentation of time, 73–83

self-consciousness, 70–71, 142, 147

self-understanding, 155

Sensorimotor Foundations of Higher Cognition (Haggard, Rossetti, & Kawato, eds.), 118

sensorimotor system, 117–18, 121, 127–28, 133

shared intentionality, 169–70, 174–76, 178–79, 182–84, 198

Shimamura, Arthur P., 47, 72

Shklar, Judith, 181

Shklovsky, Viktor, 194, 211n14

Silva, Alcino J., 84

simulation, 13, 113, 199–200, 220n6; as-relations and, 7, 128–29, 151, 163; fiction as simulation of social worlds, 163–64; paradoxes of, 117–25

simulation theory (ST), 157, 162–63, 164–65

Singer, Tania, 158, 160

sjužet, 30

sleep, 55, 87

smell, 108, 111, 112, 139

Smith, Tim, 49–50

Smollett, Tobias: *The Adventures of Ferdinand Count Fathom,* 148

social cognition, 119, 120, 151–52, 162, 165, 169, 177–80

social justice, 150, 181. *See also* injustice

social powers of narrative, 150–98,
203–4, 207; collaboration and,
169–76, 182–84; consciousness and,
186–98; distributed cognition and,
177–86; empathy and, 150, 152–69;
synchronizing cognitive activity and,
184
solipsism, 8, 90, 153–54, 156, 157, 163.
See also paradox of the alter ego
Sophocles: *Oedipus Rex,* 32
sound, 3, 20, 75, 76, 112, 115, 139.
See also music
spatial form in modern literature, 71–73,
213–14n12
speech, 60, 135–36, 183. *See also*
langue-parole distinction
Speer, Nicole, 113–14
Sperber, Dan, 216n8
Spolsky, Ellen, 80
stage fright, 142
Starr, Gabrielle, 86, 115–16
Stein, Gertrude: *Tender Buttons,* 145
Sternberg, Meir, 32, 100–101
Sterne, Laurence: *Tristram Shandy,*
51
Stevens, Catherine, 109
Stickgold, Robert, 85
structuralism, 14, 16, 41, 45, 209,
209n1, 209n4
structuralist cognitive narratology, 9,
14, 199, 200, 215n5
subjective referral, 60–64, 67, 69–72
surprise, 1, 32, 35, 55, 56, 59,
100–101
suspense, 32, 100–101
synchronization, 5, 19, 54–59, 76, 103,
171–73, 181–84

taxonomic, rule-based approach, 5, 6,
14–18, 25–26, 37–46, 202–3, 221n14.
See also categorization process; frames
and scripts
telling and following stories, 1–3, 6, 53,
117–18, 179, 184; asynchronous
temporal processes in, 55, 59, 89;
consciousness as essential to, 84;
empathy resulting from, 150–51;
evolution and, 89; memory requirements for, 84–85, 90; neurobiology of

mental functioning and, 11, 74;
participatory sense-making of, 102–3;
social powers and, 150–52; universal
grammar and, 14, 83–84; worldmaking and, 38. *See also* narrative;
narratology; reading
temporal binding, 54, 61, 89
temporality, 6, 54–104, 202; anachronies and, 12, 35, 70, 143–44, 194,
202; anticipation and retrospection,
58–73; of brain functioning, 54–63;
communal time, 103–4; endings of
stories and, 65–66, 80–81; of
integration in cognition, narrative,
and reading, 73–83; of intersubjectivity and emotion, 90–104; narrative
and, 2, 11, 13, 26, 35, 55, 199;
neuroscience of memory and forgetting, 83–90; segmentation and, 73–83;
subjective time, variations in, 94;
unity of mind and, 57
theater, 212n3
theory of mind (ToM), 151, 152, 157,
161–63, 168–69, 184, 200, 204,
219n5
Thompson, Evan, 3, 76, 211n16
to-and-fro movements, 1, 5, 9, 11, 61,
77, 86, 89, 98, 179–80, 186; of
anticipation and retrospection, 116;
collaborative sensemaking and, 102,
173, 174; of figuration and refiguration, 18, 46; of narrative interactions,
43, 175, 181; preference rules and,
19; reciprocal processes of pattern
formation, 68, 70; of shared intentionality, 177
Todorov, Tzvetan, 78
Tolstoy, Leo: *Anna Karenina,* 33–34,
91–92, 101, 138–39, 141
Tomasello, Michael, 136, 169–70,
221n12
Tomkins, Silvan, 21
Tononi, Giulio, 55, 68
top-down, bottom-up interactions, 12,
19, 70, 74
touch, 20, 106–7, 114, 189
Tourette's syndrome, 66
tragedy, 27, 36, 101, 147, 160
Trehub, Sandra, 174